Double-Outlet Right Ventricle

Konstantin V. Shatalov ·
Konstantine M. Dzhidzhikhiya
Editors

Double-Outlet Right Ventricle

Springer

Editors
Konstantin V. Shatalov
A. N. Bakulev National Medical Investigation Center for Cardiovascular Surgery
Moscow, Russia

Konstantine M. Dzhidzhikhiya
A. N. Bakulev National Medical Investigation Center for Cardiovascular Surgery
Moscow, Russia

ISBN 978-3-031-49706-3 ISBN 978-3-031-49707-0 (eBook)
https://doi.org/10.1007/978-3-031-49707-0

This Springer imprint is published by the registered company Springer Nature Switzerland AG
The registered company address is: Gewerbestrasse 11, 6330 Cham, Switzerland

Paper in this product is recyclable.

Acknowledgement

We gratefully acknowledge Dr. Khoren Abelian, Specialty Registrar in Clinical Radiology, MRCGP, Liverpool, UK, for his help in revising and preparation the manuscript.

Contents

Description

History

S. P. Glyantsev

Abstract Although the term «double-outlet right ventricle» was coined in 1957, description of anatomical specimens of the hearts with aortic root connected to both ventricles in literature accounts more than 200 years. The first anatomical correction of DORV performed in 1950s opened a new chapter in surgical correction of complex cyanotic congenital heart defects. Nowadays, surgical techniques used for treatment of DORV are the most variable compared to other congenital heart defects. This chapter describes main historical milestones in surgical correction and understanding of DORV since its first clinical description.

Keywords Double-outlet right ventricle · History

In 1814, the English physician J. R. Farre in his book «On Malformation of the Human Heart» collected all clinical and anatomical cases on a congenital heart defect (CHD) which he called *«aortic ostium attached to both ventricles»* published in the literature over the previous 30 years. According to Farre, the first scientist who observed a patient with this malformation and described the autopsy specimen in 1778 was a professor of anatomy and surgery at Leiden University E. Sandifort in a thesis entitled «Observationes Anatomico-pathologicæ». A 12-year-old child complained on exertional shortness of breath, during which his face became swollen and cyanotic, his eyes bulged, with visible pulsation of jugular veins on his neck. He suffered with frequent colds, and in winter, he shivered from cold, even if he was near the hearth. Sometimes he had nosebleeds, which brought relief. He developed these symptoms in the 3rd year of his life. At the autopsy, the foramen ovale was open, the ostium of the pulmonary valve was severely narrowed, which caused the right atrium and ventricle to be significantly dilated, and the aorta was communicating with both ventricles through the opening in the interventricular septum (IVS).

S. P. Glyantsev (✉)
Department of Cardiac Surgery History, A. N. Bakulev National Medical Investigation Center for Cardiovascular Surgery, Moscow, Russia
e-mail: spglyantsev@mail.ru

K. V. Shatalov and K. M. Dzhidzhikhiya (eds.), *Double-Outlet Right Ventricle*,
https://doi.org/10.1007/978-3-031-49707-0_1

A more detailed description of the malformation was published in 1784 by the London anatomist W. Hunter. The child lived to the 13 years old. He was thin, with a dark blue face. He had shortness of breath and palpitation. During the attack, the child's face turned almost black. He fell backwards and seemed to be dead. He usually came out of such attacks, sobbing, yawning and feeling tired. Any haste or rapid movement of the body, aggravated the symptoms, and in order to prevent it or reduce its severity, the child lay down on the left side and remained motionless for about ten minutes. On autopsy, the pulmonary artery originated from the right ventricle, but it was so narrowed that it barely let in a thin probe. The upper part of the IVS was perforated, which allowed the thumb to pass through it. The aortic opening was located so close to this perforation that during contractions of the heart it received blood from both ventricles.

A similar case was reported in 1785 by R. Pulteney. The appearance of this adolescent was the opposite of the patient described by W. Hunter. He often experienced a feeling of despondency, dizziness and shortness of breath during physical exertion. Gradually, these symptoms intensified so that he could not cross the room without the skin of his face and hands becoming black. At this time, he was abruptly weakening, and his breathing almost stopped. At the age of 13 years and 9 months, he died. On autopsy, the ostium of the pulmonary valve was smaller than usual. When examining the heart, the biventricular connection of the aorta was found, so it could let in the tip of the finger to pass through the aorta to the left ventricle.

J. Abernethy, a surgeon at St. Bartholomew's Hospital in London, described and illustrated DORV in «Surgical and Physiological Essays» in 1793. He wrote about the child who lived for two years. His skin was cyanotic and, as a rule, cold, breathing was irregular due to paroxysms, during which he often lay face down. The heart specimen was distinguished by the large foramen ovale and the aorta was located almost exclusively above the right ventricle instead of being to the left to the IVS. Also, pulmonary artery stenosis, dilation of the right heart and a hole in the upper part of the IVS were noted.

In addition to E. Sandifort (1778), W. Hunter (1784), R. Pulteney (1785) and J. Abernethy (1794), the aortic origin from both ventricles, according to J. R. Farre, was described by professor of College de France J.-N. Corvisart (1806), who along with his own observation mentioned two cases of professor Cailott, as well as A. Burns (1809), Ring (1809) and Travers (1810). The last observation is particularly noteworthy for the detailed description of the clinical picture of the malformation and the autopsy specimen of the heart.

Mr. V., aged 14, visited Dr. Travers on August 4, 1809. He was tall, but very thin and weak. There were practically no muscles on his arms and legs, the fingers and toes were thin and long with thickened ends and nail clubbing. His dark blue skin was covered with sticky sweat. The young man was suffering with shortness of breath on moderate exertion, turning into yawning, a strong cough caused by running or quickly climbing stairs, strong but regular heartbeats at rest and palpitations during physical exertion. The radial pulse was 80 beats per minute, was regular, but weak. Sometimes, the young man felt a sharp pain and burning in his chest. At night, he often woke up with a feeling of suffocation, beginning in a dream, after which he assumed a pose with his head held high. Even in warm weather he felt chilly. Mr. V. suffered from poor eyesight, and the conjunctiva quickly filled with blood during physical exertion.

February 20, 1810 V. died suddenly from pulmonary hemorrhage. Before that, he had suffered from coughing, nausea and extreme weakness. An autopsy was performed the next day. The heart was large, especially the right ventricle, which walls were as thick as the left ventricle one. The pulmonary artery was narrowed to half its normal size. The left atrium and the left ventricle were very small. The aorta was larger than usual and there was a large hole in the upper part of the IVS. The ductus arteriosus was obliterated and the foramen ovale was open.

J. R. Farre demonstrated two of his own cases of DORV. The first case dating from 1812 was notable for the fact that although the aorta originated from both ventricles the man lived with this disease for 40 years. In the second case, thanks to colleagues of J. R. Farre, doctors A. Cooper, J. Cannon and Wheelwright, clinical picture, the actions taken by the doctor, anatomy of the malformation were well described. Nothing unusual was noted at the birth of the child, but after a few months, the mother noticed that his face was darker than that of her other children. At 2 years of age, she clearly noticed that the cheeks and lips of the child were dark blue, almost black, which intensified in cold and after psycho-emotional exertion. From this period until his death, not only mental, but even a slight physical exertion aggravated the condition, especially in cold weather. At the age of 5, the child began to complain of frequent nausea and severe headache.

On October 15, 1812, at the age of 9 years and 5 months, the boy was examined by Mr. Wheelwright because the left thumb was not moving properly. The child was thin and very weak. Since he had no visible injuries, the doctor gave him medicine. After 17 days, the child developed paralysis of the left arm and leg, accompanied by short-term seizures, severe headache and frequent nausea. His skin was hot, his tongue was covered with plaque, his pupils were dilated and his pulse reached 120 beats per minute. Given such symptoms and anamnesis, the prognosis was extremely poor, but Mr. Wheelwright was kindly asked to continue the treatment. He prescribed calomel and a solution of magnesium sulfate and hirudotherapy. On the 18th day, the irregular pulse reached 124 beats per minute, convulsions appeared, which intensified and became more prolonged by the end of the day. On the 19th day, the pulse with a frequency of 86 beats per minute was weak and irregular, the child's stamina reduced dramatically, the whole body was sweaty. On the evening of the 20th day after the first examination, the child died. After death, it became known that 6–7 days before its onset, while playing with a friend, the child fell and hit his head on the ground.

During the autopsy, an abscess was found in the right hemisphere of the brain. In the heart, there was a hole in the upper part of the IVS connecting their cavities with the aortic root. The semilunar valves of the pulmonary artery were fused, and its ostium narrowed to a small hole. The ductus arteriosus was closed. The aorta originated from both ventricles of the heart and the pulmonary artery delivered little blood to the lungs due to the stricture of its valves.

Commenting on this observation, J. R. Farre pointed out that the most remarkable thing in this malformation (from his point of view) was the pulmonary artery valve, which consisted not of three, as usual, but only of two valves, so fused that only a small round hole remained between them. On our part, we add that all the first descriptions of malformation presented by J. R. Farre are the so-called DORV «tetralogy» type or tetralogy of Fallot itself: all described the biventricular location of the aorta, a large hole in the IVS (i.e., subaortic VSD), hypertrophy of the right ventricle and severe pulmonary artery stenosis. The observation of J. R. Farre himself is similar. However, without morphometry, it is difficult to attribute these descriptions to tetralogy of Fallot, especially since this malformation was described by E.-L. A. Fallot only in 1888.

DORV is a relatively rare CHD. According to M. E. Abbott (1936), incidence of DORV is 1.1%, and according to H. Bancl (1977) in 2.7% of cases of all CHDs. In 1936, M. E. Abbott in the «Atlas of Congenital Cardiac Disease» mentioned several variants of aortic dextraposition. In seven patients, the aorta took origin from both ventricles, in three—from the right and in one the aorta originated from the right ventricle with double conus. The average life expectancy of the first 7 patients was 25 years (from 1.5 to 48 years); three patients with DORV lived for 13 weeks, 10 months and 13 months. The appropriate data of the last patients are not available. M. Abbott attributed the malformation to transposition of the great arteries (TGA), without defining it as a separate malformation.

During the XIX and up to the mid XX centuries DORV was considered as one of the forms of TGA (the so-called partial form). M. E. Abbott was the first to oppose this point of view in 1927, although in her atlas she attributed the defect to TGA. In 1939, J. S. Harris and S. Farber proposed for the first time to distinguish DORV as a separate condition.

In 1926 E. Pernkopf for the first time described a heart specimen in which the aorta and the pulmonary artery originated from the right ventricle in association with subpulmonary location of ventricular septal defect (VSD). In 1949, H.B. Taussig and R. J. Bing described a heart with a complete transposition of the aorta and left position of the pulmonary artery. The aorta originated from the right ventricle and the pulmonary valve overrode IVS. The authors described in detail the clinical symptoms and results of diagnostic tools including angiocardiography (ACG). In 1950 M. Lev and B. M. Volk observed a similar case and coined the term "*Taussig-Bing anomaly*".

In 1952, K. Braun and associates reported an autopsy finding of DORV with pulmonary artery stenosis in a 19-year-old man and called the defect «*double-outlet ventricle*». In 1957, F. C. Witham introduced the term «*double-outlet right ventricle*» to denote the defect instead of the term «*partial TGA*», which was previously used to define the malformation, with subpulmonary VSD in particular.

In most cases of DORV, there is a large VSD, equal to or larger than the aortic valve diameter. Less often, in about 10% of cases, VSD has a smaller size compared to the aortic valve. In this case, VSD is called restrictive. Multiple VSDs, according to J. Kirklin (1993), occur in 13% of cases.

In 1972, G. K. Danielson distinguished two types of the course of the arterial trunks: spiral (as in the normal heart) and parallel. In the first type, the aorta and

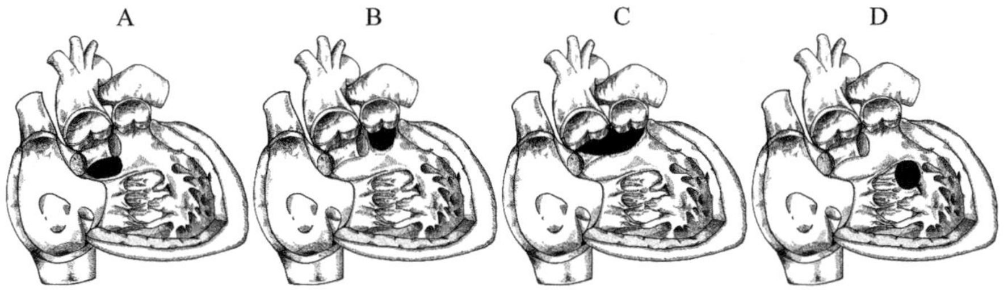

Fig. 1 Classification of DORV depending on proximity of VSD to the arterial valves: **A**–with subaortic VSD; **B**–with subpulmonary VSD; **C**–with subarterial VSD; **D**–with non-committed VSD

pulmonary artery are located normally: the aorta is to the right and slightly posterior to the pulmonary trunk so that when leaving the base of the heart, both arteries twist in a spiral manner. In the second type, the aorta locates either to the right and «side-by-side» with the pulmonary trunk, or to the right and anterior to the pulmonary artery. Finally, the aorta can be located to the left and anterior to the pulmonary artery (i.e., L-malposition), which is the rarest type.

The first classification of DORV, which was successfully used by surgeons until the 1970s, was developed by H. N. Neufeld in 1961 and included the following three main features: 1–VSD location in relation to the crista; 2–proximity of VSD to the arterial trunks; 3–presence or absence of pulmonary artery stenosis. This classification had the following form:

- **type 1**. Infracristal VSD: type 1A with subaortic VSD, with or without pulmonary artery stenosis and type 1B with VSD distant from the ostia of arterial trunks;
- **type 2**. Supracristal VSD: type 2A with subpulmonary VSD (Taussig-Bing anomaly) and type 2B with subarterial VSD.

The most popular classification widely used to date was developed in 1972 by M. Lev et al. They divided types of DORV depending on proximity of VSD to the arterial trunks (Fig. 1):

- with subaortic VSD;
- with subpulmonary VSD;
- with subarterial VSD (doubly committed);
- with non-committed VSD.

We emphasize that Lev et al. identified DORV with non-committed VSD as an independent classification unit for the first time. By this term, they understood such a location of VSD when it was not related to any of the arterial trunks. In 1972, M. Lev et al. coined the term «non-committed VSD» for this purpose. In 1999, E. Belli concretized this concept, indicating that with non-committed VSD the distance from its rim to the ostia of the aorta and pulmonary artery should exceed the diameter of the aortic valve.

Despite the more than 200-year history of describing the anatomy of DORV, there is still no consensus in the literature regarding the precise diagnostic criteria of this malformation. Many authors following M. Lev et al. consider it as a morphological syndrome with abnormal ventricular-arterial connection, in which one arterial trunk is completely, and the second one partially take origin from the right ventricle. For example, M. Lev et al. implied a position of the aorta, in which two of its leaflets and part of the third are supported by the right ventricle structures.

However, this concept, according to R. H. Anderson (1983), does not take into account anatomy of the outflow tracts and allows coexistence of DORV with other conotruncal anomalies. This underestimates the role of abnormal formation of arterial conus in ontogenesis of DORV.

In order to develop a distinguishing criterion of DORV, J. Kirklin et al. in 1973 proposed the «50% rule». According to this rule, a malformation should be considered as DORV if one of the arterial trunks completely and the second one more than «50%» take origin from the right ventricle. However, the assessment of the degree of overriding is very subjective and may vary depending on the cardiac phase as well as observer. This leads to equivocal interpretations of anatomy of the malformation by different specialists.

In 2000, D. Sidi and Y. Lecompte proposed to define DORV based on position of the outlet septum (OS). In their opinion, if the OS separates two semilunar valves, then ventricular-arterial connections are not abnormal. In cases where the same structure separates the semilunar and atrioventricular valves, there is a detachment of the arterial trunks from the corresponding ventricle. And although the authors mistakenly presented the ventriculo-infundibular fold as the OS, the idea itself turned out to be very rational. It is known that the OS separating the semilunar valves in a normal heart connects to the IVS. Its location in the right ventricle R. H. Anderson proposed to consider as a prerequisite for the diagnosis of DORV, back in 1983.

The opponents of the «50% rule» (F. J. Hallerman, 1970; M. G. Baron, 1971) considered the presence of two (subaortic and subpulmonary) infundibulums and absence of mitral-aortic fibrosa contact as typical features of DORV. Proponents of this hypothesis presented DORV not as a morphological syndrome, but as an independent entity characterized by specific embryological mechanisms, anatomical features and clinical manifestations.

Nowadays, the existence of DORV is beyond doubt. DORV is characterized by embryonic and morphological independence. The patients with this malformation require individualized surgical approach.

To date, no generally accepted definition of DORV has been proposed. After a long debate a compromise solution was achieved, according to which DORV is considered to be a type of anomalous ventricular-arterial connection, in which both arterial trunks completely or more than half of their circumferences originate from the morphologically right ventricle. Such a definition does not absolutize the exclusivity of a single feature of it, whether it is the absence of mitral-aortic fibrous continuity, the presence of double conus or 200% origin of the both vessels from the right ventricle. On the contrary, such a definition covers all the criteria characterizing DORV and makes it possible to apply them in clinical practice without any contradictions.

Table 1 Main milestones in the study and treatment of DORV

Year	Author	Event
1793	Abernethy [1]	The first description of the heart with DORV
1949	Taussig and Bing [2]	The first description of DORV with subpulmonary VSD
1952	Braun et al. [3]	The term «double-outlet ventricle» was coined
1957	Witham [4]	– The term «double-outlet right ventricle» was coined – The first description of DORV/AVSD
1957	Kirklin et al. [5]	Anatomical repair of DORV with subaortic VSD
1962	Neufeld et al. [6]	The first classification of DORV
1965	Carey and Edwards [7]	The first ACG implementation in DORV
1968	Patrick et al. [8]	Tunneling of A-aorta in DORV with subpulmonary VSD and antero-posterior arterial trunks
1969	Hightower et al. [9]	Correction of Taussig-Bing anomaly by a combination of pulmonary artery tunneling to the left ventricle and Mustard procedure
1971	Kawashima et al. [10]	Tunneling of D-aorta in DORV with subpulmonary VSD and side-by-side arterial trunks
1972	Lev et al. [11]	– Classification of DORV depending on proximity of VSD to the arterial valves – The term «non-committed VSD» was coined
1975	Zamora et al. [12]	The term «remote VSD» was coined
1977	Kirklin et al. [13]	Anatomical repair of DORV with non-committed VSD
1978	Danielson et al. [14]	Physiological repair of DORV/AVSD, atrioventricular discordance and dextrocardia
1980	Pacifico et al. [15]	Anatomical repair of DORV/AVSD
1987	Barbero-Marcial et al. [16]	Proposed multiple-patch technique for aortic tunneling in DORV with non-committed VSD
1999	Belli et al. [17]	The criterion of «non-committed VSD» was proposed
2000	Sidi et al. [18]	The term «malposition of the great arteries» was proposed
2002	Tchervenkov et al. [19]	Proposed VSD translocation technique for DORV with non-committed VSD
2006	Mair et al. [20]	Half-turned truncal switch operation for DORV with subpulmonary VSD and pulmonary artery stenosis
2006	Hu et al. [21]	Double-root translocation for DORV with subpulmonary VSD and pulmonary artery stenosis and DORV with «non-committed» VSD
2007	Yeh et al. [22]	Nikaidoh operation for DORV with subpulmonary VSD and pulmonary artery stenosis

Table 1 presents the main milestones in the study of anatomy and surgical treatment of DORV.

References

1. Abernethy J. Surgical and physiological essay. Part 11. London: James Evans; 1793. p. 162.
2. Taussig HB, Bing RJ. Complete transposition of the aorta and a levoposition of the pulmonary artery. Clinical, physiological, and pathological findings. Am Heart J. 1949;37:551–559.
3. Braun K, De Vries A, Feingold DS, Ehrenfeld NE, Feldman J, Schorr S. Complete dextoposition of the aorta, pulmonary stenosis, interventricular septal defect, and patent foramen ovale. Am Heart J. 1952;43:773–80.
4. Witham AC. Double outlet right ventricle, a partial transposition complex. Am Heart J. 1957;53:928–39.
5. Kirklin JW, Harp RA, McGoon DC. Surgical treatment of origin of both vessels from right ventricle, including cases of pulmonary stenosis. J Thorac Cardiovasc Surg. 1964;48:1026–36.
6. Neufeld HN, Lucas RV, Lester RG, Adams P, Anderson RC, Edwards JE. Origin of both great vessels from the right ventricle without pulmonary stenosis. Br Heart J. 1962;24:393–408.
7. Carey LS, Edwards JE. Roentgenographic features in cases with origin of both great vessels from the right ventricle without pulmonary stenosis. Am J Roentgenol. 1965;93:269–97.
8. Patrick DL, McGoon DC. An operation for double-outlet right ventricle with transposition of the great arteries. J Cardiovasc Surg. 1968;9:537–42.
9. Hightower BM, Barcia A, Bargeron LM, Kirklin JW. Double-outlet right ventricle with transposed great arteries and subpulmonary ventricular septal defect. The Taussig-Bing malformation Circulation. 1969;39:S207-213.
10. Kawashima Y, Fujita T, Miyamoto T, Manabe H. Intraventricular rerouting of blood for the correction of Taussig-Bing malformation. J Thorac Cardiovasc Surg. 1971;62:825–9.
11. Lev M, Bharati S, Meng CCL, Libethson RP, Paul MH, Idriss F. A concept of double outlet right ventricle. J Thorac Cardiovasc Surg. 1972;64:271–81.
12. Zamora R, Moller JH, Edwards JE. Double-outlet right ventricle Anatomic types and associated anomalies. Chest. 1975;68:672–7.
13. Kirklin JW, Castaneda AR. Surgical correction of double-outlet right ventricle with noncommitted ventricular septal defect. J Thorac Cardiovasc Surg. 1977;73:399–403.
14. Danielson GK, Tabry IF, Ritter DG, Maloney JD. Successful repair of double-outlet right ventricle, complete atrioventricular canal, and atrioventricular discordance associated with dextrocardia and pulmonary stenosis. J Thorac Cardiovasc Surg. 1978;76:710–7.
15. Pacifico AD, Kirklin JW, Bargeron LM. Repair of complete atrioventricular canal associated with tetralogy of Fallot or double-outlet right ventricle: report of 10 cases. Ann Thorac Surg. 1980;4:351–6.
16. Barbero-Marcial M, Tanamati C, Atik E, Ebaid M. Intraventricular repair of double-outlet right ventricle with non-committed ventricular septal defect: advantages of multiple patches. J Thorac Cardiovasc Surg. 1999;118:1056–67.
17. Belli E, Serraf A, Lacour-Gayet F, Hubler M, Zoghby J, Houyel L, et al. Double-outlet right ventricle with non-committed ventricular septal defect. Eur J Cardiothorac Surg. 1999;15:747–52.
18. Sidi D, Lecompte Y. Transposition and malposition of the great arteries with ventricular septal defects. In: Moller JH, Hoffman JIE, editors. Pediatric cardiovascular medicine. New York, NY: Churchill Livingstone; 2000. p. 363–373.
19. Tchervenkov CI, Korkola SJ, Be´land MJ. Single-stage anatomical repair of complete atrioventricular canal, double-outlet right ventricle and cor-triatriatum using ventricular septal defect translocation. Ann Thoracic Surg. 2002;73:1317–1320.
20. Mair R, Sames-Dolzer E, Vondrys D, Lechner E. En block rotation of the truncus arteriosus—an option for anatomic repair of transposition of the great arteries, ventricular septal defect, and left ventricular outflow tract obstruction. J Thorac Cardiovasc Surg. 2006;131:740–1.

21. Hu S, Xie Y, Li S, Wang X, Yan F, Li Y, Hua Z, Li Y. Double-root translocation for double-outlet right ventricle with noncommited ventricular septal defect of double-outlet right ventricle with subpulmonary ventricular septal defect associated with pulmonary stenosis: an optimized solution. Ann Thorac Surg. 2010;89:1360–5.
22. Yeh T, Ramaciotti C, Leonardo SR. The aortic root translocation (Nikaidoh) procedure: midterm results superior to the Rastelli procedure. J Thorac Cardiovasc Surg. 2007;133:461–9.

Anatomy

K. V. Shatalov, K. M. Dzhidzhikhiya, and M. V. Gordeeva

Abstract Understanding of DORV anatomy is one of the most complex fundamental issues in the field of CHDs. Anatomical complexity of DORV is backed by various combinations of different VSD types, arterial trunks relationship and also associated cardiac anomalies, which result in existence of multiple types of the malformation. Correct understanding of VSD morphology, relationship of the aortic and pulmonary valves, anatomy of conduction system and coronary arteries, associated cardiac anomalies, etc., is a key to successful surgical planning. Therefore, in this chapter, we provide detailed intra- and extracardiac anatomy and most important associated anomalies of all types of DORV necessary for preoperative planning and decision-making. Also, we discus on surgical and anatomical importance of the so-called transitional anatomical forms of DORV with tetralogy of Fallot and TGA which represent great anatomical challenge in understanding spectrum of conotruncal anomalies.

Keywords Double-outlet right ventricle · Anatomy · Ventricular septal defect · Committed · Non-committed · Conotruncal anomalies · Taussig–Bing anomaly · Transitional forms · Anatomical concept

1 Terminology

Understanding of DORV anatomy is based on correct identification and assessment of the following intracardiac structures (Fig. 1):

K. V. Shatalov · K. M. Dzhidzhikhiya (✉)
Department of Emergency Surgery of Congenital Heart Diseases, Cardiac Surgeon, A. N. Bakulev National Medical Investigation Center for Cardiovascular Surgery, Moscow, Russia
e-mail: d.m.konstantine@mail.ru

M. V. Gordeeva
Department of Pathology, A. N. Bakulev National Medical Investigation Center for Cardiovascular Surgery, Moscow, Russia

K. V. Shatalov and K. M. Dzhidzhikhiya (eds.), *Double-Outlet Right Ventricle*,
https://doi.org/10.1007/978-3-031-49707-0_2

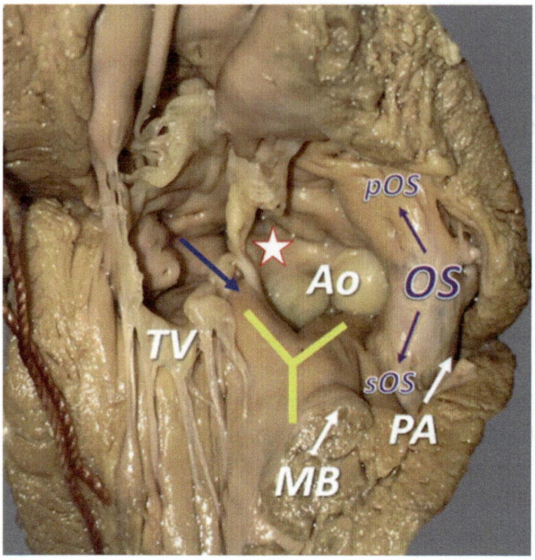

Fig. 1 DORV «tetralogy» type, view from the right ventricle (autopsy specimen). The OS with its septal (sOS) and parietal (pOS) insertions separates aortic (Ao) and pulmonary (PA) valves, forming anterior wall of the subaortic infundibulum as well as posterior wall of the subpulmonary infundibulum. The aTS and pTS (diagonal parts of the yellow figure) take origin from the body of the TS (vertical part of the yellow figure) and directed toward the OS and tricuspid valve annulus respectively. Medial papillary muscle (blue arrow) originates from the pTS to which the chordae of the tricuspid septal leaflet are attached. Moderator band (MB) origins from the body of the TS and connects the IVS with the free wall of the right ventricle

- outlet septum;
- ventriculo-infundibular fold;
- crista supraventricularis;
- trabecula septomarginalis;
- bilateral infundibulum (double conus).

Outlet septum (OS) (synonyms: «conal/conus septum», «infundibular septum», «first parietal band») is a muscle structure dividing the arterial valves. It consists of the septum itself as well as the septal (between the limbs of the trabecula septomarginalis (TS) in a normal heart) and parietal (with the right half of the VIF) insertions. The superior border of the OS is defined by the level of the arterial valves, while the inferior border is marked by the septal insertion between the limbs of the TS. In DORV, the OS is the right ventricular structure without being a part of the IVS. Not containing elements of coronary and conduction systems the OS can be safely resected during the surgery.

Ventriculo-infundibular fold (synonyms: «infundibuloventricular fold», «inner heart curvature», «bulboventricular fold», «second parietal band») is a muscle structure separating the atrioventricular and arterial valves. The VIF consists of two halves: the left (between the mitral and aortic valves) and the right (between the tricuspid and pulmonary valves). In a normal heart, the left half is completely reduced, thus causing mitral-aortic fibrotic continuity, while the right half joins the OS and thus takes part in the formation of the crista supraventricularis.

Crista supraventricularis is a muscle structure of the right ventricle formed by fusion of the OS and VIF. It takes part in separation of the inlet and outlet parts as well as of the trabecular and outlet (along with the TS and the moderator band) parts of the right ventricle. The structure also separates the pulmonary valve from the tricuspid valve. Normally, the crista supraventricularis is positioned between the limbs of the TS. In conotruncal anomalies, the crista supraventricularis is never formed.

Trabecula septomarginalis (synonyms: «septomarginal trabeculation», «septal band») is a Y-shaped structure of the IVS located on its right ventricular side. Consists of a body as well as the anterior and posterior limbs. In a normal heart, the limbs of the TS cradle the crista supraventricularis. The posterior limb gives rise to the medial papillary muscle (or papillary muscle of the conus–Lancisi muscle). The moderator band originates from the body of the TS and is directed toward free wall of the right ventricle. Since in DORV fusion of the OS and VIF is failed, the limbs of the TS cradle conoventricular VSD.

Bilateral infundibulum (synonyms: «bilateral conus», «double conus») means that both arterial valves have completely muscular basement own to the persistent VIF between the atrioventricular and arterial valves and the muscular OS separating the arterial valves. Thus, fibrous continuity between the atrioventricular and arterial valves is absent.

2 Definition

DORV is usually defined as a wide range of complex congenital heart malformations in which both arterial trunks (the aorta and pulmonary artery) predominantly originate from the right ventricle. According to such a definition, DORV is primarily a type of anomalous ventriculo-arterial connection and represented by a spectrum of various conotruncal anomalies [1].

From morphological viewpoint, the disease remains the subject of debates both from terminological perspective and common anatomical criteria. The failure of the VIF absorption (which is an embryological substrate of DORV) located between the mitral and aortic valves [2, 3] has two consequences. Firstly, it makes impossible for the aorta to shift completely to the left ventricle that explains its initial dextroposition. Secondly, the process of fusion of the OS and VIF fails, which leads to VSD formation. Thus, the anatomy of DORV is a result of embryonic heart arrest at the stage when truncus arteriosus has already been divided by the OS into two lumens (the aorta and pulmonary trunk) but both arterial trunks still originate from the right ventricle.

Nowadays, there are no common criteria for DORV definition that could help with distinguishing this malformation from other conotruncal anomalies. The presence of bilateral infundibulum when the both arterial valves have completely muscular support and lack the fibrous continuity with the atrioventricular valves was initially considered to be the main morphological feature of the disease [2–8]. Later on, double conus turned out to be unnecessary for DORV since a number of cases with predominant origin of the arterial trunks from the right ventricle in couple with mitral-aortic fibrous continuity were demonstrated [9–12]. Consequently, double conus was no longer defined as a mandatory criterion [13]. Now, bilateral infundibulum is an important feature of DORV but still not the main one.

Later for the definition of DORV, the «50%» rule has been widely accepted reflecting the degree of aortic dextroposition. The latter distinguishes simple VSD closure in tetralogy of Fallot and TGA from intraventricular tunnel construction in DORV [14]. Nevertheless, there are still no strict distinguishing criteria between tetralogy of Fallot and DORV «tetralogy» type, as well as between Taussig–Bing anomaly (DORV with subpulmonary VSD) and TGA (see below).

According to Wilcox's expression, "it is more likely that the understanding of double-outlet ventricle has suffered not from a lack of standardization but rather from too many attempts to create a standard where none should exist" [11].

However, there are features that can be counted as morphologically reliable for DORV [15], which are:

- both arterial trunks originate predominantly from the right ventricle;
- persisting VIF between the mitral valve and one of the arterial valves (bilateral infundibulum);
- interventricular communication is the solely exit from the left ventricle;
- OS is a completely right ventricular structure;
- Z-shaped egress from the left ventricle;
- left ventricle lacks its outlet component.

3 Ventricular Septal Defect

VSD is a key surgical component of all types of DORV. To understand the principle of intraventricular tunneling during a surgical repair, it is essential to correctly define the borders of VSD. In DORV, it is necessary due to existence of an extra communication between the edge of VSD and the VIF located right above and between the mitral and aortic valves. To avoid a terminological confusion, Anderson et al. suggested to define this aperture as an exit from the left ventricle. At the same time, the communication for applying a patch to tunnel the aorta to the left ventricle, limited by the crest of the IVS and right aspect of subaortic infundibulum, is defined as VSD [16] (see below). In this regard morphologically, the left ventricle in hearts with DORV lacks its outlet component consisting only of inlet and trabecular parts [11, 17]. Unintentional closure of the exit from the left ventricle instead of VSD is incompatible with life.

The exit from the left ventricle can open either between the limbs of the TS or behind pTS. In the first case, it will be located in the outlet part of the IVS causing

Table 1 Incidence of VSD types in DORV

VSD type	Oladunjoye [20]	Meng [21]	Li [22]	Bradley [23]
Subaortic	33%	48%	58%	47%
Subpulmonary	8%		4%	4%
Subarterial	25%	27%	20%	23%
Non-committed	34%	25%	18%	26%

conoventricular nature of VSD, while in the second case, it can be found in the inlet part causing inlet VSD.

Since VSD is the main characteristic of DORV, in 1972 Lev et al. based on its location and proximity (commitment) to the arterial valves proposed an anatomical classification of the disease [9]. According to their classification, the following four types of DORV were distinguished: with subaortic, subpulmonary, subarterial and non-committed VSD. The first three types are committed ones, since they are located strictly under the either arterial valves, and at the same time are conoventricular, as they open between the limbs of the TS in the outlet part of the IVS [11]. Non-committed VSD due to its location in the inlet part of the IVS and behind the pTS is remote from both arterial valves. It should be noted that the division of VSDs into committed and non-committed types pursues only surgical interest.

The existence of different types of VSD in DORV can be defined not by their various location in the IVS (since they are mostly conoventricular, encradled between the limbs of the TS), but by various arterial trunks relationship which defines the proximity of the arterial valves to VSD [17–19].

The incidence of different types of VSD in DORV according to some clinical investigations is represented in Table 1.

In committed VSDs the exit from the left ventricle to the aorta or pulmonary artery is relatively straight while in non-committed is curved (Fig. 2). Due to such a deformation of the exit from the left ventricle, the surgical repair of DORV with non-committed VSD is very challenging due to increased risk of tunnel obstruction.

Concomitant pulmonary artery stenosis is observed in 70% of subaortic, 75% of subpulmonary, 8% of subarterial and 60% of non-committed VSDs [24].

3.1 Committed VSD

Committed VSD can be found in the outlet part of the IVS strictly under one or both arterial valves between the limbs of the TS thus providing relatively straight communication between the left ventricle and the aorta/pulmonary artery [4, 11] (Fig. 3). Such a location of VSD allows to perform biventricular repair without a risk of tunnel obstruction.

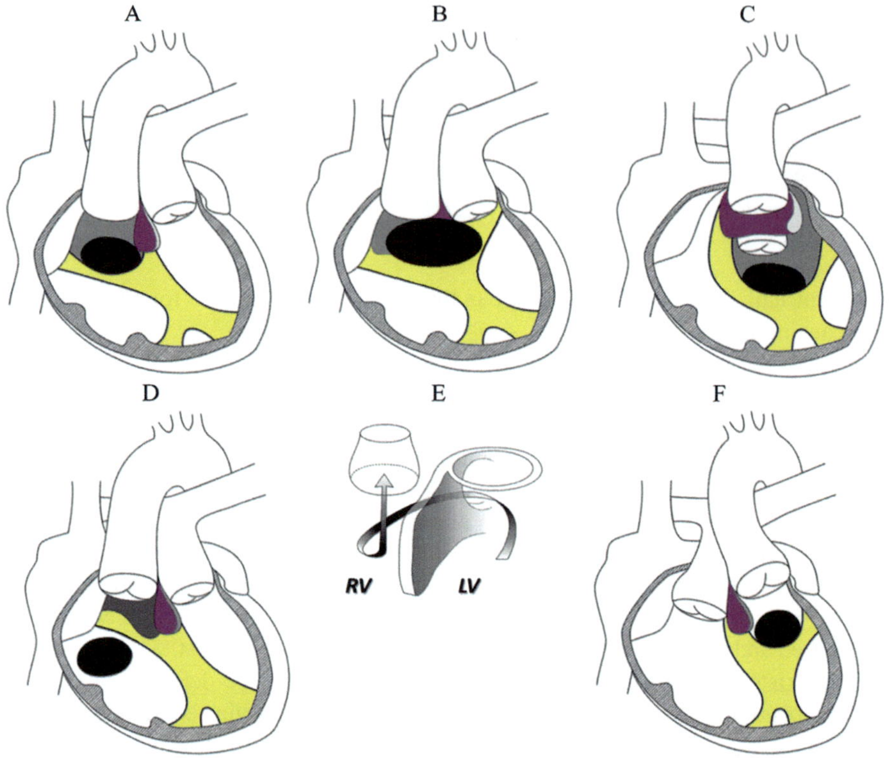

Fig. 2 Types of DORV: **A**—with subaortic VSD (relatively straight exit from the left ventricle to the aorta); **B**—with subarterial VSD (relatively straight exit from the left ventricle to the both arterial trunks); **C**—with subpulmonary VSD (relatively straight exit from the left ventricle to the pulmonary artery; the aorta is separated from VSD by the OS); **D**—with non-committed VSD (no straight exit from the left ventricle to any arterial trunks); **E**—blood flow pattern from the left ventricle to the aorta in non-committed VSD; **F**—with subaortic VSD and L-aorta (relatively straight exit from the left ventricle to the aorta located anterior and left to the pulmonary artery). *LV—left ventricle; RV—right ventricle; yellow figure—trabecula septomarginalis; violet figure—outlet septum*

Embryologically committed VSDs in fact represent a bulboventricular foramen by which the primitive ventricle communicates with the bulbus during heart development. Normally, the mechanism responsible for its closure is alignment of the OS and the IVS in the same plain. Along with this, the OS fuses with the VIF forming the crista supraventricularis. Closure of the bulboventricular foramen without aortic translocation to the left ventricle leads to formation of DORV with intact IVS [25] (see below). Malrotation of the conotruncal block disrupts alignment and fusion of the OS with the IVS and leads to persisting bulboventricular foramen—conoventricular VSD after birth.

Formation of different committed VSDs depends on the type of connection of the OS to the limbs of the TS, which in turn is conditioned by the OS orientation.

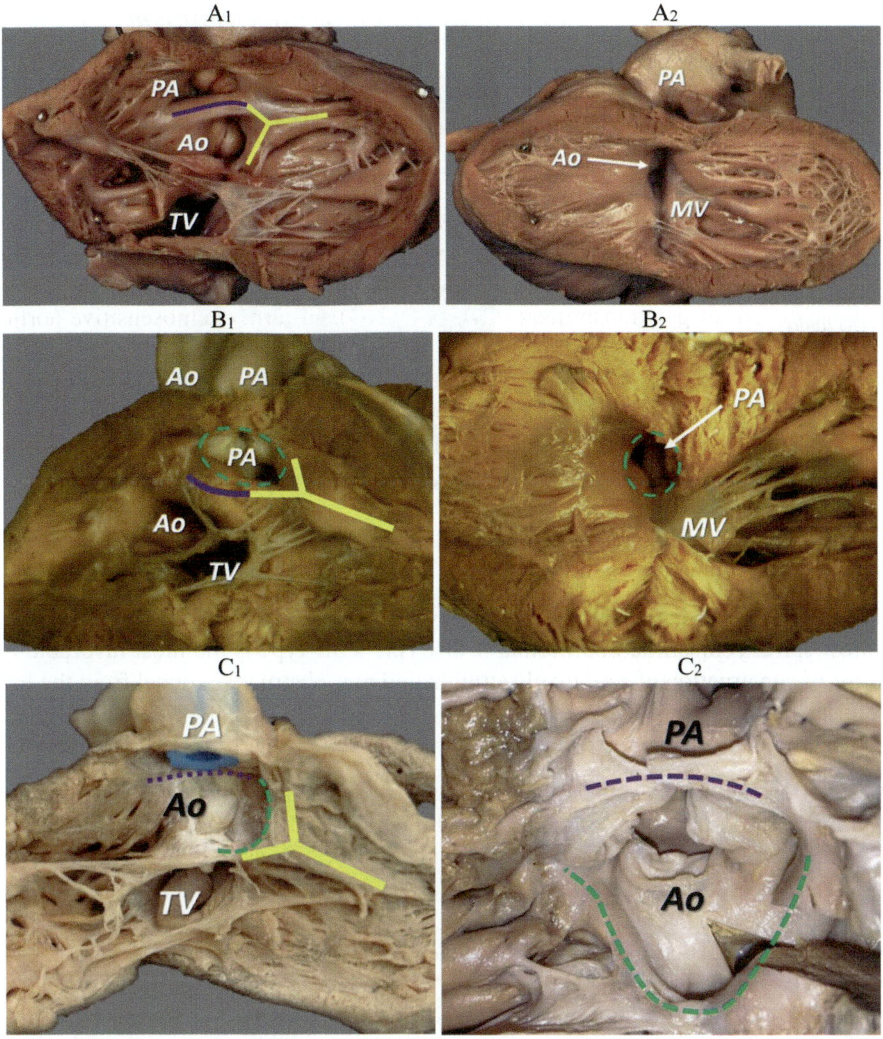

Fig. 3 Committed VSDs in DORV (autopsy specimens): **A**—subaortic VSD (the OS fuses the aTS): $\mathbf{A_1}$—view from the right ventricle; $\mathbf{A_2}$—view from the left ventricle. Muscular postero-inferior rim of VSD formed by the fusion of the pTS and the VIF protects His bundle; **B**—subpulmonary VSD (the OS fuses with the pTS): $\mathbf{B_1}$—view from the right ventricle; $\mathbf{B_2}$—view from the left ventricle; **C**—subarterial VSD: $\mathbf{C_1}$—view from the right ventricle (violet dotted line depicts absence of the OS and aortico-pulmonary fibrous continuity); $\mathbf{C_2}$—view from the right ventricle. The OS as a muscle structure is absent. *Ao—aorta; PA—pulmonary artery; TV—tricuspid valve; MV—mitral valve; yellow figure—trabecula septomarginalis; violet lines—outlet septum; green dotted figures and lines—ventricular septal defect*

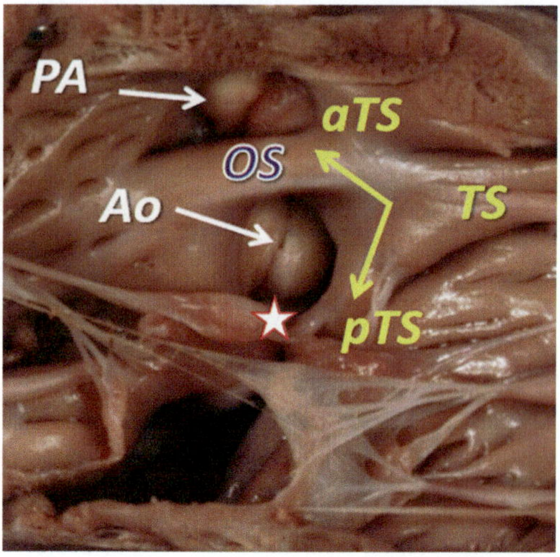

Fig. 4 DORV with subaortic VSD, view from the right ventricle (autopsy specimen). The postero-inferior rim (asterisk) is muscular (the fusion of the pTS with the VIF). *Ao–aorta; PA–pulmonary artery; OS–outlet septum; TS–trabecula septomarginalis with its anterior (aTS) and posterior (pTS) limbs*

Subaortic VSD

Subaortic VSD forms when the OS fuses with the aTS (Fig. 4). The arterial trunks follow spiral course like in a normal heart. This VSD type is the most favorable in terms of construction of a relatively straight and non-obstructive tunnel from the left ventricle to the aorta.

Anatomical rims of subaortic VSD are:

- superior–aortic valve cusps. In some cases, there is a prominent VIF between the mitral and aortic valves which leads to greater aortic dextroposition. At this point, the superior rim of VSD will be represented by the VIF itself and due to the more anterior position of the aorta the arterial trunks will follow parallel course (see below);
- anterior–the fusion of the OS with the aTS;
- inferior–the body of the TS;
- postero-inferior rim may be represented by either muscular or fibrous structure. In the first case due to fusion of the pTS with the VIF, a thick muscle band is formed which protects His bundle (that goes along the postero-inferior rim) from damage during tunneling and makes surgery safe in this area [1, 26]. Owing to this, all the rims of subaortic VSD (except the superior one) and therefore, VSD itself are muscular. In the second case, the pTS does not fuse with the VIF which causes mitral-tricuspid fibrous continuity and His bundle locates superficially and is vulnerable when placing stitches in this area during surgery. Because the postero-inferior rim is fibrous represented by the membranous septum, the nature of subaortic VSD becomes perimembranous [1, 19, 27, 28].

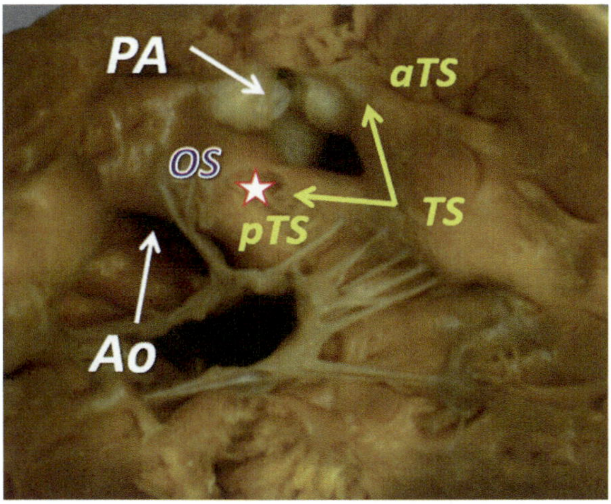

Fig. 5 DORV with subpulmonary VSD, view from the right ventricle (autopsy specimen). The postero-inferior rim of VSD is muscular formed by the fusion (asterisk) of the pTS and the OS. *Ao–aorta; PA–pulmonary artery; OS–outlet Septum; TS–trabecula septomarginalis with its anterior (aTS) and posterior (pTS) limbs*

Subpulmonary VSD

Subpulmonary VSD forms if the OS fuses with the pTS or with the VIF in the area near the pTS (Fig. 5). The arterial trunks follow parallel course with the aorta located either to the right (64–68%) or to the right-anterior to the pulmonary artery (32–36%) [29–31] (Table 2).

Anatomical rims of subpulmonary VSD are:

- superior–pulmonary valve or the VIF (in case of prominent mitral-pulmonary muscular continuity and greater shift of the pulmonary artery to the right ventricle);
- anterior–the aTS;
- inferior–the body of the TS;
- just like in subaortic VSD the postero-inferior rim can be either muscular (fusion of the OS with the pTS) or fibrous (if the OS fuses with the VIF near the pTS).

Subjectively, VSD and the TS are located more superiorly and anteriorly in the IVS than in subaortic VSD. VSD is usually perimembranous due to mitral-tricuspid fibrous continuity. The OS is entirely a right ventricle structure oriented in sagittal plane and located perpendicular to the IVS, while the IVS itself is oriented in frontal plane [34].

Table 2 Types of arterial valves relationship in Taussig–Bing anomaly

Aortic position	Vergnat [29]	Soszyn [30]	Alsoufi [31]	Hayes [32]	Sinzobahamvya [33]
D-aorta	68%	65%	64%	47%	62%
DA-aorta	32%	35%	36%	47%	38%
A-aorta	–	–	–	6%	–

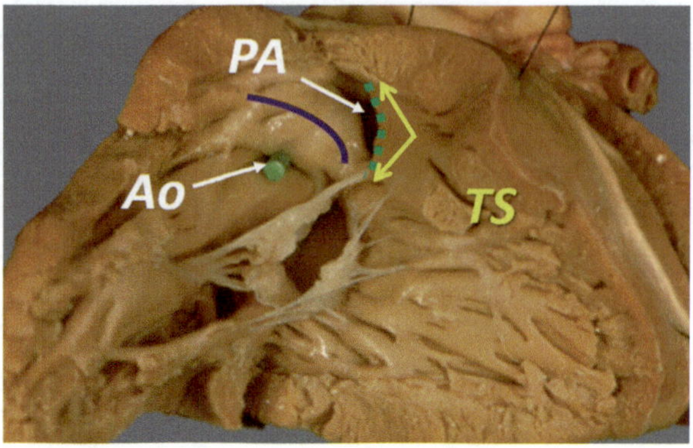

Fig. 6 Taussig–Bing anomaly with the OS deviated toward the subaortic area (violet figure) causing subaortic obstruction. Probe is passed through the aortic valve. *Ao–aorta; PA–pulmonary artery; TS–trabecula septomarginalis; green dotted line–the edge of ventricular septal defect; yellow arrows–the limbs of the trabecula septomarginalis*

In Taussig–Bing anomaly (DORV with subpulmonary VSD without pulmonary artery stenosis), the OS is usually prominent and often deviates to the subaortic area causing subaortic obstruction and hemodynamic rearrangement with predominant blood flow to the pulmonary artery and limited flow to the ascending aorta [35] (Fig. 6).

Morphology of the subpulmonary infundibulum depends on the size of VIF—the smaller the VIF, the closer the pulmonary valve to the mitral valve. If the VIF is absent, then mitral-pulmonary fibrous continuity takes place. So, if there is a prominent VIF between the mitral and pulmonary valves (double conus), the superior border of subpulmonary VSD is represented by the VIF itself within subpulmonary infundibulum. If the VIF is small or even absent, then the same border of VSD will represented by the pulmonary valve [36]. In a number of cases, the malformation may be associated with pulmonary artery stenosis [37]. In this case, the malformation cannot be considered as Taussig–Bing anomaly in its first description [38]. Cases with pulmonary artery stenosis account for 8% of DORV with subpulmonary VSD [24].

Subarterial VSD

Sometimes, the OS as a muscular structure may be completely absent that leads to the arterial valves being separated only by thin fibrous tissue causing thus aortico-pulmonary fibrous continuity [39–41]. This makes VSD being located beneath the both arterial valves which is responsible for the subarterial nature of VSD [1, 42] (Fig. 7). Thus, double-outlet both ventricles results, since the aorta and pulmonary artery communicate with the left and right ventricles [43, 44] and override conoventricular VSD between the limbs of the TS. In some cases, the VIF behind the arterial valves is also absent causing fibrous continuity between the atrioventcricular and

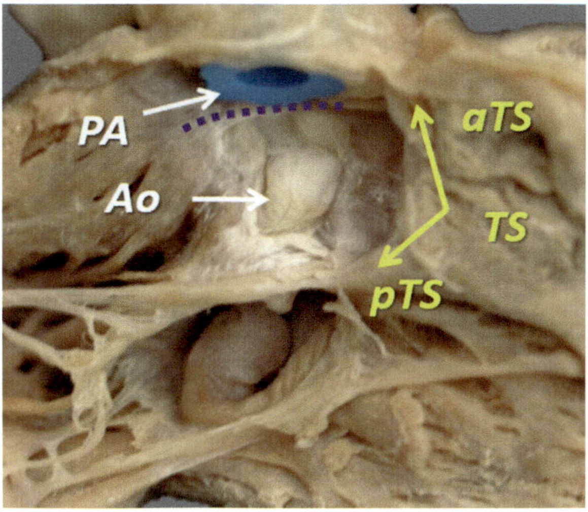

Fig. 7 DORV with subarterial VSD and fibrous OS (violet dotted line). The subarterial infundibilums are not separated. *Ao–aorta; PA–pulmonary artery; TS–trabecula septomarginalis with its anterior (aTS) and posterior (pTS) limbs*

arterial valves [45]. DORV with subarterial VSD and absent OS is featured with spiral course of the arterial trunks.

Anatomical rims of subarterial VSD are:

- superior–arterial valves;
- anterior–aTS;
- inferior–TS;
- posterior–pTS.

Consequently, the nature of committed VSD is firstly defined by the fact of fusion of the OS with the limbs of TS and secondly by the type of such a fusion. In spite of this, in rare cases, anatomy of DORV does not correspond to the traditional anatomical patterns described above. Such as, e.g., DORV with subarterial VSD and muscular OS (Fig. 8) [44].

The complexity of DORV anatomy is explained by multiple combinations of VSD types and different arterial trunks relationships. All committed VSDs are the same conoventricular VSD always located between the limbs of the TS. Hence, the proximity of conoventricular VSD is determined by which arterial valve it is located below which in turn depends on the arterial valve relationship.

In committed VSDs, one (in subaortic and subpulmonary VSD) or both (in subarterial VSD) arterial trunks are located partially in the right and left ventricles, since the superior rim of VSD is presented by one or both arterial valves. Prominent subarterial infundibulum which lifts arterial valve and remotes from subaortic or subpulmonary VSD may form superior rim of VSD. The shorter subaortic infundibulum, the closer the aortic valve to the mitral valve. As well as lack of subpulmonary infundibulum in Taussig–Bing anomaly leads to mitral-pulmonary fibrous continuity [13].

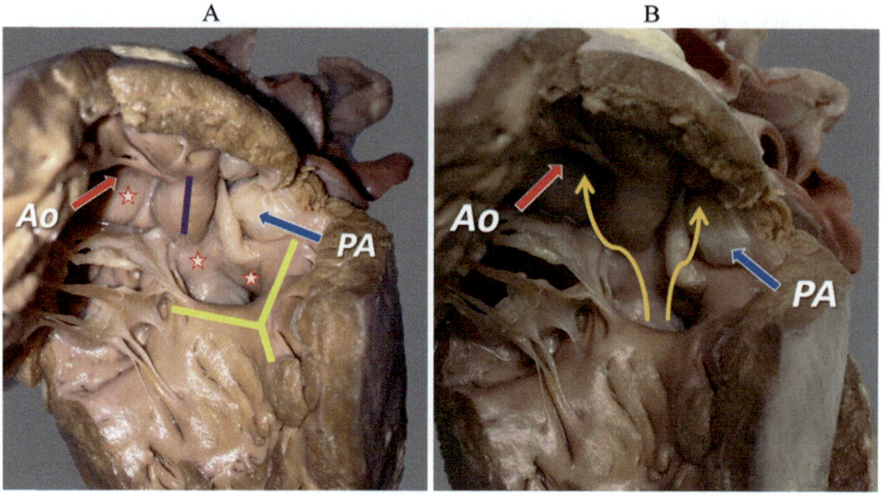

Fig. 8 DORV with subarterial VSD and muscular OS, view from the right ventricle (autopsy specimen). **A**—subarterial VSD. Narrowing of the subaortic infundibulum due to the hypertrophied OS (violet figure) and the VIF (the most left asterisk). The OS does not fuse with any limbs of the TS (yellow figure) but joins VIF to its middle part (middle asterisk); **B**—the same specimen. Despite the OS separates the aortic (red arrow) and pulmonary (blue arrow) valves VSD remains subarterial due to absence of fusion between the OS and the limbs of the TS (orange arrows) which would separate subarterial infundibulums. Thus, VSD is committed to both arterial valves. *Ao—aorta; PA—pulmonary artery*

3.2 *Non-committed VSD*

The term «non-committed» VSD was coined by Lev et al. in 1972 [9]. Zamora et al. in 1975 for such cases offered another term: «remote» VSD [25].

DORV with non-committed VSD anatomically is the most complex form of the disease which significantly impedes biventricular repair. Non-committed VSD is characterized by the fact that it is impossible to construct a straight non-obstructive tunnel from the left ventricle to any of the arterial valves.

In 1999, Belli et al. proposed a new criterion for non-committed VSD–distance between VSD and any of the arterial valves greater than the diameter of the aortic valve [46]. This approach in determining non-committed nature of VSD does not take into account its anatomical position. Based on this criterion, non-committed may be VSD located in the inlet IVS as well as conoventricular subaortic VSD with elongated subaortic conus.

In turn, if only those VSD which locate exclusively in the inlet IVS to determine as non-committed, then this contradicts the previous criterion, which can also be applied to conoventricular VSD. Thus, depending on the criterion used, both inlet and conoventricular VSDs can be non-committed, which differ in embryological, anatomical and surgical terms. In this regard, it is reasonable to divide non-committed VSDs into truly non-committed (inlet, located behind the pTS) and not directly

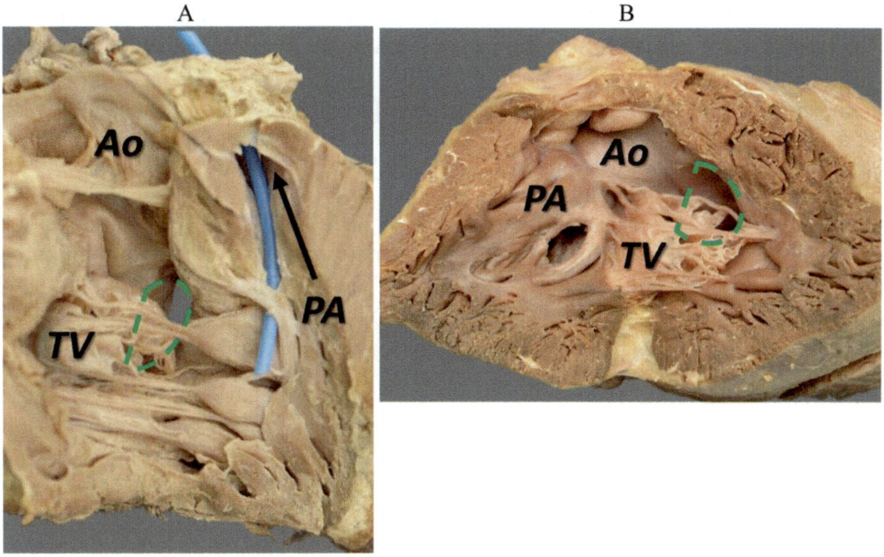

Fig. 9 DORV with non-committed VSDs (autopsy specimen): **A**–non-committed perimembranous inlet VSD («atrioventricular» type); **B**–not directly committed subaortic VSD located in the outlet IVS (L-malposition). Note the prominent VIF forming the elongated subaortic conus. *Ao–aorta; PA–pulmonary artery; TV–tricuspid valve; green dotted figure–ventricular septal defect*

committed ones (conoventricular, located between the limbs of the TS, with elongated subaortic infundibulum) [47] as it was first proposed by Beekman et al. [48].

So, the main features of DORV «non-committed» type are remoteness of VSD from the arterial valves on a distance more than aortic valve diameter, both arterial trunks arise from the right ventricle (the «200%» principle) and presence of double conus [49]. The arterial trunks are side by side and the OS is completely right ventricle structure, not IVS.

Non-committed VSD

Non-committed (or inlet) VSD locates in the inlet IVS behind the pTS [48], so the latter can serve as a reliable reference point for determining this type of VSD. Morphologically, non-committed VSDs may be represented by the following types:

– perimembranous inlet VSD («atrioventricular» type). One of the rims of such type of defect is formed by the tricuspid valve annulus (Fig. 9A). The anatomical rims of perimembranous inlet VSD:

  - superior–VIF between the mitral and the aortic valves;
  - anterior–OS;
  - inferior–muscular inlet IVS;
  - posterior–septal leaflet of the tricuspid valve.

- muscular inlet VSD. In this type of defect, there is a muscular band between the tricuspid valve and VSD. All the rims of defect are muscular represented by the inlet and trabecular IVS.
- muscular apical VSD, located near the apex [45, 50].

Among all non-committed VSDs, «atrioventricular» type (i.e., perimembranous inlet VSD) is the most common [28]. Arterial trunks relationship in DORV with non-committed VSD can be normal (57.3%) or with D- (37.3%) or L-malposition (5.3%) of the aorta. In 60% of cases the malformation is associated with pulmonary artery stenosis [51]. Due to the prominent VIF and OS, half of the patients have subaortic obstruction [28]. In 40% of cases, VSD is closer to the aortic valve, in 36% to the pulmonary valve and in 24% is equally remote from both arterial valves [51].

Not Directly Committed VSD

Not directly committed VSD (as committed ones) locates in the outlet IVS and is anatomically conoventricular [45, 48] and is usually found in subaortic area. The main feature of this type of VSD is long subaortic infundibulum own to the prominent VIF (which partially constitutes subaotric conus) that lifts the aortic valve and makes it remote from VSD [46, 52].

Surgically such a VSD is non-committed, while anatomically, being conoventricular, is committed. In fact, this type includes typical subaortic VSD with prominent VIF as well as subaortic VSD in DORV with L-aorta (Fig. 9B).

Surgical repair of not directly committed VSD unlike typical subaortic VSD requires the creation of a longer intraventricular tunnel.

So, non-committed VSDs locate behind the pTS in the inlet and trabecular IVS [53, 54], while not directly committed and committed VSDs are cradled within the limbs of the TS and locate in the outlet IVS.

In order to avoid terminological confusion in the following chapters, the term «non-committed» will be used only for those VSDs which locate in the inlet IVS.

3.3 DORV with Intact IVS

In addition to the morphological variants described above, there are also forms of DORV with intact IVS [11, 18, 25, 55, 56]. Incidence of this type of DORV is extremely low because absent exit from the left ventricle is incompatible with life. The malformation is featured with the left ventricle hypoplasia and mitral valve atresia/stenosis. Aortic diameter may approach normal size but for survival of such patients the presence of a wide interatrial communication is essential [57]. Such a set of anatomical features differs from DORV and normally is considered as a type of hypoplasia left heart syndrome.

3.4 Restrictive VSD

Stable systemic hemodynamics after biventricular repair of DORV is possible only if size of VSD is at least equal to the diameter of the aortic valve. In this regard, the important characteristic of VSD is its sufficient size to create non-obstructive exit from the left ventricle [58, 59].

Non-restrictive VSD is equal or greater than the aortic valve diameter. If defect does not meet this criterion, then it should be considered as restrictive one. Incidence of restrictive VSD in DORV is about 10% [13, 60]. Tunnel construction in this case can be fatal due to restriction of the outflow from the left ventricle and its subsequent failure immediately after repair. All restrictive VSDs without any doubt should be augmented!

An embryological prerequisite for the formation of restriction VSD is presence of prominent subaortic infundibulum which leads to convergence of subaortic conus and IVS [61] as well as the alignment of the OS and the IVS in the same plane resulting in partial closure of the embryonic bulboventricular foramen [62].

All types of committed and non-committed VSDs can be restrictive. In some cases, after pulmonary artery banding procedure, initially non-restrictive VSD may become restrictive due to compensatory right ventricle hypertrophy in response to increased afterload [63].

4 Exit from the Left Ventricle

As it was mentioned at the beginning of the chapter, VSD in DORV is a communication between the crest of the IVS and the right aspect of subaortic infundibulum. However, it should be noted that this communication, in fact, does not determine the diameter of the exit from the left ventricle. In turn, the real exit from the left ventricle on which depends normal outflow from the left heart is represented by the communication between the crest of the IVS and the VIF located between the mitral and the aortic valves (Fig. 10). The main surgical principle for construction of non-obstructive tunnel of sufficient diameter is that the size of VSD should be at least equal to the diameter of the aortic valve. Such a practical approach does not take into account the diameter of the real exit from the left ventricle. These differences become more significant with increasing of aortic dextroposition. So, instead of matching the size of VSD to the aortic diameter it will be more correct for this purpose to use the diameter of the real exit from the left ventricle [45].

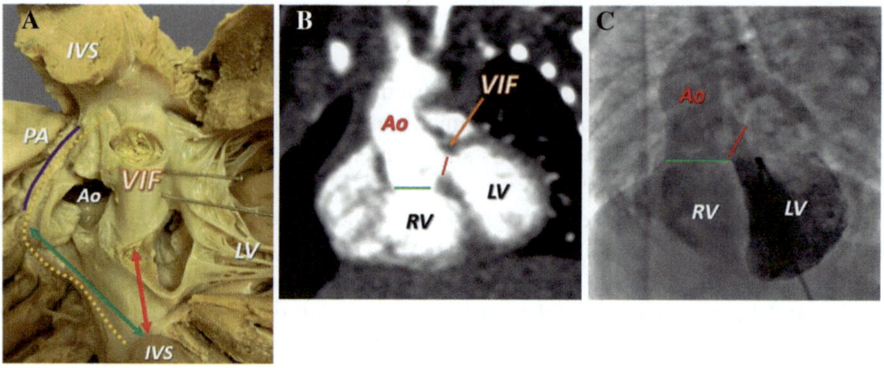

Fig. 10 Real exit from the left ventricle and VSD in DORV: **A**–DORV with subaortic VSD (autopsy specimen). The IVS is incised from the middle of its crest to the apex (view from the apex); **B**–a computed tomography scan of DORV with subaortic VSD; **C**–an angiocardiographic scan of DORV with subaortic VSD. The panels show the difference between VSD (green double-headed arrow and green lines) and real exit from the left ventricle (red double-headed arrow and red lines). Real exit from the left ventricle is limited by the crest of the IVS and the VIF between the mitral and the aortic valves, while VSD is limited by the crest of the IVS and the right aspect of subaortic infundibulum. An orange dotted line in the panel A indicates the area for applying a patch for intraventricular tunneling of the aorta. *Ao–aorta; PA–pulmonary artery; RV–right ventricle; LV–left ventricle; IVS–interventricular septum; VIF–ventriculoinfundibular fold*

5 Arterial Valves Relationship and Course of the Arterial Trunks

Arterial valves relationship is one of the main anatomical characteristics of DORV on which depends proximity of VSD to the arterial valves. This relationship is determined by the OS orientation which in turn is conditioned by different degree of truncal rotation to the right during embryogenesis.

There are the following variants of aortic and pulmonary valves relationship (Fig. 11):

- posterior aorta (P-aorta);
- right and posterior aorta (DP-aorta);
- right aorta (D-aorta);
- right and anterior aorta (DA-aorta);
- anterior aorta (A-aorta);
- left and anterior aorta (L-aorta).

In DORV, most commonly are encountered DP, D and DA types of malposition, while P and A malposition are rare.

In case of L-malposition (Figs. 2F, 9B) VSD is predominantly found in subaortic area [64–67], although it can be subpulmonary [10, 68, 69] or non-committed [70]. Due to anterior and left position of the aorta, the right coronary artery crosses the pulmonary artery in front of it, which takes place in almost all cases, while coronary

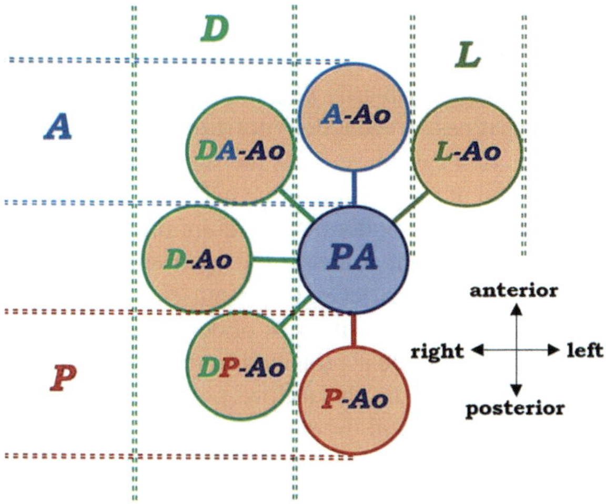

Fig. 11 Variants of arterial valves relationship in DORV

artery pattern remains normal [66]. This causes difficulties or even precludes transannular repair of right ventricular outflow tract (RVOT) if needed. In some cases, with a sufficient distance from the right coronary artery to the pulmonary annulus, it is possible to perform transannular repair by shifting incision line on RVOT to the right [71].

Course of the arterial trunks after their origin from the basement of the heart can be spiral with twisting of the pulmonary artery around the ascending aorta (as in a normal heart) or parallel [1, 5] (Fig. 12). With spiral course, VSD usually locates in subaortic or subarterial (when the OS is absent) areas, while with parallel course, VSD can be subpulmonary, subarterial (when the OS is prominent) or non-committed. It is interesting that type of DORV with subpulmonary VSD and spiraling arterial trunks has not been described in the literature until today.

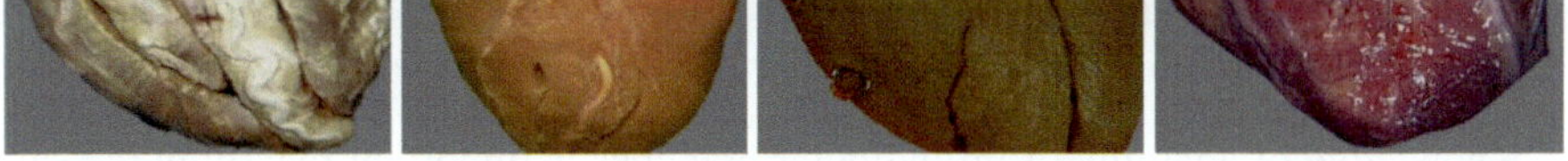

Fig. 12 Arterial valves relationship in DORV (autopsy specimen): **A**–DP-aorta; **B**–D-aorta (Taussig–Bing anomaly); **C**–DA-aorta; **D**–L-aorta

5.1 Conduction System Anatomy

Since DORV is primarily an anomaly of ventriculoarterial connection, morphology of various types of VSDs does not differ from isolated VSDs. Consequently, anatomy of conduction system remains the same.

Location of conduction tissue in DORV depends on type of VSD. In conoventricular VSD (including not directly committed subaortic VSD), His bundle follows its postero-inferior rim along the left ventricular side of the IVS. In this regard, surgical augmentation of restrictive conoventricular VSD can be safely performed in antero-superior fashion without a risk of developing heart block. If the pTS fuses with the VIF, then His bundle is protected by this muscle structure. In inlet «atrioventricular» type VSD His bundle also follows posterior rim, while in case of muscular inlet VSD along superior rim in the muscular band between the septal leaflet of the tricuspid valve and superior rim of VSD [11, 34, 44].

5.2 Coronary Artery Anatomy

Detection of coronary artery abnormalities is important for repair of various types of DORV mainly due to need for coronary arteries reimplantation during the arterial switch operation (ASO) and some other techniques requiring aortic root mobilization (see Chapter 10). In addition, preoperative diagnostics of infundibular branches crossing RVOT is very helpful for surgical planning.

During the cardiac development, coronary arteries follow the shortest pathway between aortic wall and corresponding atrioventricular grooves. Accordingly, this distance is primarily determined by relationship of the arterial trunks.

As mentioned above, preoperative assessment of coronary anatomy is most important for Taussig–Bing anomaly because ASO is a first-line option for such patients. Incidence of coronary artery abnormalities in Taussig–Bing anomaly accounts for 32–51%, which is almost one and a half times more than in TGA [30, 72].

As given in Table 2, there are three types of arterial trunks relationship in Taussig–Bing anomaly, which imply the orientation of the OS. Depending on angle formed by the OS and the IVS, these relative positions can be characterized as follows [73] (Fig. 13):

- angle > 70° with side by side arterial trunks;
- angle of 20°–70° with right and anterior aorta;
- angle < 20° with anterior aorta.

Knowledge of anatomy of infundibular branches is important regarding the safe incision when transannular RVOT reconstruction is required.

Types of coronary artery patterns and their incidence in Taussig–Bing anomaly are listed in Table 3.

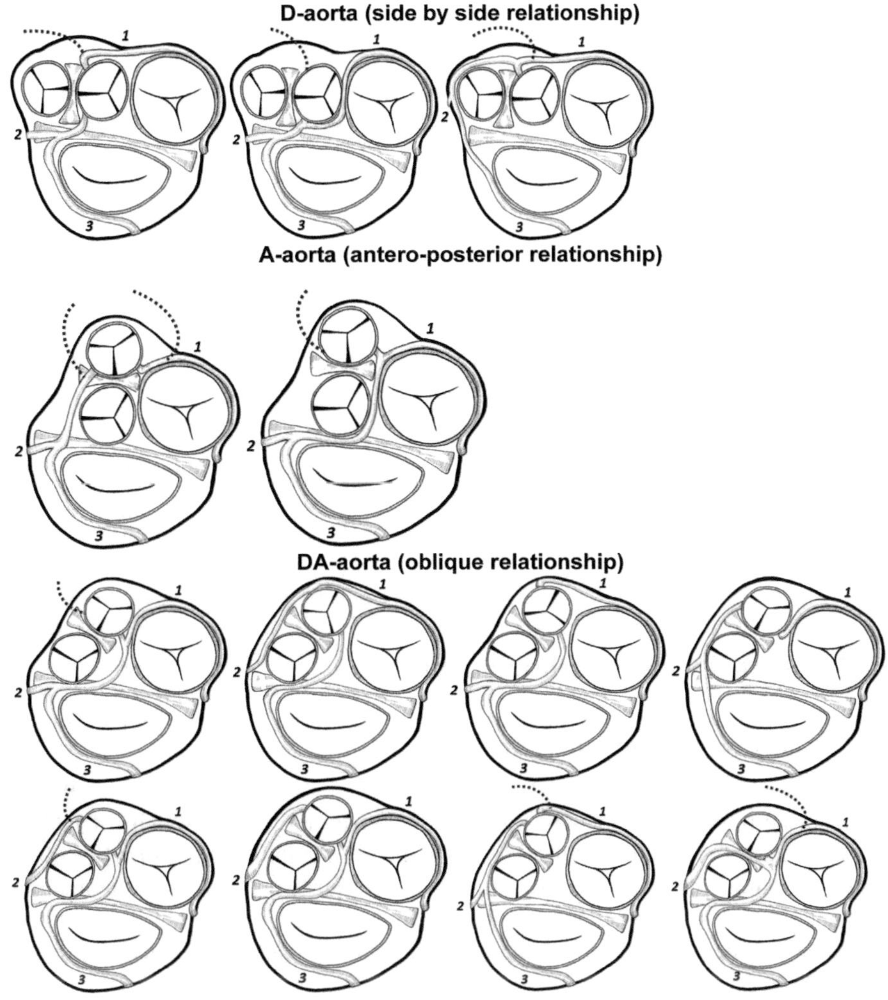

Fig. 13 Coronary artery pattern in Taussig–Bing anomaly depending on relationship of the arterial trunks according to Uemura et al. *1–right coronary artery; 2–left descending artery; 3–circumflex artery; dotted line–infundibular branch*

Table 3 Types of coronary artery patterns in Taussig–Bing anomaly according to different authors

Pattern (*Yacoub's type*)	Vergnat [29]	Patwary [74]	Hayes [32]	Soszyn [30]	Feng [75]	Griselli [76]
1LCx, 2R (A) *1LCx, 2R (C)*	35% 4%	83.3%	40%	49.1%	77.9%	42% 3%
1LCxR (B)	–	–	–	1.8%	7.6%	9%
1L, 2RCx (D)	10%	–	14%	19.3%	11.8%	30%
2RLCx	–	–	14%	7%		
1LR, 2Cx (E)	51%	–	14%	8.8%	2.9%	15%
1R, 2LCx (F)	–	–	12%	14%	–	
Intramural course	–	4.7%	2%	–	–	9%
Others	–	16.6%	7%	–	–	–

6 Associated Cardiac Abnormalities

6.1 *Atrioventricular Valve Anomalies*

Atrioventricular valve anomalies significantly affect surgical treatment of DORV regarding choice of certain technical features and even inability to perform biventricular repair. Anomalies of the atrioventricular valves can be represented by anomalous attachment of tricuspid chordae to the OS, valve straddling (when subvalvular structures attach either to the IVS or contralateral ventricle) and atrioventricular septal defect (AVSD).

Anomalous Tricuspid Valve Attachment to the Outlet Septum

Normally, all chords of the septal, anterior and posterior leaflets of the tricuspid valve are attached to the IVS and free wall of the right ventricle. With this arrangement, subvalvular structures do not hinder construction of intraventricular tunnel. Sometimes chordae may have an abnormal attachment to the OS, potentially located in the projection of a tunnel, which may cause certain difficulties when sewing a patch inside the right ventricle and affect surgical tactics (Fig. 14).

Straddling Atrioventricular Valve

Straddling atrioventricular valve is an abnormal attachment of its subvalvular structures to both sides of the IVS or to the papillary muscle of contralateral ventricle (biventricular attachment). These anatomical disorders are possible only in the

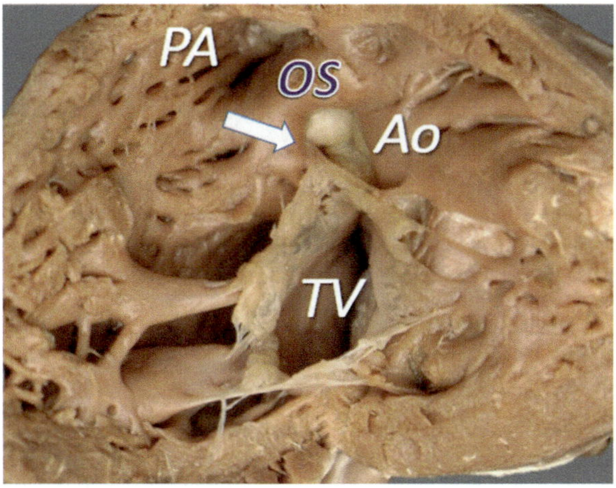

Fig. 14 DORV with subaortic VSD, view from the right ventricle (autopsy specimen). Some chords of the anterior leaflet of the tricuspid valve are attached to the OS (arrow) *Ao–aorta; PA–pulmonary Artery; OS–outlet Septum; TV–tricuspid Valve*

presence of VSD and reflect a maldevelopment of chordo-papillary apparatus of atrioventricular valve.

Depending on the site of anomalous attachment, the following types of straddling atrioventricular valves are distinguished [77] (Figs. 15, 16):

- type «A»—chords are attached to the crest of the IVS (edge of VSD) or next to it on the side of contralateral ventricle;
- type «B»—chords are attached to the IVS but on the side of contralateral ventricle and significantly further from the crest of the IVS than in type «A»;
- type «C»—chords are attached to the free wall of contralateral ventricle.

Atrioventricular Septal Defect

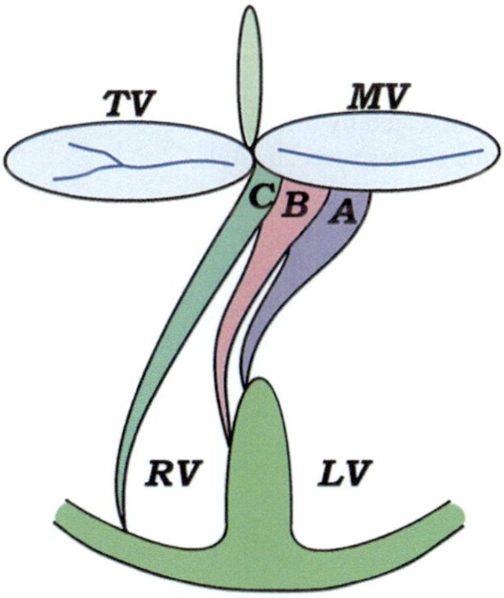

Fig. 15 Straddling types of atrioventricular valves according to Tabry classification (on mitral valve example). The chords are attached to the crest of the IVS (edge of VSD) (type «A»), to the IVS on the side of contralateral ventricle (type «B») and to the free wall of contralateral ventricle (type «C»). *MV–mitral valve; TV–tricuspid valve; LV–left ventricle; RV–right ventricle*

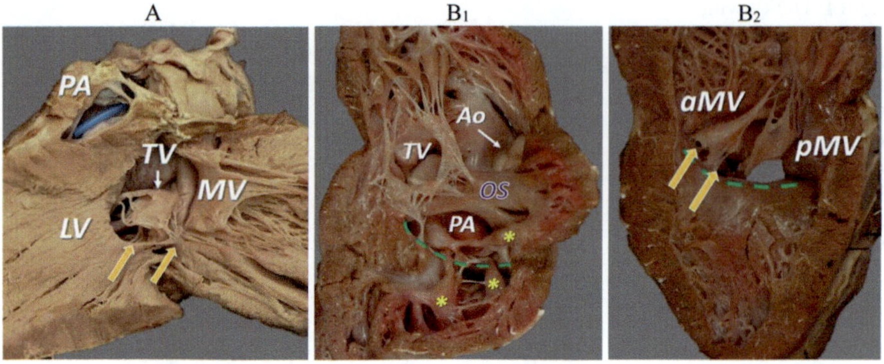

Fig. 16 DORV with straddling atrioventricular valve (autopsy specimen): **A**–straddling of the tricuspid valve type «A» (view from the left ventricle). Chords of the septal leaflet of the tricuspid valve are attached to the edge of VSD (orange arrows); **B**–straddling of the mitral valve type «C» (view from the right ventricle): $\mathbf{B_1}$–the papillary muscles of the mitral valve are attached to the free wall of the right ventricle (yellow asterisks) crossing VSD (green dotted line); $\mathbf{B_2}$–the same specimen (view from the left ventricle). The chords of the anterior leaflet of the mitral valve are attached to the edge of VSD (orange arrows)—«straddling» type «A». The posterior leaflet of the mitral valve crosses VSD edge and attaches to the free wall of the right ventricle. *Ao–aorta; PA–pulmonary artery; TV–tricuspid valve; MV–mitral valve; OS–outlet septum; aMV–anterior leaflet of the MV; pMV–posterior leaflet of the MV*

AVSD occurs in 13.6% of DORV, while in Tetralogy of Fallot, only in 1.7% [78]. In addition to the presence of common atrioventricular annulus, an important characteristic of AVSD is deficient of the inlet component of the IVS. This leads to the inlet/outlet components ratio being less than 1, while normally they are almost equal (Fig. 17).

Fig. 17 DORV/AVSD. Lack of inlet component of the IVS. The inlet/outlet components ratio is less than 1 (indicated by the red and blue arrows respectively)

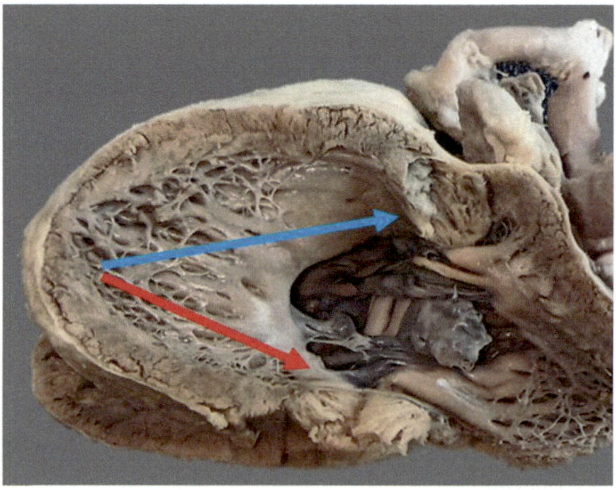

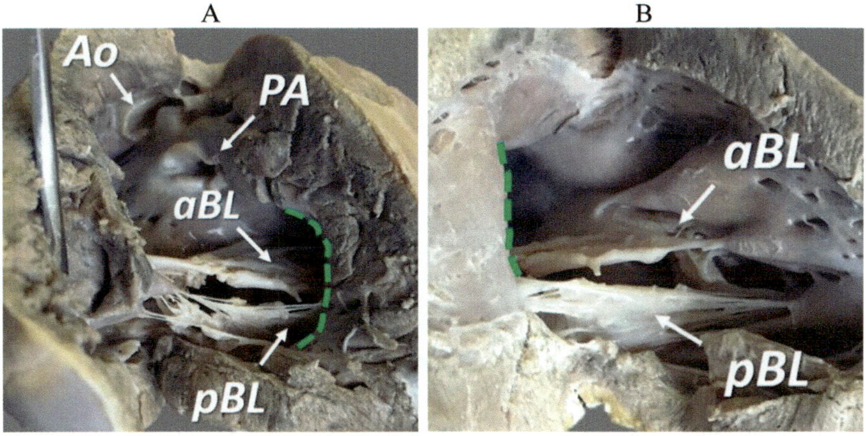

Fig. 18 DORV/AVSD and right ventricle hypoplasia (autopsy specimen): **A**–view from the right ventricle; **B**–view from the left ventricle. *Ao–aorta; PA–pulmonary artery; aBL–anterior bridging leaflet; pBL–posterior anterior bridging leaflet; green dotted line–the edge of ventricular septal defect*

DORV/AVSD is divided into balanced and unbalanced types depending on morphology of the ventricles with dominant right or left ventricle as in isolated form of AVSD. In the presence of hypoplasia of any of the ventricles, biventricular repair is contraindicated and univentricular palliation is the only possible option of surgical treatment (Fig. 18).

DORV/AVSD is often associated with heterotaxy syndrome, genetic abnormalities, as well as anomalous drainage of systemic, pulmonary and hepatic veins, which significantly complicate or even preclude biventricular repair. Heterotaxy syndrome occurs in 42–75% of DORV/AVSD [79–82], Down syndrome is observed in 44–60% of cases [78, 79].

Most often in DORV is observed «C» type of AVSD [78, 81–86] according to the Rastelli classification [87], in which the anterior bridging leaflet floats over the IVS and the posterior one is attached to the edge of VSD (Fig. 19).

There may be fibrous (which contributes to the extension of VSD to the subaortic area) or muscular continuity between the anterior bridging leaflet and the aortic valve depending on the absence or presence of VIF between them respectively [28]. Within some rare cases, the anterior bridging leaflet may have fibrous continuity between both arterial valves and then VSD has subarterial extension [88].

Thus, depending on extension of inlet VSD to subarterial infundibulums DORV/AVSD can be with subaortic–44%, subarterial–9%, subpulmonary–3% extension as well as non-committed type in 44% of cases. The last two types are the most difficult in surgical terms. Arterial trunks relationship may be normal (36%), with D-aorta (26%), DA-aorta (26%), A-aorta (6%) and L-aorta (6%) [89].

Concomitant pulmonary artery stenosis is observed in 62–100% of patients with DORV/AVSD [83, 84, 89].

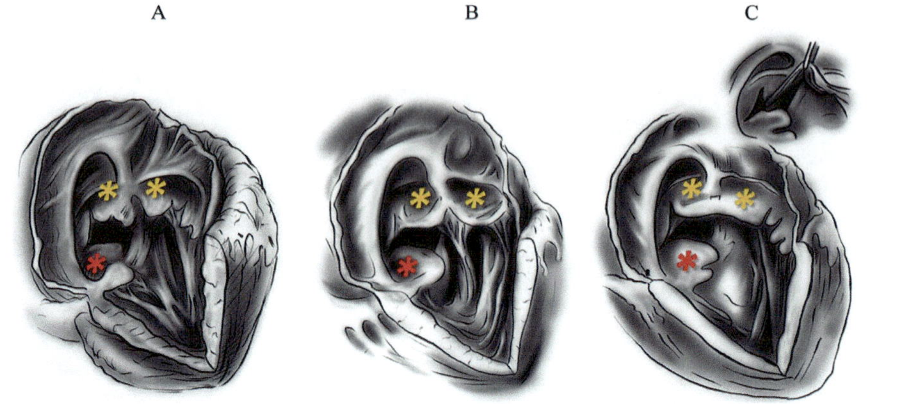

Fig. 19 Classification of AVSD proposed by Rastelli [adapted [88]: **A**—«A» type. The anterior bridging leaflet is divided by the commissure into the tricuspid and mitral components both of which are attached to the edge of VSD; **B**—«B» type. Both components of the anterior bridging leaflet have attachment in the right ventricle by means of an abnormal muscle; **C**—«C» type. The anterior bridging leaflet is not divided, floats freely over the edge of VSD and attaches near the apex of the right ventricle. *Orange asterisks—anterior bridging leaflet; red asterisks—posterior bridging leaflet*

6.2 Aortic Arch Obstruction

Aortic arch obstructive lesions among all anatomical variants of DORV are most often found in Taussig–Bing anomaly and «non-committed» type.

Taussig–Bing anomaly is characterized by prominent OS which if deviated toward the subaortic area contributes to the development not only of subaortic obstruction, which takes place in 14–82% of patients [29–33], but also of various aortic arch obstructions that occur in 23–70% of cases [29–32, 90–92]. For comparison, in TGA, aortic arch obstruction occurs in about 5% of patients [93]. The morphological elements of subaortic obstruction are represented by the OS and the VIF.

Aortic arch diameter less than «patient's weight + 1» is a criterion for its hypoplasia [90]. In the presence of arch obstruction, pulmonary valve in Taussig–Bing anomaly is larger than the aortic valve. The greater pulmonary valve/aortic valve ratio the more frequent aortic arch obstruction [29].

Morphologically obstruction of the aortic arch can be represented by coarctation (64%), hypoplasia (57%) and interruption (21%) or their combination. In most cases, coarctation and hypoplasia are associated with each other [94] (Fig. 20).

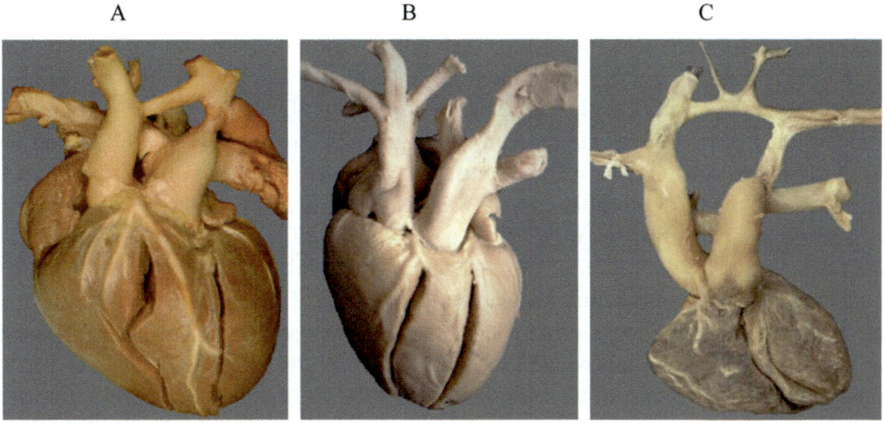

Fig. 20 Types of aortic arch obstructive lesions in DORV: **A**–Taussig–Bing anomaly with coarctation and arch hypoplasia; **B**–Taussig-Bing anomaly with interrupted aortic arch type «A»; **C**–subarterial VSD (without the OS) with arch hypoplasia

6.3 Transitional Anatomical Forms of DORV

As it was already mentioned above, there is still no generally accepted definition as well as clear anatomical concept of DORV. From embryological viewpoint, DORV engages middle position in the spectrum of conotruncal anomalies between tetralogy of Fallot and TGA depending on degree of rotation of the conotruncal block, which causes certain difficulties in determining distinctive morphological features of DORV.

DORV is characterized by a wide spectrum of morphological forms mainly depending on VSD location and arterial trunks relationship. Since there are no clear anatomical criteria for DORV today, it is inevitable that the so-called «transitional anatomical forms» in the spectrum of conotruncal anomalies are exist, which in some cases cannot be distinguished from each other. There are following two transitional anatomical forms of DORV between:

- tetralogy of Fallot and DORV «tetralogy» type;
- TGA with VSD and Taussig–Bing anomaly.

6.4 Transitional Form with Tetralogy of Fallot

The main criteria that can serve to distinguish tetralogy of Fallot and DORV with subaortic VSD and pulmonary artery stenosis are:

- mitral-aortic fibrous or muscular continuity;
- degree of aortic dextroposition.

As mentioned, presence of mitral-aortic muscular continuity (due to which bilateral conus is formed) was initially considered as a defining anatomical criterion of DORV. However, as it was shown later, in some hearts with DORV, there is mitral-aortic fibrosis continuity with aortic origin more than 50% from the right ventricle. This, on the one hand, leads to a certain ambiguity in terminology of DORV, and on the other hand, complicates its differentiation from tetralogy of Fallot. That is why subsequently the term «double conus» was rejection as a key feature of DORV [9].

Embryological substrate of DORV is a persistence of the VIF between the mitral and aortic valves. Resorption of the VIF here (which takes place in a normal heart) leads not only to posterior and leftward translocation of the aortic valve toward the left ventricle, but also to its clockwise rotation (when viewed from above). Based on this from embryological viewpoint, all hearts with the presence of mitral-aortic muscular continuity should be considered as DORV, regardless of degree of aortic dextroposition.

Lev et al. in their study noted that in tetralogy of Fallot mitral-aortic fibrosis continuity was formed mainly with non-coronary aortic cusp rather than with left coronary cusp, while in DORV they observed the opposite picture [9]. Thus, we can assume greater degree of clockwise rotation of the conotruncal block in tetralogy of Fallot compared to DORV.

Considering mitral-aortic muscular continuity as a main criterion of DORV, the following question inevitably arises: how to determine hearts with muscular continuity, but in which the greater part of aorta originates from the left ventricle and there is pulmonary artery stenosis [95]? In this case, the malformation is likely to be named tetralogy of Fallot, embryogenesis of which is completely different from that of DORV. But if consider as a main criterion of DORV the "50%" rule, then another question is brought up: should we consider a heart with a displacement of the aorta to the right ventricle by more than 50%, but with the presence of mitral-aortic fibrous continuity as DORV?

These uncertainties suppose existence of DORV with mitral-aortic fibrous continuity, on the one hand, and tetralogy of Fallot with mitral-aortic muscular continuity, on the other hand. This, in turn, causes certain anatomical contradictions. Thus, the use of these two criteria separately from each other leads to the failure of each of them in distinguishing DORV and tetralogy of Fallot.

As it is known anterolateral deviation of the OS serves as an embryological substrate of tetralogy of Fallot [96, 97], which results in pulmonary artery stenosis: valvular (due to hypoplasia of annulus) and subvalvular (due to the OS with its septal and parietal insertions). At the same time, the OS itself remains a part of the IVS. However, without RVOT obstruction and pulmonary artery stenosis, «tetralogy of Fallot» can never be diagnosed. Thus, tetralogy of Fallot is an anomaly of the deviated OS, which entails RVOT obstruction. In turn, DORV (if use «50%» rule), first of all, is a type of ventriculoarterial connection with predominant origin of both arterial trunks from the right ventricle regardless of presence of pulmonary artery stenosis and RVOT obstruction. In this regard, some authors without finding any contradictions allow coexistence of tetralogy of Fallot and DORV [27, 45, 98]!

Such an assumption is not paradoxical and can be logically explained. When determining tetralogy of Fallot an anatomical criterion is used–anterolateral deviation of the OS which causes RVOT obstruction. At the same time, DORV is determined on the basis of a functional criterion–degree of aortic dextroposition (overriding). It is very important to notice that both of these criteria are not mutually exclusive! Thus, the anatomical criterion of tetralogy of Fallot of the OS deviation can be applied to DORV, and vice versa–the functional criterion of DORV can be applied to tetralogy of Fallot. Hence, it becomes clear that it is impossible to establish clear anatomical boundaries between the two malformations when using these criteria. For this purpose, it is necessary to use mutually exclusive criteria, but not coexisting!

From surgical viewpoint, the presence of mitral-aortic muscular continuity in context of aortic tunneling to the left ventricle has a great practical importance. First, since the hole limited by the VIF (between the mitral and aortic valves) and the edge of VSD is an exit from the left ventricle (in other words the entrance to the intraventricular tunnel) the presence of mitral-aortic muscular continuity can significantly contribute to development of subaortic obstruction after surgery. This fact is confirmed by the study of Li et al., in which the presence of subaortic conus (mitral-aortic muscular continuity) was revealed as a risk factor for subaortic obstruction in long-term period after biventricular repair of DORV [22]. Considering that development of subaortic obstruction after repair of tetralogy of Fallot is not as actual as in DORV, differentiation of the malformations by the presence of mitral-aortic muscular continuity seems to be fundamental and important. Secondly, aortic dextroposition depends on size of the VIF, which eventually determines patch size and therefore length of intraventricular tunnel.

6.5 *Transitional Form with TGA*

For its part, the main distinguishing criteria for Taussig–Bing anomaly and TGA with VSD are:

- morphology of mitral-pulmonary continuity (fibrous or muscular);
- extend of deviation of the OS to the right and degree of pulmonary artery origin from the ventricles;
- arterial trunks relationships.

According to some authorities the term «Taussig–Bing» anomaly can only be used in the presence of mitral-pulmonary muscular continuity [99–101]. But if consider DORV as a type of ventriculoarterial connection, then this contradicts the definition of Taussig–Bing anomaly in the presence of such mitral-pulmonary muscular continuity, but with origin of the major part of the pulmonary artery from the left ventricle. Then, the second contradiction arises when determining cases with mitral-pulmonary fibrosis continuity, but when pulmonary artery predominantly takes origin from the right ventricle.

TGA as DORV is an anomaly of ventriculoarterial connection regardless of VSD type in which both arterial trunks are transposed. At the same time, in Taussig–Bing anomaly the aorta is transposed while the pulmonary artery locates above VSD in its normal anatomical position [102].

In TGA with aligned OS, the latter connects to the anterior edge of IVS. As the OS deviates to the right, pulmonary artery shifts toward the right ventricle. With this displacement of the pulmonary artery, the left aspect of the VIF proportionally becomes more expressed between the mitral and pulmonary valves, as well as the disconnection of the OS and the anterior edge of IVS (Figs. 21, 22). The problem that arises in this case (as with the transitional form with tetralogy of Fallot) is the following; which of the two criteria should be considered as the main for distinguishing DORV "TGA" type and TGA—the «50%» rule or the presence of mitral-pulmonary fibrous or muscular continuity? As already mentioned, these criteria—one being anatomical, and the other functional—are not mutually exclusive! As a result, on the one hand, it is possible to assume the existence of Taussig–Bing anomaly with mitral-pulmonary fibrous continuity and origin of the major part of the pulmonary artery from the right ventricle, as well as, on the other hand, TGA with mitral-pulmonary muscular continuity and origin of the major part of the pulmonary artery from the left ventricle.

6.6 Anatomical and Surgical Considerations of the Transitional Forms of DORV

According to the figurative expression of Edwards: «If we are asked how we know that this is Aunt Minnie walking toward us, we may say, «Because she *looks like* Aunt Minnie». Similarly, if we are asked how we know that a certain heart should be classified as double-outlet right ventricle or as tetralogy of Fallot, we often reply (in so many words), «Because it *looks like* cases we have seen before» [27].

Existence of transitional forms of DORV contributes great confusion into the anatomical terminology of conotruncal anomalies and, thereby, their differentiation from each other which is necessary not only for correct systematization of conotruncal malformations, but also for the correct report of surgical results. Thus, hearts with the same anatomical features can be considered by different authors as two different diseases, which to a certain extent leads to errors and drawbacks in the description and comparison of surgical results. Also, the presence of transitional forms once again proves the fact that all conotruncal anomalies represent a single spectrum.

From the surgical perspective, the existing uncertainties and contradictions regarding the transitional forms are less significant than in anatomical terms. Thus, the only difference between DORV "tetralogy" type from tetralogy of Fallot in terms

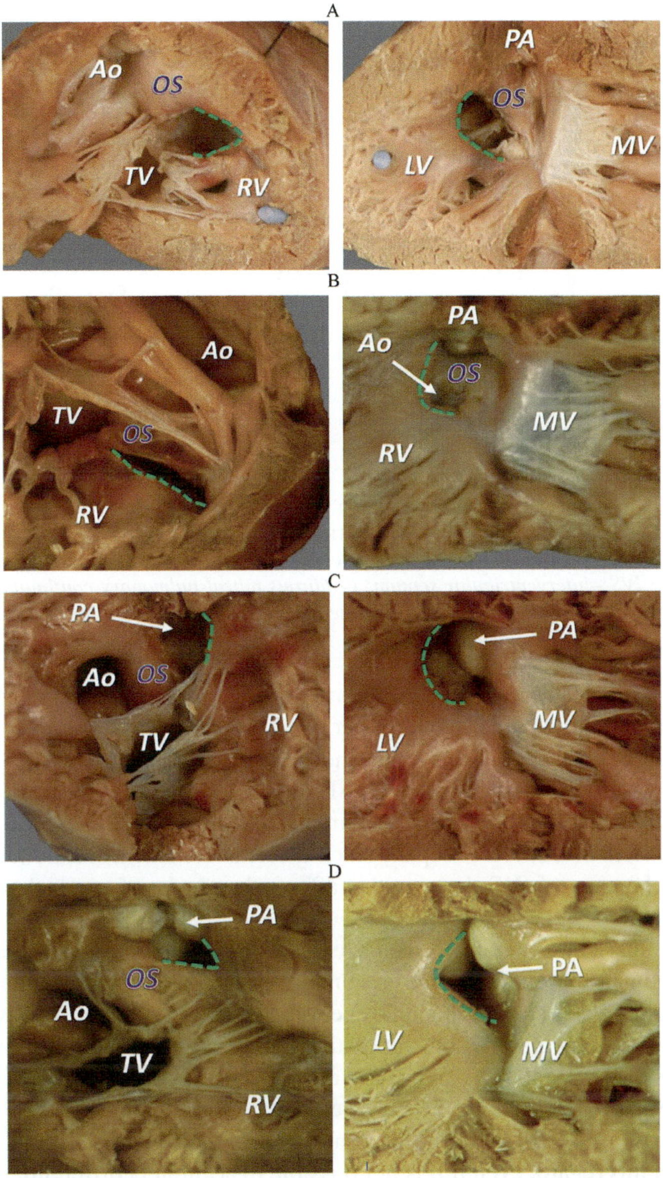

Fig. 21 Transitional anatomical forms of TGA and DORV «TGA» type (autopsy specimen). Change in the position of the OS and arterial valves with gradual shifting of the pulmonary valve toward the right ventricle. The left vertical row represents views from the right ventricle; the right vertical row represents views from the left ventricle. **A**—TGA with perimembranous VSD with aligned OS; **B**—TGA with perimembranous VSD and the OS deviated to the right ("malalignment"); **C**—TGA with subpulmanary VSD; **D**—Taussig–Bing anomaly. Note that the more the OS shifts to the right the more pulmonary artery originates from the right ventricle

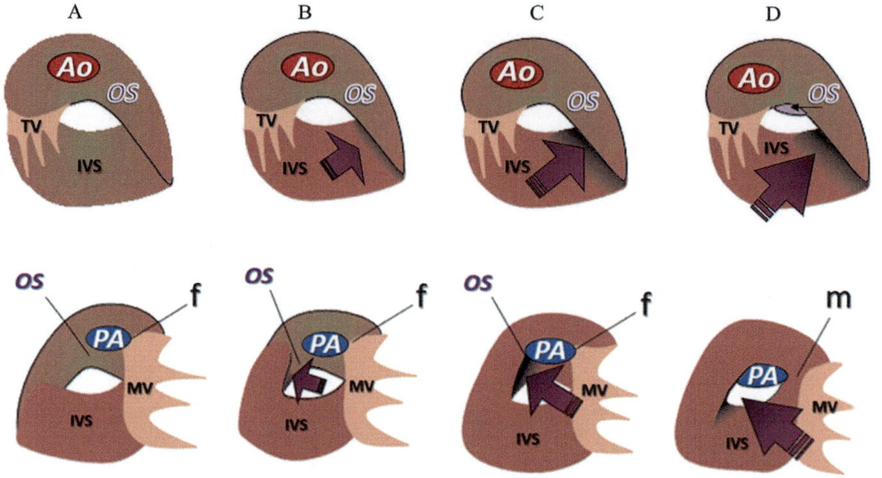

Fig. 22 Supplemented schematic representation of changes in the position of the OS shown in the Fig. 21. The upper row represents views from the right ventricle; the lower row represents views from the left ventricle. *Ao—aorta; PA—pulmonary artery; MV—mitral valve; TV—tricuspid valve; OS—outlet septum; IVS—interventricular septum; f—fibrous mitral-pulmonary continuity; m—muscle mitral-pulmonary continuity. The arrows indicate the direction and extend of OS displacement*

of surgical repair is a need to create an intraventricular tunnel instead of simple VSD closure, which requires the use of a larger patch.

It should be taken into account that the presence of the VIF between the mitral and aortic (in DORV with subaortic VSD) and mitral and pulmonary (in DORV with subpulmonary VSD) valves plays important role in development of subaortic obstruction after biventricular repair, since it forms the exit from the left ventricle along with the crest of IVS. In turn, this affects the results of surgical treatment of such patients.

From the surgical viewpoint, it seems reasonable not to divide conotruncal anomalies with anomalous ventriculoarterial connection into separate anatomical entities, but rather to represent them as a single spectrum of malformations. This approach is supported by the fact that the same operation can be performed in different anatomical variants of DORV and TGA [103]. In other words, for the surgeon, the main goal is to restore anomalous ventriculoarterial connection, which is achieved by intraventricular tunneling of the aorta or pulmonary artery (followed by ASO) to the left ventricle. In this regard, even if it is not possible to accurately differentiate the exact type of a conotruncal malformation with anomalous ventriculoarterial connection the main criteria for a decision-making are the following:

- VSD location;
- tricuspid-to-pulmonary valve distance;
- presence of pulmonary artery stenosis.

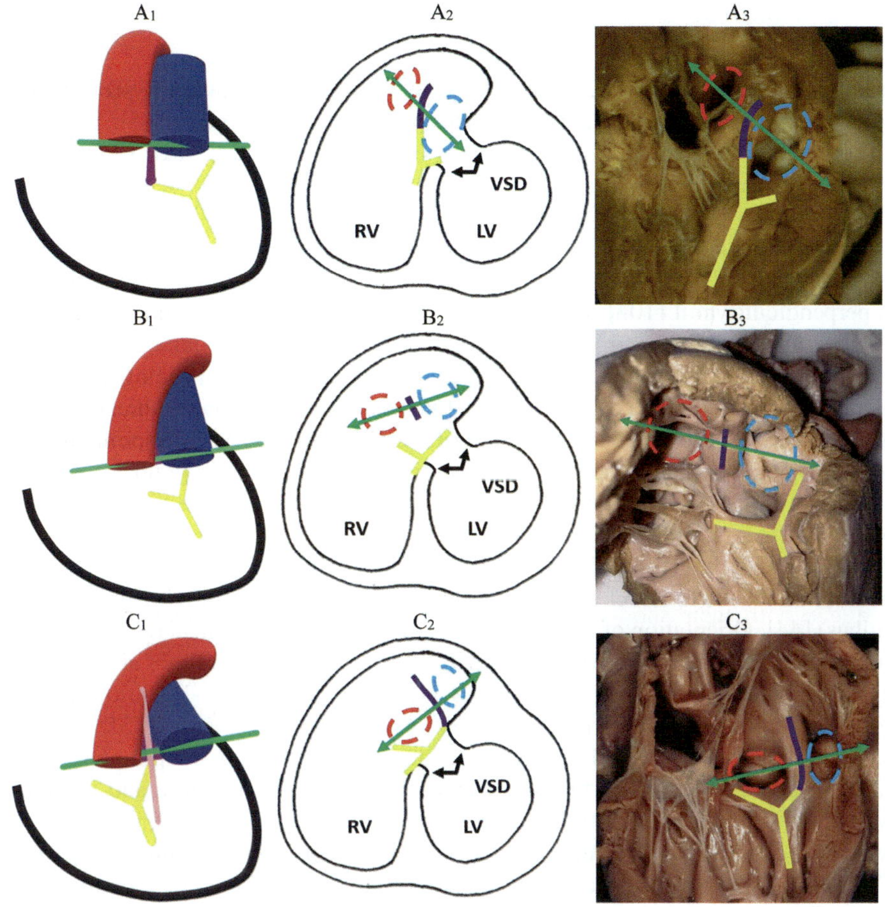

Fig. 23 Dependence of VSD type formation and course of the arterial trunks on OS orientation: **A**—parallel course of the arterial trunks with D-aorta (**A_1**). The axis of the arterial valves is oriented perpendicular to the IVS (**A_2**). The OS is fused with the pTS, thereby committing conoventricular VSD (i.e., bulboventricular foramen) to the subpulmonary area (**A_3**); **B**—with the start of the conotruncal rotation and OS reorientation the arterial trunks begin to twist (**B_1**). The axis of the arterial valves is oriented at an acute angle to the IVS (**B_2**). As a result of the reorientation, the OS shifts away from the pTS and fuses with the VIF in its middle part (**B_3**); **C**—with higher degree of conotruncal rotation spiral twisting of the arterial trunks occurs (**C_1**). The axis of the arterial valves is oriented parallel to the IVS (**C_2**). The OS fuses with the aTS, committing VSD to the subaortic infundibulum (**C_3**) *VSD—ventricular septal defect; LV—left ventricle; RV—right ventricle; yellow figure—trabecula septomarginalis; violet figure—outlet septum; green figure—arterial valve axis; blue figure—pulmonary valve; red figure—aortic valve; pink figure—outlet septum axis*

7 Anatomical Concept of DORV

It is believed that in DORV, there is no strict dependence between VSD type and course of the arterial trunks, and there are only certain tendencies [45]. So, if the arterial trunks are spirally twisted, as it happens in a normal heart, then VSD is more likely to be found in subaortic area while if they have parallel course subpulmonary VSD is usually detected [12].

In normal relationship of the arterial trunks with right and posterior aorta, the axis of the arterial valves is oriented almost parallel to the IVS, and the OS respectively is perpendicular to it [104]. In this regard, the process of fusion of the OS with the aTS becomes possible, and VSD locates under the aortic valve. Course of the arterial trunks is spiral in this case. With parallel course and side by side trunks, the opposite picture is observed: the axis of the arterial valves is perpendicular to the IVS, while the OS is parallel to it. Thus, the fusion of the OS with the aTS is impossible, and VSD opens under the pulmonary valve.

Formation of particular type of VSD and arterial valves relationship in DORV is based on the following principles. First of all, it is necessary to take as a basis that development of the OS, dividing of truncus and its rotation are independent processes without reference to development of ventricular complex (primitive ventricle and bulbus) [44]. Orientation of the OS depends on the degree of truncal rotation during embryogenesis. The IVS and the TS with its anterior and posterior limbs are relatively fixed structures of the developing heart and do not change their initial position after the complete formation of ventricular complex. Type of conoventricular VSD depends on how the OS is connected to the TS (subaortic, subarterial or subpulmonary). In case of subaortic VSD, the OS forms anterior wall of the subaortic and posterior wall of the subpulmonary infundibulum, while in subpulmonary VSD, it forms right wall of the subpulmonary and left wall of the subaortic infundibulum (Fig. 1 in Chapter 3). Thus, the OS is a structure that, when connected to one or another limb of the TS, separates subaortic and subpulmonary infundibulums which indicates a direct influence of the degree of truncal rotation on VSD type.

During embryogenesis truncal cushions that appear on the inner surface of the truncus grow toward each other and merge in a vertical plane, thus dividing the truncus into the aortic and pulmonary components. Immediately after separation, the truncal components (i.e., ascending aorta and pulmonary artery) are oriented in parallel fashion with aorta located to the right to the pulmonary artery. At this stage, anatomy of a developing heart corresponds to Taussig–Bing anomaly with side by side arterial trunks. This stage of embryogenesis determines DORV or TGA formation depending on direction of further conotruncal block rotation. Clockwise rotation (to the right if viewed from above) leads to DORV spectrum formation while anticlockwise (to the left) to TGA spectrum.

7.1 *Clockwise Rotation of the Conotruncus–DORV Formation*

Formation of Subpulmonary VSD

Normally, after dividing the truncus into the aortic and pulmonary components, it begins to rotate clockwise. Initially both components of the truncus are oriented parallel to each other, while the OS separating them locates in the sagittal plane closer to the pTS (Fig. 23A1). If there is no further truncal rotation, the OS fuses with the pTS (or with the VIF near the area of pTS), bulboventricular foramen remains open under the pulmonary valve, course of the arterial trunks is parallel, and the aorta completely originates from the right ventricle (Fig. 23A2). Subpulmonary and subaortic infundibulums are side by side and are in fibrous or muscular continuity with the atrioventricular valves. Such a morphological arrangement is typical for Taussig-Bing anomaly (Fig. 23A3).

Formation of Subarterial VSD with the Outlet Septum

When the conotruncus begins clockwise rotation, the posterior aspect of the OS shifts away from the pTS and begins to «slide» along the VIF to the left and locates just above and in the middle of the bulboventricular foramen (i.e., VSD) between the limbs of the TS not connecting to any of them (Fig. 23B1). In this case, the only anatomical structure with which the OS remains fused is the middle part of the VIF, located between the atrioventricular valves. As the OS «slides» along the VIF, the conotruncus rotates to the right and the aorta moves posteriorly to the pulmonary artery. Due to disconnection of the OS with the limbs of the TS, bulboventricular foramen opens both in subaortic and subpulmonary infundibulums (Fig. 23B2). This morphological arrangement corresponds to rare form of DORV with subarterial VSD with muscular OS (Fig. 23B3).

Formation of Subaortic/Subarterial VSD Without the Outlet Septum

If there is a further rotation of the truncus to the right (as viewed from above), then the aorta moves more posterior to the pulmonary artery and is positioned between the atrioventricular valves, communicating with both ventricles. The OS approaches the aTS, the pulmonary artery shifts anteriorly completely losing contact with the atrioventricular valves and is situated as in its normal anatomical position (Fig. 23B1). Thus, subaortic and subpulmonary infundibulums are oriented in antero-posterior fashion (Fig. 23B2). For complete translocation of the aorta to the left ventricle, resorption of the VIF between the mitral and aortic valves is necessary, which leads to additional truncal rotation. Since this process is failed in DORV, the OS fuses with the aTS and bulboventricular foramen opens in subaortic area. Such a morphological arrangement corresponds to DORV with subaortic VSD (Fig. 23B3). If such a scenario is accompanied by fibrotic or severely hypoplastic OS, then subarterial VSD without OS is formed.

Spiral Twisting of the Arterial Trunks

With the rightward truncal rotation, OS reorientation and shifting of the aorta, spiral twisting of the arterial trunks occurs. This can explain parallel course of the arterial trunks in Taussig-Bing anomaly and spiral course in DORV with subaortic VSD. Thus, degree of conotruncal rotation (and OS reorientation, respectively) determines relationship between the type of VSD and course of the arterial trunks. This concept is backed by the fact that in a number of anatomical studies DORV with subpulmonary VSD and spiraling arterial trunks has never been described [1, 45]. Also, there were no any cases of DORV with subpulmonary VSD with right and posterior aorta [98].

7.2 Anticlockwise Rotation of the Conotruncus–TGA Formation

If at the «Taussig–Bing» stage of embryogenesis, the conotruncal block and the OS rotate anticlockwise (i.e., to the left), then the further formation of a heart represents a «mirror-imaged» scenario of those changes that occur when the conotruncus rotates to the right.

As the conotruncal block rotates to the left, the pulmonary artery moves left and posterior to the aorta toward the left ventricle, crosses the crest of IVS and at the same time gradually loses its subpulmonary infundibulum between the mitral and pulmonary valves. It is this kind of anatomy that is a variant of the transitional anatomical form between Taussig–Bing anomaly and TGA. In this case, according to the «50%» rule, if the pulmonary valve still predominantly takes origin from the right ventricle, then the malformation is defined as Taussig–Bing anomaly. Otherwise, TGA with VSD will be diagnosed.

Extreme rotation of the conotruncus to the left leads to mitral-pulmonary fibrosis continuity and pulmonary artery origin predominantly or entirely from the left ventricle. We should note here that in TGA course of the arterial trunks is always parallel!

Such an anatomical concept combines all morphological types of DORV and TGA into a single spectrum of conotruncal malformations, between which there are no clear anatomical boundaries. Isolation of DORV and TGA into separate malformation is conditional (Fig. 24). Based on the all above mentioned the following conclusions can be drawn:

- the stage of heart embryogenesis when the aorta and pulmonary artery are parallel and side by side, completely originate from the right ventricle (due to the lack of truncal rotation and OS reorientation), and bulboventricular foramen opens under the pulmonary artery corresponds to Taussig–Bing anomaly («Taussig–Bing» stage of embryogenesis);
- during embryogenesis the «Taussig–Bing» stage is the preceding morphological stage of DORV and TGA;

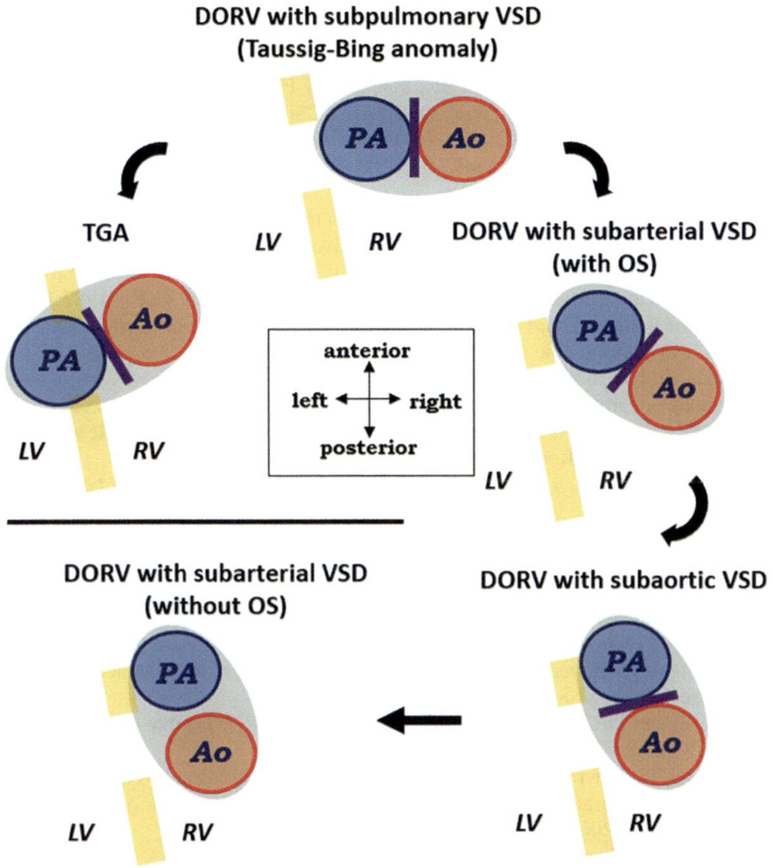

Fig. 24 Influence of the direction of conotruncal rotation at the «Taussig–Bing» stage of embryogenesis on the type of malformation formed (view from above). See text. *Ao—aorta; PA—pulmonary artery; RV—right ventricle; LV—left ventricle; OS—outlet septum*

- clockwise conotruncal rotation at the «Taussig–Bing» stage leads to formation of DORV spectrum and gradual twisting of the arterial trunks, while anticlockwise rotation leads to TGA formation;
- spiral twisting of the arterial trunks takes place only as a result of clockwise (rightward) rotation of the conotruncus.

References

1. Anderson RH, Becker AE, Wilcox BR, Macarthney FJ, Wilkinson JL. Surgical anatomy of double-outlet right ventricle—a reappraisal. Am J Cardiol. 1983;52:555–9.
2. Anderson RH, Wilkinson JL, Arnold R, Becker AE, Lubkiewicz K. Morphogenesis of bulboventricular malformations. II. Observations on malformed hearts. Br Heart J. 1974;36:948–70.
3. Baron MG. Angiographic differentiation between tetralogy of Fallot and double-outlet right ventricle: relationship of the mitral and aortic valves. Circulation. 1971;43:451–55.
4. Van Praagh S, Davidoff A, Van Praagh R. Double outlet right ventricle: anatomic types and developmental implications based on a study of 101 autopsied cases. Coeur. 1982;13:389–440.
5. Sridaromont S, Ritter DG, Feldt RH, Davis GD, Edwards JE. Double-outlet right ventricle: anatomic and angiographic correlations. Mayo Clinic Proceed. 1978;53:555–77.
6. Hallerman FJ, Kincaid OW, Ritter DG, Titus J.L Mitral-semilunar valve relationships in the angiography of cardiac malformations. Radiology. 1970;94:63–8.
7. Dayem MKA, Preger L, Goodwin JF, Steiner RE. Double outlet right ventricle with pulmonary stenosis. British Heart Kournal. 1967;29:64–77.
8. Carey LS, Edwards JE. Roentgenographic features in cases with origin of both great vessels from the right ventricle without pulmonary stenosis. Am J Roentgenol. 1965;93:269–97.
9. Lev M, Bharati S, Meng CCL, Libethson RP, Paul MH, Idriss F. A concept of double outlet right ventricle. J Thorac Cardiovasc Surg. 1972;64:271–81.
10. Stewart S. Double-outlet right ventricle: a collective review with a surgical viewpoint. J Thoracic Cardiovascul Surg. 1976;71:355–65.
11. Wilcox BR, Ho SY, Macartney FJ, Becker AE, Gelis LM, Anderson RH. Surgical anatomy of double-outlet right ventricle with situs solitus and atrioventricular concordance. J Thorac Cardiovasc Surg. 1981;82:405–17.
12. Ebadi A, Spicer DE, Backer CL, Fricker FJ, Anderson RH. Double-outlet right ventricle: revisited. J Thorac Cardiovasc Surg. 2017;154:598–604.
13. Walters HL III, Mavroudis C, Tchervenkov CI, Jacobs JP, Lacour-Gayet F, Jacobs ML. Congenital heart surgery nomenclature and database project: double outlet right ventricle. Ann Thorac Surg. 2000;69:S249-263.
14. Lacour-Gayet F, Haun C, Ntalakoura K, Belli E, Houyel L, Marcsek P, et al. Biventricular repair of double outlet right ventricle with non-committed ventricular septal defect (VSD) by VSD rerouting to the pulmonary artery and arterial switch. Euro J Cardiothoracic Surg. 2002;21:1042–8.
15. Kupryashov AA. Double-outlet right ventricle: a chapter in the book Pediatric Cardiac Surgery (Bockeria L.A. Shatalov K.V.). Bakulev Scientific Center of Cardiovascular Surgery. Moscow. 2016—864 c.
16. Anderson RH, Spicer DE, Hlavacek AM, Cook AC, Backer CL. Wilcox's surgical anatomy of the Heart. Cambridge Academ. 4th edn. p. 388
17. Bockeria LA, Berishvili II. Surgical anatomy of the heart, vol. 3. Congenital heart defects—conotruncal anomalies and pathophysiology of hemodynamics. Bakulev Scientific Center of Cardiovascular Surgery; Moscow; 2006. p. 312
18. Sridaromont S, Feldt RH, Ritter DG, Davis GD, Edwards JE. Double-outlet right ventricle: hemodynamic and anatomic correlations. Am J Cardiol. 1976;38:85–94.
19. Capuani A, Uemura H, Ho SY, Anderson RH. Anatomic spectrum of abnormal ventriculoarterial connections: surgical implications. Ann Thorac Surg. 1995;59:352–60.
20. Oladunjoye O, Piekarski B, Baird C, Banka P, Marx G, del Nido PJ, Emani SM. Repair of double outlet right ventricle: midterm outcomes. J Thorac Cardiovasc Surg. 2019. https://doi.org/10.1016/j.jtcvs.2019.06.120.
21. Meng H, Pang K, Li S, His D, Yan J, Hu S, Hua Z, Wang H. Biventricular repair of double-outlet right ventricle: preoperative echocardiography and surgical outcomes. World J Pediatric Congenital Heart Surg. 2017;3:354–60.

22. Li S, Ma K, Hu S, Hua Z, Yang K, Yan J, Chen Q. Surgical outcomes of 380 patients with double outlet right ventricle who underwent biventricular repair. J Thorac Cardiovasc Surg. 2014;147:817–24.
23. Bradley TJ, Karamlou T, Kilik A, Mitrovic B, Vigneswaran T, Jaffer S, Glasgow PD, Williams WG, Van Arsdell GS, McCrindle BW. Determinants of repair type, reintervention, and mortality in 393 children with double-outlet right ventricle. J Thorac Cardiovasc Surg. 2007;134:967–73.
24. Musumeci F, Shumway S, Lincoln C, Anderson RH. Surgical treatment for double-outlet right ventricle at the Brompton Hospital, 1973 to 1986. J Thorac Cardiovasc Surg. 1988;96:278–87.
25. Zamora R, Moller JH, Edwards JE. Double-outlet right ventricle anatomic types and associated anomalies. Chest. 1975;68:672–7.
26. Hosseinpour A-R, Jones TJ, Barron DJ, Brawn WJ, Anderson RH. An appreciation of the structural variability in the components of the ventricular outlets in congenitally malformed hearts. Euro J Cardiothoracic Surg. 2007;31:888–93.
27. Edwards WD. Double-outlet right ventricle and tetralogy of Fallot. Two distinct but not mutually exclusive entities. J Thoracic Cardiovascul Surg. 1981;82:418–22.
28. Stellin G, Ho SY, Anderson RH, Zuberbuhler JR, Siewers RD. The surgical anatomy of double-outlet right ventricle with concordant atrioventricular connection and noncommitted ventricular septal defect. J Thorac Cardiovasc Surg. 1991;102:849–55.
29. Vergnat M, Baruteau A, Houyel L, Ly M, Roussin R, Capderou A, Lambert V, Belli E. Late outcomes after arterial switch operation for Taussig-Bing anomaly. J Thorac Cardiovasc Surg. 2015;149:1124–32.
30. Soszyn N, Fricke TA, Wheaton GR, Ramsay JM, d'Udekem Y, Brizard CP, Konstantinov IE. Outcomes of the arterial switch operation in patients with Taussig-Bing anomaly. Ann Thorac Surg. 2011;92:673–9.
31. Alsoufi B, Cai S, Williams WJ, Coles JG, Caldarone CA, Redington AM, Van Arsdell GS. Improved results with single-stage total correction of Taussig-Bing anomaly. Euro J Cardiothoracic Surg. 2008;33:244–50.
32. Hayes DA, Jones S, Quaegebeur JM, Richmond ME. Andrews HF, Glickstein JS, Chen JM, Bacha E, Liberman L. Primary repair switch operation as a strategy for total correction of Taussig-Bing anomaly. A 21-year experience. Circulation. 2013;128:S194–198.
33. Sinzobahamvya N, Blaschzok HC, Asfour B, Arenz C, Jussli MJ, Schnidler E, Photiadis J, Yrban AE. Right ventricular outflow tract obstruction after arterial switch operation for Taussig-Bing anomaly. Eur J Cardiothorac Surg. 2007;31:873–8.
34. Stellin G, Zuberbuhler JR, Anderson RH, Path MRC, Siewers R. The surgical anatomy of the Taussig-Bing anomaly. J Thorac Cardiovasc Surg. 1987;93:560–9.
35. Rudolph AM, Heymann MA, Spitznas U. Hemodynamic considerations in the development of narrowing of the aorta. Am J Cardiol. 1972;30:514–25.
36. Luo K, Zheng J, Wang S, Zhu Z, Gao B, Xu Z, Liu J. Single-stage correction for Taussig-Bing anomaly associates with aortic arch obstruction. Pediatric Cariol. 2017;38:1548–55.
37. Bret J, Torner-Soler M. Complete transposition of the aorta: levoposition of the pulmonary artery with pulmonary stenosis: clinical and pathological findings in three cases. Am Heart J. 1957;54:385–95.
38. Taussig HB, Bing RJ. Complete transposition of the aorta and a levoposition of the pulmonary artery. Clinical, physiological, and pathological findings. Am Heart J. 1949;37:551–59.
39. Griffin ML, Sullivan ID, Anderson RH, Macartney FJ. Doubly committed subarterial ventricular septal defect: new morphological criteria with echocardiographic and angiocardiographic correlation. Br Heart J. 1988;59:474–9.
40. Freedom RM, Mawson J, Yoo S-J, Bemson LN. Congenital Heart Disease: Textbook of Angiocardiography. Armonk, New-York, Futura; 1997. pp. 1119–161.
41. Anderson RH, Brown NA, Mohun TJ. Insights regarding the normal and abnormal formation of the atrial and ventricular septal structures. Clin Anat. 2016;29:290–304.
42. Freedom RM, Yoo SL. Double-outlet right ventricle: pathology and angiocardiography. Pediatric Cardiac Surg Ann Semin Thoracic Cardiovascul Surg. 2000;3:3–19.

43. Brandt PWT, Calder AL, Barratt-Boyes BG, Neutze JM. Double outlet left ventricle, morphology, cineangiocardiographic diagnosis and surgical treatment. Am J Cardiol. 1976;38:897–909.
44. Aiello VD, Spicer DE, Anderson RH, Brown NA, Mohun TJ. The independence of the infundibular building blocks in the setting of double-outlet right ventricle. Cardiol Young. 2017;27:825–36.
45. Anderson RH, Ho SY, Wilcox BR. The surgical anatomy of ventricular septal defect Part 4: double outlet ventricle. J Card Surg. 1996;11:2–11.
46. Belli E, Serraf A, Lacour-Gayet F, Hubler M, Zoghby J, Houyel L, et al. Double-outlet right ventricle with non-committed ventricular septal defect. Euro J Cardiothoracic Surg. 1999;15:747–52.
47. Basarab YS. Surgical anatomy of double-outlet right ventricle. Bullakulev Scien Center Cardiovascul Surg. 2005;5:58–65.
48. Beekman RP, Bartelings MM, Hazekamp MG, Gittenberger-de Groot AC, Ottenkamp J. The morphologic nature of noncommitted ventricular septal defects in specimens with double-outlet right ventricle. J Thorac Cardiovasc Surg. 2002;124:984–90.
49. Lacour-Gayet F. Biventricular repair of double outlet right ventricle with noncommitted ventricular septal defect. Pediatric Cardiac Surg Ann Semin Thoracic Cardiovascul Surg. 2002;5:163–72.
50. Barbero-Marcial M, Tanamati C, Atik E, Ebaid M. Intraventricular repair of double-outlet right ventricle with non-committed ventricular septal defect: advantages of multiple patches. J Thorac Cardiovasc Surg. 1999;118:1056–67.
51. Li S, Ma K, Hu S, Hua Z, Yan J, Pang K, Wang X, Yan F, Liu J, Zhang S, Chen Q. Biventricular repair for double outlet right ventricle with non-committed ventricular septal defect. Eur J Cardiothorac Surg. 2015;48:580–7.
52. Beekman RP, Roest AAW, Helbing WA, Hazekamp MG, Schoof PH, Bartelings MM, Sobotka MA, de Roos A, Ottenkamp J. Spin echo MRI in the evaluation of hearts with a double-outlet right ventricle: usefulness and limitations. Magn Reson Imaging. 2000;18:245–53.
53. Freedom RM, Yoo SL. DORV: pathology and angiocardiography. Semin Thorac Cardiovasc Surg. 2000;3:3–19.
54. Mostefa-Kara M, Bonnet D, Belli E, Fadel E, Hiuyel L. Anatomy of the ventricular septal defect in outflow tract defects: similarities and differences. J Thorac Cardiovasc Surg. 2014;3:682-688.e1.
55. Ainger LE. Double outlet right ventricle, intact ventricular septum, mitral stenosis and blind left ventricle. Am Heart J. 1965;70:521–5.
56. Ikemoto Y, Nogi S, Teraguchi M, Imamura H, Kobayashi Y. Double-outlet right ventricle with intact ventricular septum. Acta Paediatr Jpn. 1997;39:233–6.
57. Menon S, Ashok Kumar CJ, Mathew T, Venkateshwarn S, Jayakumar K, Dharan BS. Double outlet right ventricle with intact ventricular septum: avulsion or exclusion. World J Pediatric Congen Heart Surg. 2016;7:220–2.
58. Mason DT, Morrow AG, Elkins RC, Friedman WF. Origin of both great vessels from the right ventricle associated with severe obstruction to left ventricular outflow. Am J Cardiol. 1967;24:118–24.
59. Matsuoka Y, Akimoto K, Sennari E, Hayakawa K. Double outlet right ventricle with severe left ventricular outflow tract obstruction due to small ventricular septal defect and anomalous adherence of the mitral valve to the ventricular septum. Japanese Circul J. 1987;1335–40.
60. Tchervenkov CI, Marelli D, Beland MJ, Gibbons JE, Paquet M, Dobell ARC. Institutional experience with a protocol of early repair of double-outlet right ventricle. Ann Thorac Surg. 1995;60:S610-613.
61. Serratto M, Arevalo F, Goldman EJ, Hastreiter A, Miller RA. Obstructive ventricular septal defect in double outlet right ventricle. Am J Cardiol. 1967;19:457–63.
62. Lavoie R, Sestier F, Gilbert G, Chameides L, Van Praagh R, Grondin P. Double outlet right ventricle with left ventricular outflow tract obstruction due to small ventricular septal defect. Am Heart J. 1971;3:290–9.

63. Freed M, Rosenthal A, Plauth WH, Nadas AS. Development of subaortic stenosis after pulmonary artery banding. Circulation. 1973;48:S7-10.
64. Lincoln C. Total correction of d-loop double-outlet right ventricle with bilateral conus, l-transposition, and pulmonic stenosis. J Thorac Cardiovasc Surg. 1972;64:435–40.
65. Danielson GK, Ritter DG, Coleman N, DuShane JW. Successful repair of double-outlet right ventricle with transposition of the great arteries (aorta anterior and to the left), pulmonary stenosis, and subaortic ventricular septal defect. J Thorac Cardiovasc Surg. 1972;63:741–6.
66. Van Praagh R, Perez-Trevino C, Reynolds JL, Moes CAF, Keith JD, Roy DL, Belcourt C, Weinberg PM, Parisi LF. Double outlet right ventricle (S, D, L) with subaortic ventricular septal defect and pulmonary stenosis. Pediatr Cardiol. 1975;35:42–53.
67. Awasthy N, Radhakrishnan S, Sharma R. Anatomically corrected malposition of the great arteries (S, D, L,) with left juxtaposition of the atrial appendages in DORV: influence on surgical approach. World J Pediatric Congen Heart Surg. 2013;4:217–9.
68. Shaffer AB, Lopez JF, Kline IK, Lev M. Truncal inversion with biventricular pulmonary trunk and aorta from right ventricle (variant of Taussig-Bing complex). Circulation. 1967;37:783–8.
69. Yamaguchi M, Horikoshi K, Toriyama A, Kimura K, Mito H, Tei G, Kaneda H, Ogawa K, Asada S. Successful repair of double-outlet right ventricle with bilateral conus, l-transposition of great arteries (S, D, L), and subpulmonary ventricular septal defect. J Thorac Cardiovasc Surg. 1976;71:366–70.
70. Wu Q, Yu Q, Yang X. Modified Rastelli procedure for double outlet right ventricle with left-malposition of the great arteries: report of 9 cases. Ann Thorac Surg. 2003;75:138–42.
71. Kaneko Y, Murakami A, Imanaka K, Okabe H, Takamoto S. Transannular patch repair of double-outlet right ventricle, (S, D, L), and single right coronary artery. J Thorac Cardiovasc Surg. 1999;117:622–3.
72. Wang C, Chen S, Zhang H, Liu J, Xu Z, Zheng J, Yan Q, Huang H, Huang M. Anatomical classification of the coronary arteries in complete transposition of the great arteries and double outlet right ventricle with subpulmonary septal defect. Thoracic Cardiovascul Surg. 2017;65:26–30.
73. Uemura H, Yagihara T, Kawashima Y, Nishigaki K, Kamiya T, Ho SY, Anderson RH. Coronary arterial anatomy in double-outlet right ventricle with subpulmonary VSD. Ann Thorac Surg. 1995;59:591–7.
74. Patwary ME, Khan MS, Marwah A, Singh V, Shekhawat S, Sharma R. Arterial switch for transposition of the great arteries with large ventricular septal defect and for Taussig-Bing anomaly: experience from a tertiary care center in the developing world. World J Pediatric Congen Heart Surg. 2005;6:413–21.
75. Feng B, Liu Y, Hu S, Shen X, Wang X, Wang H, Ming B. Arterial switch for transposition of the great vessels and Taussig-Bing anomaly after six months of age. Ann Thorac Surg. 2009;88:1948–51.
76. Griselli M, McGuirk SP, Ko C, Clarke AJB, Barron DJ, Brawn WJ. Arterial switch operation in patients with Taussig-Bing anomaly—influence of staged repair and coronary anatomy on outcome. Euro J Cardiothoracic Surg. 2007;31:229–35.
77. Tabry IF, McGoon DC, Danielson GK, Wallace RB, Tajik AJ, Seward JB. Surgical management of straddling atrioventricular valve. J Thorac Cardiovasc Surg. 1979;77:191–201.
78. Ong J, Brizard CP, d'Udekem Y, Weintraub R, Robertson T, Cheung M, Konstantinov IE. Repair of atrioventricular septal defect associated with tetralogy of Fallot of double-outlet right ventricle: 30 years of experience. Ann Thorac Surg. 2012;94:172–8.
79. Oshima Y, Yamaguchi M, Yoshimura N, Oka S, Ootaki Y. Anatomically corrective repair of complete atrioventricular septal defects and major cardiac anomalies. Ann Thorac Surg. 2001;72:424–9.
80. Takeuchi K, McGowan FX, Moran AM, Zurakowski D, Mayer JE, Jonas RA, del Nido PJ. Surgical outcome of double-outlet right ventricle with subpulmonary VSD. Ann Thorac Surg. 2001;71:49–53.
81. Devaney EJ, Lee T, Gelehrter S, Hirsch JC, Ohye RG, Anderson RH, Bove EL. Biventricular repair of atrioventricular septal defect with common atrioventricular valve and double-outlet right ventricle. Ann Thorac Surg. 2010;89:537–43.

82. Raju V, Myers PO, Quinonez LG, Emani SM, Mayer JE, Pigula FA, del Nido P, Baird CW. Aortic root translocation (Nikaidoh procedure): intermediate follow-up and impact of conduit type. J Thorac Cardiovasc Surg. 2015;149:1349–55.
83. Sridaromont S, Feldt RH, Ritter DG, Davis GD, McGoon DC, Edwards JE. Double-outlet right ventricle associated with persistent common atrioventricular canal. Circulation. 1975;52:933–42.
84. Pacifico AD, Kirklin JW, Bargeron LM. Repair of complete atrioventricular canal associated with tetralogy of Fallot or double-outlet right ventricle: report of 10 cases. Ann Thorac Surg. 1980;4:351–6.
85. Toussaint M, Planche C, Graff WC, Royon M, Ribierre M. Double-outlet right ventricle associated with common atrioventricular canal: report of nine anatomic specimens. J Am Coll Cardiol. 1986;2:396–401.
86. He G, Mee RBB. Complete atrioventricular canal associated with tetralogy of Fallot or double-outlet right ventricle and right ventricular outflow tract obstruction: a report of successful surgical treatment. Ann Thorac Surg. 1986;41:612–5.
87. Rastelli GC, Kirklin JW, Titus JL. Anatomic observations on complete form of persistent common atrioventricular canal with special references to atrioventricular valves. Mayo Clin Proc. 1966;41:293–308.
88. Bockeria LA, Shatalov KV. Pediatric cardiac surgery. bakulev scientific center of cardiovascular surgery. Moscow. 2016—864 c.
89. Bharati S, Kirklin JW, McAllister HA, Lev M. The surgical anatomy of common atrioventricular orifice associated with tetralogy of Fallot, double-outlet right ventricle and complete regular transposition. Circulation. 1980;61:1142–9.
90. Comas JV, Mignosa C, Cochrane AD, Wilkinson JL, Karl TR. Taussig-Bing anomaly and arterial switch operation: aortic arch obstruction does not influence outcome. Euro J Cardiothoracic Surg. 1996;10:1114–9.
91. Aoki M, Forbess JM, Jonas RA, Mayer JE, Castaneda AR. Results of biventricular repair for double-outlet right ventricle. J Thorac Cardiovasc Surg. 1994;2:338–50.
92. Erek E, Suzan D, Aydin S, Yildiz O, Kirat B, Demir H, Odemis E. Outcomes of arterial switch operation for Taussig-Bing anomaly versus transposition of great arteries and ventricular septal defect. Turkish J Thoracic Cardiovascul Surg. 2019;27:266–73.
93. Fricke TA, Konstantinov IE. Arterial switch operation: operative approach and outcomes. Ann Thorac Surg. 2019;107:302–10.
94. Fricke TA, Donaldson S, Schneider JR, Menahem S, d'Udekem Y, Brizard CP, Konstantinov IE. Outcomes of the arterial switch operation in patients with aortic arch obstruction. J Thoracic Cardiovascul Surg. 2020;159.592–99.
95. Dickinson DF, Wilkinson JL, Smith A, Hamilthon DI, Anderson RH. Variations in the morphology of the ventricular septal defect and disposition of the atrioventricular conduction tissue in tetralogy of Fallot. J Thorac Cardiovasc Surg. 1982;5:243–9.
96. Van Mierop LH, Wigelsworth FW. Pathogenesis of transposition complexes. II. Anomalies due to faulty transfer of the posterior great artery. Am J Cardiol. 1963;12:226–32.
97. Goor DA, Lillehei CW, Edwards JE. Ventricular septal defects and pulmonic stenosis with and without dextroposition anatomic features and embryologic implications. Chest. 1971;60:117–28.
98. Howell CE, Ho SY, Anderson RH, Elliot MJ. Fibrous skeleton and ventricular outflow tracts in double-outlet right ventricle. Ann Thorac Surg. 1991;51:394–400.
99. Van Praagh R. What is the Taussig-Bing malformation? Circulation. 1968;38:445–9.
100. Goor DA, Ebert PA. Left ventricular outflow obstruction in Taussig-Bing malformation. J Thorac Cardiovasc Surg. 1975;70:69–75.
101. Bharati S, Lev M. The conduction system in double outlet right ventricle with subpulmonic ventricular septal defect and related hearts (the Taussig-Bing group). Circulation. 1976;3:459–67.
102. Beuren A. Differential diagnosis of the Taussig-Bing heart from complete transposition of the great vessels with a posteriorly overriding pulmonary artery. Circulation. 1960;21:1071–87.

103. Sakata R, Lecompte Y, Batisse A, Borromee L, Durandy Y. Anatomic repair of anomalies of ventriculoarterial connection associated with ventricular septal defect. I. Criteria of surgical decision. J Thoracic Cardiovascul Surg. 1988;95:90–5.
104. Arteaga M, de la Cruz MV, Sanchez C, Diaz GF. Double outlet right ventricle: experimental morphogenesis in the chick embryo heart. Pediatr Cardiol. 1982;3:219–27.

Classification

K. V. Shatalov and K. M. Dzhidzhikhiya

Abstract Because of its anatomical complexity, classification of DORV allows to simplify surgical and therapeutic approaches. Initially proposed classification by division of VSDs into infra- and supracristal types is now obsolete and no longer used. In these chapter, we provide actual classifications of DORV by VSD location, infundibular anatomy and anatomico-clinical presentation which are helpful not only in therapeutic management, but also in surgical decision-making.

Keywords Double-outlet right ventricle · Types · Classification · Ventricular septal defect · Infundibulum

Since the beginning of study of DORV, several classifications have been proposed, each of which corresponded to a certain understanding of anatomy and methods of surgical correction of the disease existed at that time. The earliest one is the anatomical classification suggested by Neufeld et al. in 1961 [1–3], according to which the following variants of DORV were distinguished:

- with pulmonary artery stenosis;
- without pulmonary artery stenosis:
  - **type I**–with infracristal VSD located closer to the aorta and remote from the pulmonary artery (subaortic VSD);
  - **type IIa**–with supracristal VSD located closer to the pulmonary artery and remote from the aorta (Taussig-Bing anomaly);
  - **type IIb**–with supracristal VSD located under the both arterial valves (subarterial VSD).

Over the past decades, evolving understanding of DORV anatomy is significant, and such terminology now looks outdated. Thus, above-mentioned classification has lost its initial clinical value and currently has only historical interest.

K. V. Shatalov · K. M. Dzhidzhikhiya (✉)
Department of Emergency Surgery of Congenital Heart Diseases, A. N. Bakulev National Medical Investigation Center for Cardiovascular Surgery, Moscow, Russia
e-mail: d.m.konstantine@mail.ru

K. V. Shatalov and K. M. Dzhidzhikhiya (eds.), *Double-Outlet Right Ventricle*,
https://doi.org/10.1007/978-3-031-49707-0_3

The most important anatomical classifications that are relevant to today include the classification of DORV by VSD location proposed by Lev et al. [4] in 1972, as well as classification by the relationship of subarterial infundibulums developed by de la Cruz et al. [5] in 1992.

In 2000, the Society of Thoracic Surgeons and the European Society of Cardiovascular Surgery in the joint project «The Congenital Heart Surgery Nomenclature and Database Project Committee» proposed anatomico-hemodynamic classification of DORV which is generally accepted over the world [6].

1 Classification by VSD Location

The classification is based on the proximity of VSD to the arterial valves, according to which the following types of DORV are distinguished:

- with subaortic VSD;
- with subpulmonary VSD;
- with subarterial VSD;
- with non-committed VSD.

2 Classification by Relationship of Subarterial Infundibulums

This classification is based on the relationship of subarterial infundibulums, depending on which, there are variants of DORV with antero-posterior and side-by-side infundibulums.

DORV with antero-posterior infundibulums is formed when the OS fuses with the aTS (i.e., DORV with subaortic VSD) and only the posterior (subaortic) infundibulum has contact with atrioventricular valves (Fig. 1A).

The anatomical walls of the anterior (subpulmonary) infundibulum are:

- OS;
- right ventricle free wall;
- outlet component of the IVS.

The anatomical walls of the posterior (subaortic) infundibulum are:

- OS;
- right ventricle free wall;
- right half of the VIF;
- on the left, the posterior infundibulum opens to the left ventricle through subaortic VSD located between the limbs of the TS.

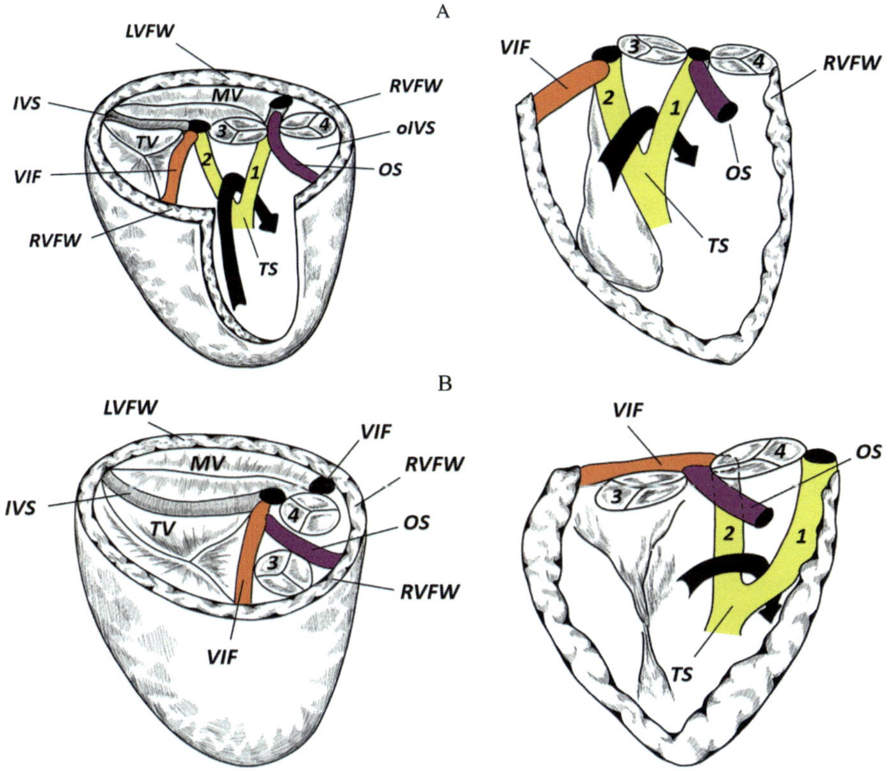

Fig. 1 DORV with antero-posterior (**A**) and «side-by-side» (**B**) infundibulums according to de la Cruz et al. *1–anterior limb of the trabecula septomarginalis; 2–posterior limb of the trabecula septomarginalis; 3–aortic valve; 4–pulmonary valve; LVFW–left ventricle free wall; RVFW–right ventricle free wall; IVS–interventricular septum; MV–mitral valve; oIVS–outlet part of the interventricular septum; TS–trabecula septomarginalis; TV–tricuspid valve; OS–outlet septum; VIF–ventriculo-infundibular fold*

DORV with side-by-side infundibulums is formed when the OS fuses with the pTS, (i.e., DORV with subpulmonary VSD) and both infundibulums have contact with atrioventricular valves (Fig. 1B).

The anatomical walls of the left (subpulmonary in D-malposition) infundibulum are:

- OS;
- right ventricle free wall;
- left half of the VIF;
- on the left side, the left infundibulum opens to the left ventricle through subpulmonary VSD located between the limbs of the TS.

The anatomical walls of the right (subaortic in D-malposition) infundibulum are:

- OS;

- right ventricle free wall;
- right half of the VIF.

The practical value of this classification is backed by the fact that the knowledge of the anatomical boundaries of subaortic and subpulmonary infundibulums in their different relationships allows to correctly recognize the intracardiac structures (mainly of the right ventricle) during the intracardiac revision as well as accurately differentiate anatomical structures responsible for subaortic or subpulmonary stenosis which must be eliminated during the repair.

3 Anatamico-Hemodynamic Classification

Depending on the clinical, hemodynamic and anatomical features, the following types of DORV may be distinguished:

- «VSD» type (with subaortic/subarterial VSD). Features:
  - no cyanosis due to direct flow of arterial blood from the left ventricle to the ascending aorta;
  - pulmonary overcirculation and hypertension.
- «tetralogy» type (with subaortic/subarterial VSD) and pulmonary artery stenosis. Features:
  - cyanosis due to mixed arterio-venous blood in the ascending aorta;
  - pulmonary undercirculation.
- «TGA» type (with subpulmonary VSD). Features:
  - severe cyanosis due to predominant flow of arterial blood from the left ventricle to the pulmonary artery and venous blood from the right ventricle to the ascending aorta;
  - pulmonary overcirculation and hypertension.
- «non-committed» type with or without pulmonary artery stenosis. Features:
  - hemodynamics and clinical presentation depend on the proximity of VSD to the arterial valves and presence or absence of pulmonary artery stenosis.

References

1. Neufeld HN, Dushane JW, Wood EH, Kirklin JW, Edwards JE. Origin of both great vessels from the right ventricle I without pulmonary stenosis. Circulation. 1961;23:399–412.
2. Neufeld HN, Dushane JW, Edwards JE. Origin of both great vessels from the right ventricle II without pulmonary stenosis. Circulation. 1961;23:603–12.

3. Neufeld HN, Lucas RV, Lester RG, Adams P, Anderson RC, Edwards JE. Origin of both great vessels from the right ventricle without pulmonary stenosis. Br Heart J. 1962;24:393–408.
4. Lev M, Bharati S, Meng CCL, Libethson RP, Paul MH, Idriss F. A concept of double outlet right ventricle. J Thorac Cardiovasc Surg. 1972;64:271–81.
5. de la Cruz MV, Cayre R, Martinez OA, Sadowinski S, Serrano A. The infundibular interrelationships and ventriculoarterial connection in double outlet right ventricle. Clinical and surgical implications. Int J Cardiol 1992;5:153–164
6. Walters HL III, Mavroudis C, Tchervenkov CI, Jacobs JP, Lacour-Gayet F, Jacobs ML. Congenital heart surgery nomenclature and database project: double outlet right ventricle. Ann Thorac Surg. 2000;69:S249–63.

Arterial Hypoxemia

A. K. Kade, P. P. Polyakov, S. A. Zanin, and Z. M. Dzhidzhikhiya

Abstract Arterial hypoxemia is a leading clinical syndrome, especially in DORV with subpulmonary and non-committed VSD. The syndrome develops as a result of blood mixing at the ventricular level and significantly affects quality of life. It this chapter we describe arterial hypoxemia from pathophysiological standpoint as a non-specific syndrome associated with all cyanotic CHDs, in particular with DORV. Acute episodes of severe arterial hypoxemia are potentially life-threatening conditions and require urgent care. In patients with long standing arterial hypoxemia, hypoxia-inducible factor initiates different mechanisms (molecular, cellular, etc.) of adaptation which play crucial role in supporting relatively stable clinical condition. Despite its direct influence arterial hypoxemia is also responsible for secondary erythrocytosis and coagulation abnormalities as well as angiogenesis and osteoarthropathy which complicate medical and surgical treatment.

Keywords Double-outlet right ventricle · Cyanotic congenital heart defects · Arterial hypoxemia · Coagulation · Hypoxia-inducible factor

Complex and at the same time diverse intracardiac anatomy of the entire spectrum of DORV determines the existence of a wide range of hemodynamic scenarios of the disease. Intracardiac hemodynamics, specific for each morphological type of DORV, triggers pathophysiological mechanisms, by which the adverse effects of the disease occur and which determine the clinical symptoms. Knowledge of the main pathophysiological processes as well as the mechanisms of their manifestation at different levels of the organism contributes to a more thorough planning for both therapeutic and surgical treatment. For example, in cyanotic patients with DORV, hypoxemia triggers a number of pathological processes in almost all tissues, which must be taken into account not only during the hospital period, but also in the long-term after

A. K. Kade · P. P. Polyakov (✉) · S. A. Zanin
Departement of Pathophisiology, Kuban State Medical University, Krasnodar, Russia
e-mail: palpal.p@yandex.ru

Z. M. Dzhidzhikhiya
Research Institute – Ochapovsky Regional Clinical Hospital №1, Krasnodar, Russia

K. V. Shatalov and K. M. Dzhidzhikhiya (eds.), *Double-Outlet Right Ventricle*,
https://doi.org/10.1007/978-3-031-49707-0_4

surgical correction, which can significantly reduce the incidence of complications and improve the effectiveness of treatment and patients' quality of life.

The main pathophysiological syndromes accompanying DORV are:

- arterial hypoxemia;
- myocardial remodeling and heart failure;
- pulmonary hypertension.

Pulmonary hypertension in CHDs is widely discussed in a literature. The pathophysiological mechanisms and influence on the organism of arterial hypoxemia and remodeling of the heart, which are characteristic of all cyanotic CHDs, will be described below.

Partial pressure of O_2 in dry atmospheric air at sea level is 0.21 (FiO_2—21%) × 760 mmHg = 156 mmHg (21.2 kPa). In upper airways at 37 °C, taking into account humidification (and partial pressure of water vapor equal to 47 mmHg), the partial pressure of O_2 (PiO_2) is 150 mmHg (0.21 × (760–47)) or 20 kPa. At the alveolar level, the partial pressure (P_AO_2) decreases, in particular, due to the dilution with carbon dioxide. This indicator can be calculated using the simplified alveolar gas equation: $P_AO_2 = PiO_2$—(P_aCO2/RQ), where P_aCO_2 is the partial pressure of CO_2 in arterial blood (can be measured in the laboratory), RQ is the respiratory coefficient, which approaches 0.8 (characterizes tissue metabolism, namely the ratio of CO_2 produced to O_2 consumed). Thus, this formula can be written as follows: $P_AO_2 = 150$ mmHg—($P_aCO2/0.8$) [1].

The difference between the oxygen content in the alveoli and pulmonary arteries (in other words, in venous blood, which is 32 mmHg or 4.3 kPa), the so-called pressure gradient, ensures the diffusion of oxygen into the blood, an increase in the oxygen pressure in the pulmonary veins (denoted as P_aO_2, the normal value is 75–100 mmHg or 10–13.3 kPa) and arterial blood. In an «ideal» lung, P_AO_2 and P_aO_2 are equal, but in a real situation, there is a limited diffusion rate and an imperfect ventilation-perfusion ratio in different parts of the lungs (in other words, change of the V/Q ratio–an increase in dead space and an increasing shunt fraction) [1].

Using the above-mentioned formula and results of the analysis of arterial blood gases, it is possible to calculate the value of A-a gradient, that is, the difference between the oxygen pressure in the alveolar air (P_AO_2, estimated by the equation) and in arterial blood (P_aO_2, measured in the laboratory). A-a gradient is a convenient tool for differential diagnosis of the etiology of hypoxemia. The A-a gradient increases within lung diseases and remains normal within extrapulmonary pathologies with the exception of right-to-left shunt, which also increases the A-a gradient [2].

The intracellular oxygen pressure is 8–10 mmHg in the cytoplasm and 6–8 mmHg in the mitochondria [3]. The gradual decrease in oxygen pressure in the alveoli, blood, cytoplasm and mitochondria is known as «oxygen cascade».

Oxygen delivery (DO_2) to tissues depends on two factors and can be expressed by the following formula: DO_2 = cardiac output (liter per min.) × oxygen content in arterial blood (CaO_2, ml/dl). Cardiac output depends on the heart rate and stroke volume, while CaO_2 depends on the amount of oxygen combined with Hb (98.5%), as well as dissolved in blood plasma (1.5%). Thus, the total oxygen content in arterial

Fig. 1 Oxyhemoglobin dissociation curve

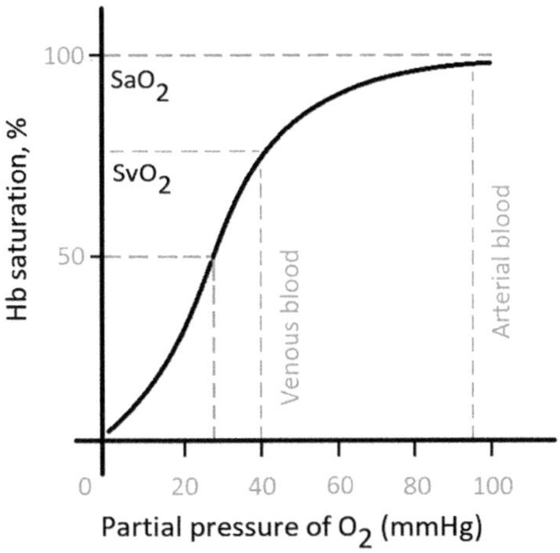

blood can be expressed as follows: $CaO_2 = Hb(g/l) \times 1.34 \times S_aO_2\ (\%) + P_aO_2 \times 0.003$, where 1.34 is Hüfner's constant, reflecting the oxygen-binding capacity of hemoglobin [1, 4].

S_aO_2 depends on P_aO_2, which is graphically expressed as oxygen-hemoglobin dissociation curve (Fig. 1). The initial nonlinear part of the curve is explained by the phenomenon of positive cooperation—when one of the four hemoglobin subunits binds oxygen, the affinity of the others increases. The middle ascending part reflects the direct linear dependence of S_aO_2 on P_aO_2, while the plateau-saturation of hemoglobin. At a level of about 60 mmHg, S_aO_2 approaches the level of plateau ($> 94\%$).

The dissociation curve of oxyhemoglobin shifts to the right with a decrease in the affinity of hemoglobin to oxygen, which can be observed with an increase in the level of 2,3-diphosphoglycerate (a natural regulator of the affinity of hemoglobin to oxygen produced during glycolysis in the erythrocyte), hyperthermia, acidosis (Bohr effect) and high carbon dioxide content. An increase in affinity and a shift of the curve to the left, on the contrary, is observed with a decrease in the level of 2,3-diphosphoglycerate, hypothermia, alkalosis and low carbon dioxide content [3].

Indicators of S_aO_2 (measured by CO-oximeter), S_pO_2 (measured by pulse oximeter) and P_aO_2 are not informative enough without taking into account the clinical context. So, in a patient on oxygen therapy (e.g., with $FiO_2 = 0.5$), the P_aO_2 value equal to 100 mmHg (saturation is close to 100%) reflects the presence of a serious pathology. The oxygenation index (P_aO_2/FiO_2), which depends on numerous factors, in this case is much less than it should be [5]. At the same time, $SpO_2 > 94\%$ can be observed in a patient who is in a state of hypoxia [6]. This may be due to a shift in the dissociation curve of oxyhemoglobin to the left in alkalosis, low carbon dioxide content, hypophosphatemia (lowers the level of 2,3-diphosphoglycerate), sepsis (lowers the level of 2,3-diphosphoglycerate) etc.

Incorrect results of pulse oximetry can be explained by the presence of endogenous and exogenous pigments in the blood, the patient's motor activity (trembling, convulsions, screaming, crying of a child, etc.), reduced perfusion of peripheral tissues (circulatory insufficiency, inflating of the cuff for measuring blood pressure), increased venous pulsation (tricuspid regurgitation), carboxyhemoglobinemia, methemoglobinemia, sulfhemoglobinemia, and possibly a significant amount of fetal hemoglobin (HbF). Devices that have protection against interference and artifacts, as well as the use of CO-oximetry that recognizes inactivated forms of hemoglobin, allow to avoid false results [7, 8].

The capabilities of pulse oximetry in detecting «normal» forms of hemoglobin are apparently comparable to those of CO-oximetry at S_aO_2 greater than 91%. However, with more pronounced hypoxemia, pulse oximetry may overestimate ($S_pO_2 > S_aO_2$) the amount of oxygenated hemoglobin (false negative result) [8]. This is due to the fact that the calibration of devices is carried out on healthy volunteers under normal conditions, as well as with some other causes [7, 9]. This problem, in particular, has been studied in newborn children with heart defects and patients after surgery with cardiopulmonary bypass [10–12].

The effect of erythrocytosis on pulse oximetry is not entirely clear. According to Schmidt et al., erythrocytosis does not distort the measurement result in children with CHD and saturation less than 80% [10].

A striking clinical sign of an increase in the amount of deoxyhemoglobin and a decrease in S_aO_2 is central cyanosis, which is clinically manifested at a deoxyhemoglobin level of 50 g/l. At the same time, a decrease or increase in the total hemoglobin content affects the occurrence of this symptom. For example, with anemia and a hemoglobin concentration of 60 g/l, even the presence of 60% deoxyhemoglobin (36 g/l) will not be accompanied by cyanosis, while with erythrocytosis and a hemoglobin concentration of 180 g/l, already 28% of deoxyhemoglobin will manifest as cyanosis [13].

The oxygen delivered is consumed by tissues, the intensity of which can be represented as oxygen extraction ratio using the following formula: $O_2ER = (CaO_2—CvO_2)/CaO_2$, where CaO_2 is the oxygen content in arterial blood and CvO_2 is the oxygen content in venous blood. Normally, the extraction coefficient is 20–30% ($O_2ER = 0.2–0.3$). This indicator varies depending on the metabolic needs of tissues (e.g., myocardial O_2ER is 0.6). With a decrease in oxygen delivery (Fig. 2), organs can compensatorily increase its extraction, but this mechanism works up to a certain limit, after which aerobic metabolism is no longer possible and lactic acidosis develops. Organs with high metabolic needs cannot significantly increase oxygen uptake from the blood, since O_2ER is normally high enough [4].

Oxygen consumption may increase with excitation, convulsions, hyperventilation, fever, sepsis, etc., and decreases with sedation, muscle relaxation, hypothermia, inactivation of electron transport chain respiratory enzymes, etc. [4].

At each of the above-mentioned levels, from the external environment to the mitochondria, disturbances are possible that lead to the development of hypoxia. Hypoxia is a typical pathophysiological process, in which all (generalized form) or

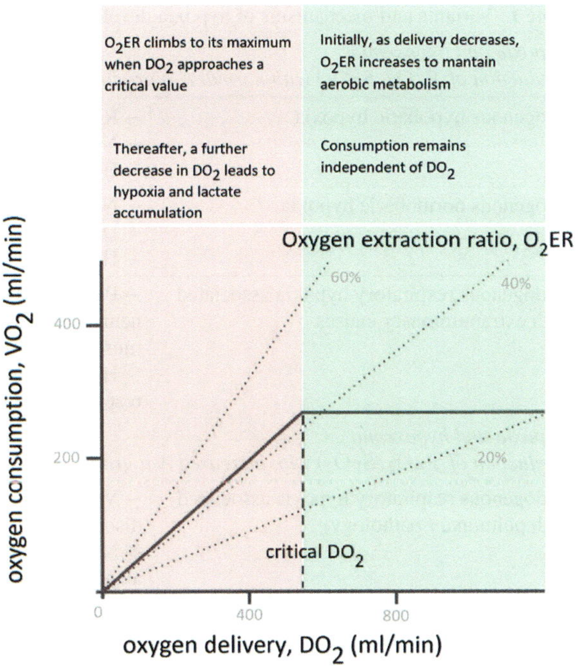

Fig. 2 Decrease in oxygen consumption can be compensated by its enhanced extraction ratio (dotted lines), e.g., from 30 to 40%, but up to a certain limit after which lactate acidosis develops

some (local form) organs and tissues of the body do not receive or are unable to use oxygen in an amount sufficient for normal intracellular metabolism.

According to the etiology, hypoxia can be divided into:

- exogenous: hypobaric, normobaric;
- endogenous: respiratory, hemic, circulatory, tissue.

Depending on the type of hypoxia, the indicators of FiO_2, P_aO_2, A-a gradient, S_aO_2 and DO_2 may differ (Table 1).

Hypoxemia is characterized by a decrease in partial oxygen pressure in arterial blood. As follows from the CaO_2 calculation equation, the partial oxygen pressure is not identical to the oxygen content in the blood and even more so to the delivery and consumption of it by tissues. The partial pressure determines the solubility of oxygen in the blood (according to Dalton's law of partial pressures) and S_aO_2, but not the amount of hemoglobin. A patient with severe anemia may have normal P_aO_2 and S_pO_2 values.

The main mechanisms of hypoxemia include:

- low-pressure oxygen in the inhaled air;
- hypoventilation not related to lung diseases;
- ventilation, perfusion and diffusion in the lungs;
- venoarterial (right-left) blood shunt.

The last two groups are characterized by an increase in the A-a gradient.

Table 1 Variants and mechanisms of hypoxia development [2, 14]

Hypoxia and hypoxemia (Reduction of P_AO_2, S_PO_2*) with normal A-a gradient*	
Exogenous hypobaric hypoxia	– Reduced atmospheric pressure; – Normal FiO_2; – Hypocapnia, respiratory alkalosis
Exogenous normobaric hypoxia	– Normal atmospheric pressure; – Decrease in FiO_2 (<0.21); – Hypercapnia, respiratory acidosis
Endogenous respiratory hypoxia associated with extrapulmonary causes	– Pathology of the nervous system, neuromuscular transmission, respiratory muscles, pleura, thorax; – Hypercapnia, respiratory acidosis (type II respiratory failure)
Hypoxia and hypoxemia (Reduction of P_AO_2, S_PO_2*) with increased A-a gradient*	
Endogenous respiratory hypoxia associated with pulmonary pathology	– Ventilation, perfusion and/or diffusion disorders; – Normocapnia/hypocapnia and respiratory alkalosis in type I respiratory failure, hypercapnia and acidosis in type II
Endogenous circulatory hypoxia with venoarterial shunt	– Cyanotic CHD, pulmonary arteriovenous malformations (e.g., Osler-Weber-Rendu disease), etc
Hypoxia without hypoxemia (Normal P_AO_2*, normal or falsely normal* S_PO_2*)*	
Endogenous circulatory hypoxia without venoarterial shunt	– Ischemia, venous hyperemia
Endogenous hemic hypoxia	– Anemia
	– Inactivation of hemoglobin by carbon monoxide, methemoglobinemia, sulfhemoglobinemia
Endogenous tissue hypoxia	– Inactivation of electron transport chain enzymes (cyanides, carbon monoxide, barbiturates, rotenone), uncouplers of oxidative phosphorylation (salicylates, dinitrophenol); – Hyperoxia, which increases free radical oxidation and mitochondrial dysfunction; – Normal DO_2.value

Thus, the terms hypoxia and hypoxemia are not synonymous. For example, conditions in which tissues do not consume oxygen due to mitochondrial dysfunction (tissue hypoxia) are not accompanied by a decrease in P_aO_2 and S_aO_2.

Table 1 combines both presented classifications.

1 Hemodynamic Bases of Hypoxemia in DORV

In patients with DORV «VSD» type arterial hypoxemia is not typical. Due to subaortic/subarterial location of VSD and absence of pulmonary artery stenosis, blood from the left ventricle predominantly goes to the ascending aorta minimally mixing with venous blood in the right ventricule.

In DORV «tetralogy» type, hypoxemia develops as a result of limited pulmonary circulation due to multilevel RVOT and pulmonary artery stenosis (Q_s>Q_p) which leads to an increase in proportion of venous blood (coming from venae cavae) compared with arterial blood (coming from the pulmonary veins) when two flows are mixed at the ventricular level. In addition, pulmonary artery stenosis contributes to a greater mixing of arterial and venous blood in the right ventricle.

In DORV «TGA» type hypoxemia is caused by predominant flow of venous blood from the right ventricle into the aorta and arterial blood from the left ventricle into the pulmonary artery.

In DORV with non-committed VSD hypoxemia develops because arterial blood from the left ventricle does not enter the aorta directly, but only after shunting to the right ventricle and significantly mixing with venous blood. Additional pulmonary artery stenosis leads to greater mixing of flows in the right ventricle.

Thus, two general mechanisms of arterial hypoxemia can be distinguished in DORV: limited pulmonary blood flow and venoarterial shunting (Table 2).

Hypoxemia in patients with DORV (with the exception of «VSD» type) takes place from the moment of transition from placental to pulmonary respiration starting from the first breath of the child. The most severe clinical manifestations of hypoxemia that occur immediately after birth are seen in DORV «TGA» type without pulmonary artery stenosis (Taussig-Bing anomaly). In such cases, balloon atrioseptostomy is urgently performed to stabilize the child's condition and results in greater mixing of systemic and pulmonary venous flows at the atrial level, so the more oxygenated blood enters the right ventricle and aorta (see Chap. 10). In Taussig-Bing anomaly surgical intervention is indicated in the first weeks of life due to the risk of pulmonary hypertension. However, in some cases, such patients may undergo pulmonary artery banding as a first stage of surgical treatment. In DORV

Table 2 Mechanisms and severity of arterial hypoxemia in various types of DORV

DORV type	Hypovolemia of pulmonary blood flow	Venoarterial shunting	Cyanosis
«VSD»	–	–	–
«Tetralogy»	+/++/+++	+/++/+++	+/++/+++
«TGA» (without pulmonary artery stenosis-Taussig-Bing anomaly)	–	+++	+++
«Non-committed»: without pulmonary artery stenosis with pulmonary artery stenosis	– +	+/++ ++/+++	+/++ ++/+++

«tetralogy» and «non-committed» types, the optimal age for anatomical correction is 6–12 months. In younger children, palliative surgery imply either modified systemic-to-pulmonary artery shunt or pulmonary artery banding (for non-committed VSD without pulmonary artery stenosis).

2 Mechanisms of Adaptation to Acute Hypoxemia

2.1 Adaptation at the Level of Organs and the Organism

Episodes of acute hypoxemia in DORV mainly occur in patients with «tetralogy» type and manifest as spells due to right ventricular infundibulum spasm with severe restriction of pulmonary circulation.

The most sensitive and the earliest structures reacting in response to acute hypoxia are carotid chemoreceptors located in carotid bifurcation (the so-called carotid glomus). Type I glomus cells are activated in response to hypoxemia (but not hypoxia without hypoxemia, e.g., with anemia and hemoglobin inactivation!) using the intracellular system of gas transmitters (CO, H_2S, NO). In turn, chemosensitive aortic arch tissue reacts to hypoxic stimuli in the absence of hypoxemia.

Stimulation from chemoreceptors via afferent fibers is transmitted to the central nervous system (to the nucleus tractus solitarii) and further to efferent structures (including the rostral ventrolateral medulla) where sympathoactivating neurons activity increases [15].

The main adaptive reaction which occurs in response to acute hypoxia at the levels of organs and the organism as a result of activation of chemoreceptors is the activation of sympathetic nervous system. The effects of the latter include [16, 17]:

- bronchodilation (β_2-adrenergic receptors);
- tachycardia (β_1-adrenoreceptors);
- increased myocardial contractility (β_1-adrenoreceptors);
- arterial vasoconstriction (α-adrenoreceptors) and increased afterload on the heart (with possible subsequent post-hypoxic vasodilation due to the development of lactate acidosis);
- renin secretion by the juxtaglomerular apparatus of the kidneys (β_1-adrenoreceptors);
- retention of Na^+ ions (α-adrenergic receptors) and water in proximal renal tubules, increase in blood volume and preload;
- contractions of the spleen capsule with the release of blood cells from the «depot» (α_1-adrenoreceptors), an increase in hematocrit, leukocytosis;
- increased cleavage of glycogen (β_2-adrenoreceptors, activation of glycogen phosphorylase, suppression of glycogen synthase, inhibition of insulin secretion (α-adrenoreceptors), hyperglycemia;
- reduction of motility (α- and β-adrenoreceptors) and secretion (α-adrenoreceptors) of the gastrointestinal tract;
- secretion of antidiuretic hormone (β_1-adrenergic receptors).

2.2 Cellular and Tissue Levels

A short-term response to hypoxia at the cellular level is provided by allosteric regulation of enzyme activity (phosphofructokinases react to the level of ATP, AMP, citrate) and activation of hypoxia-inducible factor–HIF. HIF-1α activity is manifested mainly in the early stages of hypoxia (up to 24 h). In deep acute hypoxia, these factors are responsible for the regulation of glycolysis and apoptosis. With prolonged non-critical hypoxia (more than 48 h), a switch to HIF-2α occurs, which is expressed in tissues involved in long-term adaptation (kidneys, liver, endothelium) (see below).

In normoxia, HIF-α is inactivated by prolyl hydroxylase and von Hippel-Lindau protein factor. In hypoxia, HIF-α stabilizes, binds to constitutively expressed oxygen-independent HIF-β, attracts coactivators (CREB-binding protein (CBP)/p300) and interacts with hypoxia response element (HRE, 5′-(A/G) CGTG-3′). In addition, many target genes are indirectly controlled by HIF, which affects other transcription factors, epigenetic mechanisms and RNA interference (Fig. 3).

Cellular glucose uptake is enhanced due to HIF-dependent increase in glucose transporters GLUT-1 and GLUT-3. Increased glycolysis, inhibition of oxidative decarboxylation of pyruvate, the Krebs cycle and oxidative phosphorylation occur due to the effect of HIF on a number of enzymes involved in these processes. Compensation of intracellular acidosis is regulated by HIF by increasing the expression of IX Carbonic anhydrase, Na^+/H^+-exchangers and monocarboxylate transporters (MCT-1, -4) that secrete lactate.

The main adaptation reactions in response to acute hypoxia at the cellular and tissue levels as a result of HIF activation are:

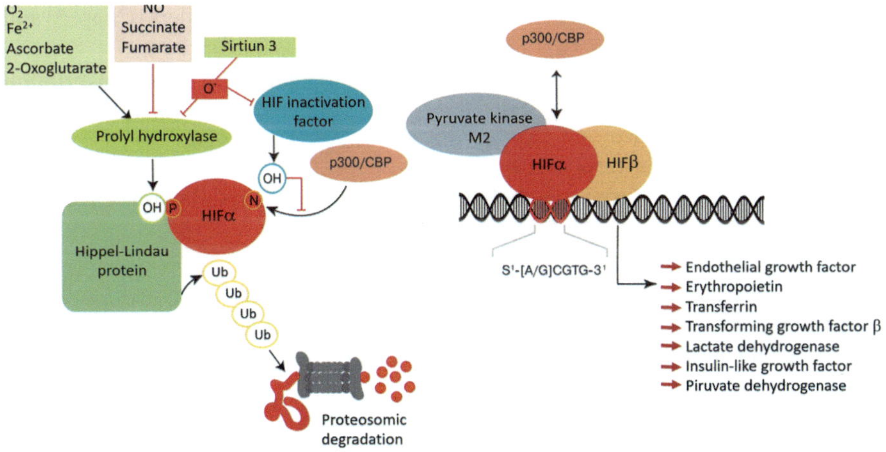

Fig. 3 Molecular mechanisms of HIF activation [adapted from [18]]. *HIF—hypoxia-inducible factor; Ub—ubiquitin*

- increased glucose uptake by cells;
- increased glycolysis;
- accumulation of lactate (Pasteur effect) in cells and its enhanced excretion along with H^+ ions into the extracellular environment, which leads to lactate acidosis;
- inhibition of mitochondrial metabolism.

When the intracellular partial oxygen pressure decreases to 1 mmHg, HIF induces apoptosis, stimulating the work of pro-apoptotic proteins (Noxa, BAX, BID) [3].

Developing metabolic acidosis (lactate acidosis type A, with an increase in anion gap) promotes stimulation of central chemoreceptors in the medulla oblongata, causing hyperventilation, as well as type I glomus cells and activation of chemoreceptor reflex (see above). Simultaneous decrease of myocardial contractility, bronchoconstriction and vasodilation counteracts the effects of sympathetic nervous system. The development of acidosis contributes to a decrease in the affinity of hemoglobin to oxygen (a shift of the dissociation curve to the right–the Bohr effect). In addition, at the intracellular level, the work of enzymes with the appropriate pH-optimum (including phosphofructokinase, which limits the rate of glycolysis) is inhibited, thus causing the positive feedback and aggravating the energy deficit.

3 Mechanisms of Adaptation to Chronic Hypoxemia

Chronic exposure to hypoxia and hypoxemia leads to myocardial hypertrophy and increased blood pressure, increased pressure in the pulmonary artery, secondary erythrocytosis, changes in iron metabolism, increased angiogenesis, as well as changes in intracellular metabolism. These processes are described in more detail in the relevant sections on myocardial remodeling, angiogenesis disorders (Chap. 5) and hematological complications (see below).

These processes are also controlled by HIF acting together with other transcription regulators. HIF targets are (Table 3):

- erythropoietin and erythropoietin receptor;
- proteins regulators of iron metabolism (see «Secondary erythrocytosis and other pathology of the blood system»);
- proangiogenic factors (see «Angiogenesis disorder»);
- pro-inflammatory (non-specific TLR4 receptors, cytokines, enzymes) and anti-inflammatory factors (ecto-5'-nucleotidase, adenosine receptors);
- growth and proliferation stimulators (cyclin D1), as well as anti-proliferative (proteins p53, p21) factors;
- extracellular matrix modifiers (matrix metalloproteinases, lysyl oxidase, β transforming growth factor (TGF- β).

Thus, the reaction to hypoxia at the cellular, tissue and organ levels depends on many factors and mainly on the amount of residual oxygen and macroergic compounds. With an absolute energy deficit, the implementation of very complex

Table 3 HIF molecular targets [19–25]

Changes at the cellular, organ or organismal levels necessary for adaptation to hypoxia		HIF targets
Increased oxygen delivery to cells	Blood oxygen-carrying capacity increase	Erythropoietin The erythropoietin receptor (EpoR) in the bone marrow Transferrin receptors in the bone marrow Ferrochelatase (combines iron ions and protoporphyrin IX)
	Changes in iron metabolism	Duodenal cytochrome b (reduction of Fe^{3+} to Fe^{2+}) Divalent metal transporter (absorption of Fe^{2+} by enterocytes) Ferroportin (transports iron ions from enterocytes, macrophages of the spleen and other cells into the blood) Transferrin (transports iron ions through the blood) Heme oxygenase
	Increased angiogenesis	VEGF PDGFB IL-6 Tie-2 Angiopoietin 2 ANGPTL4 L1CAM Cyclooxygenase 2 Inducible NO synthase Matrix metalloproteinases SCF, KIT-ligand SDF1
Glucose metabolism	Increased glucose uptake by cells	GLUT-1 GLUT-3
	Increased glycolysis, inhibition of mitochondrial metabolism (oxidative decarboxylation of pyruvate, Krebs cycle, respiratory chain)	Hexokinases 1,2 Phosphofructokinase L Aldolases A,C Alpha-enolase Phosphoglycerate kinase 1 Phosphoglycerate mutase Pyruvate decarboxylase kinase 1 Cytochrome c oxidase
Compensation of acidosis (resulting from the accumulation of lactate)	CO_2 production from H^+ and bicarbonate	IX Carbonic anhydrase
	Transport of H^+	Na^+/H^+—transporter (Na^+/H^+ exanger, NHE)
	Lactate transport	Monocarboxylate transporter MCT-1, MCT-4

(continued)

Table 3 (continued)

Changes at the cellular, organ or organismal levels necessary for adaptation to hypoxia		HIF targets
Inflammation (HIF in close interaction with NF-kB, JAK-STAT)	Receptors	TLR4
	Cytokines	TNF-α, IL-6, CCL5, CXCL12
	Other mediators	Endothelins 1,2
	Enzymes	Cyclooxygenase 2 Inducible NO synthase
Metabolism of the extracellular matrix	Extracellular matrix degradation	Matrix metalloproteinase 2,9,14
	Synthesis of the extracellular matrix	Collagen prolyl 4-hydroxylase Lysyl oxidase Inhibitor of TIMP-1 TGF-β1 Smad2/3, Smad4
Metabolism of extracellular ATP/ADP	Conversion to adenosine	Ecto-5'-nucleotidase (CD73)
	Effects of adenosine (anti-ischemic, anti-inflammatory)	Adenosine Receptors 2A, 2B
Cell survival	Growth factors, mitogens	VEGF, EPO, IGF
	Signal transduction	MAPK, PI3K
	Cell cycle regulators	p21, p27, cyclin D1
	Tumor suppressors genes	p53, PTEN
	Effect on apoptosis (at O2 0–0.5%—induction of apoptosis, 1–3%—inhibition of apoptosis)	MCL1 BNIP BNIP3L PPP5C Noxa BAX BID Survivin
	Autophagy regulation	BNIP BNIP3L Beclin-1
	Telomerase activity regulation	hTERT
Effect on non-coding RNAs	microRNA	microRNA-155, 429, 155, 210, 204, 19a etc
	Long non-coding RNAs	lincRNA-p21
Epigenetic changes	Histone methylation/ demethylation	H3JI4 methyltransferase TET1 (hydroxylates cytosines as a part of HRE, contributing to demethylation) demethylases JmjC (Jumonji C)
	Histone acetylation and deacetylation	HDAC3 (deacetylates H3K4)

genetic programs is difficult. Disruption of the transmembrane ATP-dependent electrolyte transport leads to cell overload with Na^+ and water as well as Ca^{2+} ions, which activate intracellular proteases, phospholipases, endonucleases, proteases, endonucleases and other enzymes and exacerbates mitochondrial dysfunction, which leads to necrosis at the tissue level [26].

If hypoxia has not led to an absolute depletion of cellular energy carriers, HIF and the «colleagues» launch an adaptation program. The latter may be manifested by stopping the cell cycle (e.g., with the help of the p21 protein at the G0/G1 stage) and triggering apoptosis (at an O_2 level of less than 1 mmHg) or, conversely, increased growth and proliferation, accompanied by corresponding changes in metabolism. Together with disorders of connective tissue production and stimulation of angiogenesis, these changes at the tissue level manifest as hypertrophy, hyperplasia, dystrophy, atrophy, fibrosis or malignization.

HIF dysfunction underlies secondary erythrocytosis, hemostasis disorders and other hematological disorders, increased tissue vascularization, as well as the progression of heart failure.

4 Secondary Erythrocytosis and Other Pathology of the Blood System

One of the consequences of chronic hypoxia and hypoxemia is a HIF-dependent increase in erythropoietin synthesis. This glycoprotein with a molecular weight of 34–39 kDa is produced by the peritubular cells of the kidneys (to a lesser extent in the liver and brain). Erythropoietin interacts with erythropoietin receptors, the intracellular signal from which is transmitted by the enzyme JAK2 and STAT5 factor. As a result of stimulation, apoptosis of bone marrow red blood cell precursors is suppressed (in particular, the synthesis of the anti-apoptotic molecule BCL-X_L increases), and the count of circulating red blood cells increases [27].

Additional effects of HIF in relation to hematopoiesis are [22]:

- increased density of erythropoietin receptors;
- enhanced reduction of trivalent iron to divalent (Fe^{3+} to Fe^{2+}) in the gastrointestinal tract by duodenal cytochromes b;
- increased absorption of Fe^{2+} by divalent metal transporters;
- enhanced transport of Fe^{2+} from enterocytes, splenic macrophages and hepatocytes into the blood by ferroportins;
- increasing the amount of transferrin;
- enhancement of Fe^{2+} capture by bone marrow by transferrin receptors;
- increased activity of ferrochelatase connecting Fe^{2+} and protoporphyrin ring.

Secondary erythrocytosis in cyanotic CHDs can be compensated and decompensated. During decompensation, an increase in hematocrit is not accompanied by an improvement in tissue oxygenation due to the predominance of negative effects such as increased blood viscosity, poor microcirculation, platelet activation and thrombocytopenia as well as intensive iron utilization and iron deficiency [28]. Venoarterial shunt of blood contributes to an even greater decrease in the adaptive value of secondary erythrocytosis.

In compensated secondary erythrocytosis, there is no excess blood viscosity, iron deficiency does not develop, and an increased hemoglobin level improves tissue oxygenation (according to the formula Broberg et al., the amount of hemoglobin (g/dl) of adults with cyanotic CHD, sufficient for normal tissue oxygenation, is equal to 61—$SaO_2/2$, if the saturation is not lower than 75%) [28, 29].

Increased bilirubin metabolism is also associated with erythrocytosis, which leads to increased risk of gallstones formation twice as much as in patients with acyanotic CHD [30].

Some other diseases of the erythrocyte system pathogenetically associated with CHD and its complications (hemoptysis with pulmonary hypertension, heart failure, protein-losing enteropathy and malabsorption, etc.), and possible concomitant diseases, including hereditary, are listed in Table 4.

Microcytosis is associated with change of the mechanical properties of erythrocytes (deformability) and increased viscosity regardless of hematocrit [34]. In adult patients with cyanotic CHD, microcytosis is an independent risk factor for ischemic stroke, arterial hypertension and atrial fibrillation [35]. Iron deficiency in addition to the development of anemia contributes to the dysfunction of a number of proteins (myoglobin, respiratory chain enzymes, etc.), e.g., sideropenic syndrome (weakness of smooth muscles, sphincters, lesions of skin, mucous membranes, Plummer-Vinson syndrome). Intracellular metabolism is regulated by iron through its binding to special iron-regulating proteins IRP. Cardio specific «shutdown» of these proteins in the experiment with mice leads to mitochondrial dysfunction and contractile disorders [36]. Other possible causes of microcytosis are listed in Table 4.

Anemia in patients with cyanotic CHD has a complex genesis, therefore, the most accurate diagnostic methods should be used to detect its causes. Thus, a decrease in MCV and MCHC in iron deficiency can be «masked» by macrocytosis and hyperchromia, which is explained by concomitant vitamin B_9/B_{12} deficiency, the presence of which in 50% of adult patients with cyanotic CHD is assumed on the basis of hyperhomocysteinemia [34, 37]. Other possible causes of macrocytosis are listed in Table 4. MCV and MCHC are thus unreliable indicators of iron deficiency, as is serum iron, which decreases in anemia of chronic diseases. In this respect, the level of ferritin (which, however, is an acute phase protein and is intensively synthesized during inflammation), total iron binding capacity, transferrin concentration, soluble transferrin receptors are more preferable [34].

In children and adult patients with cyanotic CHD, diseases caused by venous or arterial thrombosis (e.g., cerebrovascular) are described. However, for secondary erythrocytoses, these complications are not typical [38, 39]. The described cases are probably explained by a combination with other risk factors that should be paid attention to (Table 5).

Antiphospholipid syndrome, hyperhomocysteinemia (homozygous homocystinuria, hypovitaminosis B_6, B_9, B_{12}), Anderson-Fabry disease, immune complex

Table 4 Possible disorders of the erythrocyte system in patients with cyanotic CHD [27, 31–33]

Pathogenetically related disorders	Possible concomitant disorders
Erythrocytosis	
• Secondary erythrocytosis due to hypoxia and hypoxemia	– Erythrocytosis in chronic myeloproliferative disease (Osler-Vaquez disease and other diseases, often associated with a mutation of the JAK2 gene); – Erythrocytosis due to mutations of EpoR genes, von Hippel-Lindau protein, prolyl hydroxylase-2, HIF-2α; – Erythrocytosis in hypoxia of other etiologies; – Autonomous production of EPO by tumors (kidney, liver, brain)
Microcytosis (MCV < 80 fL)	
• Iron deficiency due to increased erythropoiesis and increased need for iron; • Iron deficiency due to enteropathy and malabsorption; • Anemia of chronic diseases due to chronic heart failure	– Iron deficiency anemia of other etiologies: blood loss, poor nutrition, malabsorption, iron-refractory iron deficiency anemia (mutations of matriptase-2 genes, divalent metallotransporters, transferrin, ceruloplasmin); – Anemia of chronic diseases of other etiology (rheumatological diseases, infections, tumors); – Hereditary sideroblastic anemias (Kearns-Sayre syndrome, etc.); – Acquired sideroblastic anemias (lead poisoning and etc.); – Some hemoglobinopathies (thalassemia, HbC, HbE and etc.)
Macrocytosis (MCV > 100 fL)	
• Deficiency of B_9 or B_{12} due to malabsorption; • B_9 deficiency due to hepatic dysfunction/ cardiac cirrhosis in CHF; • Myelodysplastic syndrome (Down syndrome, Noonan syndrome); • Copper deficiency due to malabsorption; • Macrocytosis in liver lesions; • Hypothyroidism (hypoxemia, Down syndrome,)	– Imerslund-Gräsbeck syndrome; – Transcobalamin II gene mutation; – Orotic aciduria; – Lesch–Nyhan syndrome; – Myelodysplastic syndrome (refractory cytopenia in childhood, chromosome 7q deletion, etc.); – Aplastic anemia (Fanconi, Diamond-Blackfan) – Congenital dyserythropoietic anemia; – Other causes of B_9 and B_{12} deficiency; – Liver lesions of other origin; – Hypothyroidism due to other causes; – Medications intake

Table 5 Risk factors for venous thrombosis and thromboembolism [27]

Hereditary	Non-hereditary
• Hereditary resistance of factor V to protein C (Factor V Leiden); • Mutations of protein C, protein S, anti-thrombin, prothrombin (G20210A) genes	– Primary erythrocytosis (chronic myeloproliferative diseases); – Antiphospholipid syndrome; – Tumors (chronic DIC, Trousseau's syndrome); – Spinal cord injury; – Immobilization; – Nephrotic syndrome; – Paroxysmal nocturnal hemoglobinuria; – Medications intake (heparin-induced thrombocytopenia, thalidomide, estrogen-containing drugs, selective estrogen receptor modulators, recombinant erythropoietins)

diseases, atherosclerosis, atrial fibrillation and others predispose to arterial thrombus formation and systemic embolism [27].

5 Hemorrhagic Syndrome

In patients with cyanotic CHD secondary erythrocytosis contributes more to the development of hemorrhagic syndrome than thrombosis. Erythrocytosis is pathogenetically associated with the most common variant of hemostasis disorders in cyanotic CHD–thrombocytopenia. Increased blood viscosity impairs microcirculation and leads to excessive activation of platelets. This mechanism is presumably supplemented by the followings [40]:

- decrease in platelet production;
- impaired platelet pool replenishment;
- sequestration and a relative decrease in platelets count (see below).

Decrease in platelet production. Hypoxemia and circulatory hypoxia directly affect thrombopoiesis in the bone marrow. In the experiment, under the influence of these factors, the proliferation and maturation of megakaryocyte progenitor cells is inhibited as well as a decrease in platelet circulation time [41, 42]. It is possible that insufficient production of thrombopoietin in the liver also contributes due to ischemic lesions and venous congestion [40].

Impaired platelet pool replenishment. Venoarterial shunting leads to increased platelet destruction by the following mechanism. Megakaryocytes normally leave the bone marrow and their fragmentation occurs in the lungs. With venoarterial shunting, fragmentation of megakaryocytes occurs in systemic circulation (see «Hypertrophic osteoarthropathy»), which does not lead to replenishment of the circulating platelet pool [40, 43].

In addition, there is also impairment of the functional activity of platelets, which can be restored after surgical correction of cyanotic CHD [44, 45]. According to other data, platelet function is preserved, and coagulation disorders play a leading role in the development of hemorrhagic complications [46] (Table 6).

Apparently, impaired fibrinogen activation is also associated with erythrocytosis. Thus, in children with cyanotic CHD and Ht>54 with preoperative thromboelastography, a lower than normal maximum amplitude (MA) index is achieved (MA– reflects the best density and «quality» of clot before fibrinolysis and depends on the properties of platelets, fibrinogen and factor XIII). At the same time, the functional

Table 6 Causes and mechanisms of hemorrhagic syndrome development in patients with cyanotic CHD [27, 28, 50]

Pathogenetically related to the disease	Possible associated lesions
Vascular level	
• Increased tissue vascularization	– Hereditary hemorrhagic telangiectasia (HHT), (Osler–Weber–Rendu disease); – Anderson–Fabry disease; – Marfan syndrome, Ehlers-Danlos Syndrome, Loeys-Dietz Syndrome, etc.; – Vasculitis; – Drug-induced and endogenous hypercortisolism
Platelet level	
• Thrombocytopenia associated with erythrocytosis; • Platelet consumption in DIC syndrome (debatable); • Thrombocytopenia within liver lesions; • Thrombocytopathy (debatable); • Acquired von Willebrand syndrome (hypothyroidism, turbulent flow)	– Other thrombocytopenias and thrombocytopathies; – Von Willebrand disease; – Acquired Von Willebrand disease and similar conditions (hypothyroidism, aortic stenosis, paraproteinemia, myeloproliferative disorders, Wilms' tumor, medications intake)
Coagulation hemostasis	
• Fibrinogen dysfunction due to erythrocytosis; • Deficiency of factors II, V, VII, IX, X due to liver dysfunction and vitamin K deficiency; • Consumption coagulopathy in DIC syndrome (debatable); • Dysfibrinogenemia due to liver dysfunction	– Other causes of deficiency factors, including early (first 24 hours after birth, phenytoin, coumarins, rifampin phenytoin, coumarins, rifampicin and other medications intake by the patient's mother during pregnancy), classical (2–7 day, nutritional) and late vitamin K deficiency (cholestasis, malabsorption, prolonged antibiotic therapy); – Acquired inhibitors of coagulation; – Anticoagulation therapy

fibrinogen assay in the same patients shows a greater contribution of fibrinogen activation disorders (reduced MAfibrinogen index), but not thrombocytopathy (slightly reduced MAplt). The maximum amplitude, MAfibrinogen, MAplt were the lower, the higher the hematocrit. In the control group, in children with Ht<54, these indicators were close to normal before surgery [46].

In a study by Jensen et al., Ht level negatively correlated with platelet count, maximum amplitude and α-angle value (another indicator of clotting dynamics) during thromboelastography in patients with normal hepatic function. Correction of iron deficiency worsened the laboratory parameters of hypocoagulation. Such results illustrate a difficult situation, because iron deficiency and microcytosis are associated with serious complications and require treatment, possibly negatively affecting hemostasis [47]. However, it should be noted that some authors regard these results as laboratory artifacts. Arguments in favor of the «artifact point of view» and counterarguments to it are described in the literature [48, 49].

In patients with cyanotic CHD, there may also be a decrease in the level of blood clotting factors (Table 6), possible causes of which are liver dysfunction (hypoxia, hypoxemia and venous congestion) and vitamin K deficiency. Some patients show laboratory signs of increased fibrinolysis: increased D-dimers [28]. Most of the changes described above (thrombocytopenia, coagulation disorders and fibrinolysis) could be explained by the presence of non-overt disseminated intravascular coagulation (in the terminology of the International Society on Thrombosis and Haemostasis) induced by increased blood viscosity, but not all studies confirm this hypothesis [28].

The complex genesis of hemostasis disorders in cyanotic CHD requires dynamic assessment using thromboelastography (TEG) or Rotational Thromboelastometry (ROTEM) [28, 50].

Hemostasis disorders associated with perioperative stress and cardiopulmonary bypass are a particular problem. Severe blood loss, massive infusion therapy, acidosis (reduces the activity of vitamin K-dependent coagulation factors), hypothermia can contribute to the development of hemodilution-induced coagulopathy. The latter reversibly affects fibrinolysis, as well as the activity and relative number of platelets (induces hepatic sequestration) [50, 51]. Cardiopulmonary bypass contributes to hemostasis disorders due to non-pulsatile blood flow, exposure to perfusate components and blood contact with the «non-endothelial» surface of the contour of bypass itself, which leads to activation of plasma proteases (kinin-kallikrein system, coagulation system, fibrinolytic system, complement system). The mediators released in this case trigger inflammation, increase vascular permeability and damage the endothelium, activate platelets.

These processes lead to increased consumption of coagulation factors and platelets, the number of which decreases by 25–60% after the first passage of blood through the extracorporeal circuit of bypass, but rarely falls to a critical level (if initially normal). A decrease in platelet concentration to $20–100 \times 10^9$ or less (or more than 50%) should be alarming primarily in relation to heparin-induced thrombocytopenia type 2 (production of antibodies against heparin/platelet factor 4 (PF4), as well as other causes of thrombocytopenia.

Consumption coagulopathy and thrombocytopenia underlie the pathogenesis of hemorrhagic syndrome. Thrombocytopathy (due to mechanical action, the influence of adsorbed fibrinogen, loss of receptors, etc.) resolves relatively quickly and probably does not play a leading role [52].

6 Angiogenesis Disorders

Angiogenesis disorders play a key role in the pathogenesis of at least two pathophysiological manifestations of DORV:

- increased tissue vascularization and bleeding risk due to increased angiogenesis due to hypoxia, hypoxemia and HIF hyperactivation;
- remodeling of the heart due to local inhibition of angiogenesis and capillary rarefaction associated with a decrease in HIF activity.

Hypoxia, as mentioned above, leads to the stabilization of HIF, which stimulates the synthesis of proangiogenic molecules, the key of which is vascular-endothelial growth factor (VEGF). Some other HIF targets with proangiogenic properties include: platelet-derived growth factor (PDGF), interleukin-6, angiopoietins, angiopoietin receptors (Tie-2), cyclooxygenase-2, inducible NO synthase, chemokine CXCL12 (or SDF1), etc.

First of all, angiogenesis, unlike vasculogenesis, implies the development of vessels from already existing ones. Depending on the mechanism of development, sprouting and intussusception angiogenesis can be distinguished.

The onset of angiogenesis is preceded by an increase in the permeability of the vascular wall (due to the influence of NO, VEGF, angiopoietin-2), and degradation of the extracellular matrix (under the influence of matrix metalloproteinases and angiopoietin-2). This is followed by the process of proliferation and collective migration of endotheliocytes-sprouting angiogenesis (Fig. 4).

The tip cells have filopodia and move along the VEGF concentration gradient due to the VEGFR2 receptor. At the same time, they prevent neighboring cells moving behind them from acquiring the tip phenotype (by acting on their Notch receptor with the Dll4 membrane molecule). These cells, called «stalk cells», form the lumen of the future vessel. They synthesize membrane and soluble forms of the VEGF1 receptor, which performs the function of a VEGF «trap», and help apical cells acquire their phenotype (by acting on them with the Jagged1 molecule-another ligand of the Notch receptor). Thus, the first phase of germinal angiogenesis—tip/stalk differentiation—is completed.

The second phase (stabilization phase) is characterized by the involvement of mural cells (pericytes and vascular smooth muscles) and the synthesis of extracellular matrix. This phase is controlled by PDGFB (responsible for migration and proliferation of mural cells), TGF-β (suppresses proliferation of endotheliocytes, promotes differentiation of mural cells, formation of basal membrane),

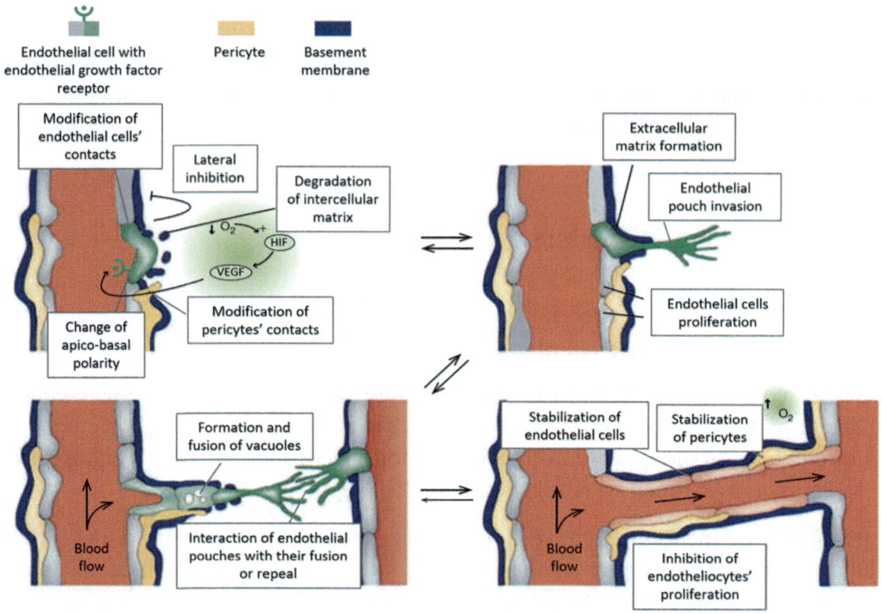

Fig. 4 Mechanism of germinal angiogenesis [adapted from [18]]. *HIF—hypoxia-induced factor; VEGF—vascular-endothelial growth factor*

angiopoietin-1 (strengthens intercellular contacts) and other molecules [53–56] (Fig. 5).

The next stage of angiogenesis is followed by arteriovenous differentiation, in which VEGF, its VEGFR2 receptor and neuropilins 1 and 2 coreceptors also play a leading role. If the signal from this receptor, which is «assisted» by neuropilin-1, is transmitted by the mitogen-activated protein kinases system, then the Dll4-Notch signaling pathway is activated and B2 ephrins appear on the cell surface. This is the axial sequence of events of arterial vessel formation. When acquiring a venous phenotype, the processes described above are inhibited, for example, by the COUP-TFII factor (chicken ovalbumin upstream promoter transcription factor II). Venous cells interact with arterial cells via the EphB4 receptor for ephrin B2. Ephrins and their receptors work in this and other cases when it is necessary to sort initially «mixed» cells at the border of compartments formed in this way (arterial and venous) [57, 58].

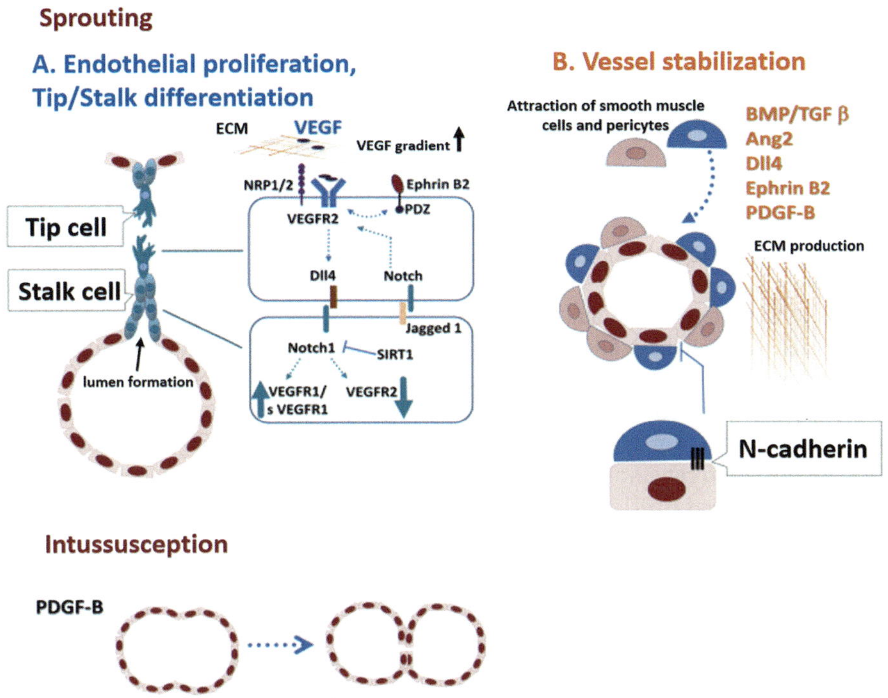

Fig. 5 Mechanisms and types of angiogenesis. *BMP—bone morphogenetic protein; Ang2—angiopoietin-2; NRP—neuropilins; SIRT1—sirtuin-1; ECM—extracellular matrix; PDGF—platelet-derived growth factor*

The pathogenesis of increased vascularization in cyanotic CHD is not completely clear [59]. For example, children with tetralogy of Fallot have high plasma levels of VEGF, CXCL12, of circulating endothelial progenitor cells and their functional activity (ability to migration, adhesion, proliferation) [60]. Other studies in children with CHD (including those with single ventricle physiology) also revealed a high concentration of proangiogenic molecules (CXCL12, VEGFR1), which, however, had a weak correlation with the severity of aortopulmonary collateral vessels [59, 61].

6.1 *Mechanisms of Vascular Rarefication*

In a healthy heart, each cardiomyocyte is separated from the endothelial cell of the microcirculatory bed by no more than 2–3 microns. With the progression of heart failure, the capillary density of the myocardium decreases—the so-called rarefication process. Rarefication is one of the main mechanisms of myocardial remodeling and the most important difference between pathological and physiological hypertrophy (see below). Vascular rarefication leads to increased ischemia and energy deficiency, cell death, fibrosis, an even greater drop in myocardial contractility and aggravation of circulatory hypoxia [62, 63].

The most studied and, perhaps, the main mechanism of rarefication is the inhibition of the function of HIF and the corresponding target proteins [62, 64], and therefore this aspect of myocardial remodeling will be considered in this section.

With an increase in the load on the heart and/or its damage, HIF and proangiogenic growth factors have mainly protective functions, the main of which is to stimulate angiogenesis and maintain normal blood supply sufficient for the increasing needs of hypertrophied myocardium. These same molecules, being growth factors, trigger the process of hypertrophy, which, with sufficient supply of oxygen and nutrients to the heart, is also likely to have adaptive significance. However, as heart failure progresses, the function of HIF and VEGF decreases, the main cause of which is considered to be the p53 protein [62, 64]. Stimuli for its synthesis are damage to the genetic apparatus of cells (e.g., free radicals or Ca^{2+}-dependent enzymes), hemodynamic stress, exposure to catecholamines and angiotensin II (which enhance the production of free radicals and overload cells with Ca^{2+} ions), as well as hypoxia [65, 66]. In hypoxia, HIF stimulates p53 protein synthesis. The relationship between these two transcription regulators is quite complex. Both mechanisms of mutual reinforcement and weakening of the function are known. On the other hand, HIF and p53 have many common targets, such as glucose transporter GLUT-1, cell cycle regulator protein p21, pro-apoptotic proteins Noxa and BAX. The p53 protein is known as the «guardian of the genome», since its main function is to recognize damage to the genetic apparatus by means of sensor proteins, as well as to stop the cell cycle (with the help of p21) at the G1 stage and start apoptosis [67, 68].

According to the Sermeus and Michiels model with moderate hypoxia, the effects of HIF-1α that promote cell survival prevail (among them, perhaps, proteasome-dependent and calpain-dependent degradation p53). With the aggravation of hypoxia due to an increase in concentration, the effects of p53 prevail, which competes with HIF for transcriptional coactivators (p300), inhibits HIF synthesis, causes its degradation and stimulates apoptosis. This scheme however does not take into account the combined effect of both factors [67, 68].

All new functions of the p53 protein as a key participant in the molecular mechanisms of myocardial remodeling are becoming known. Being a transcription regulator, it enhances inflammation (increases the synthesis of intercellular adhesion molecules ICAM-1), endothelial dysfunction (inhibits the production of NO, stimulates the production of endothelin-1), controls return to the fetal gene program by acting on the proteins PGC1α, PPARα, GATA4, Mef2a/d, Nkx-2.5, etc. [69, 70] (see below).

In addition to the suppression of the effects of HIF by p53 protein, a number of other mechanisms of vascular rarefication have been described, in particular: an increase in the production of anti-angiogenic factors (VEGFR1, some matricellular proteins, matricryptins and matrikines, endothelin-1, TGF-β, etc.), impaired signal transmission from growth factor receptors by phosphatase enzymes, the work of anti-angiogenic microRNAs, etc. [62]

Arterial hypoxemia negates the positive proangiogenic effects of HIF, VEGF, PDGF and other growth factors while maintaining their prohypertrophic and profibrogenic potential.

7 Hypertrophic Osteoarthropathy. Venoarterial Shunt and Failure of Non-respiratory Lung Functions

The pathogenesis of nail clubbing (Hippocratic fingers) symptoms in cyanotic CHD is not entirely clear, especially if we take into account their diverse etiology. The combination of these symptoms with ossifying periostitis and arthralgias is called hypertrophic osteoarthropathy (Marie-Bamberger syndrome). Hypertrophic osteoarthropathy may be hereditary (15-hydroxyprostaglandin dehydrogenase and SLCO2A1 transporter metabolizing prostaglandin E). In this case, there are also pachydermia (thickened, folded skin, especially in the forehead and scalp), enteropathy, etc. Paraneoplastic variants of pachydermoperiostosis are also known [71, 72]. Non-hereditary variants of osteoarthropathy are divided into localized (with hemiplegia, aneurysms, infectious arthritis, patent ductus arteriosus) and generalized. The latter can occur in various diseases of the lungs, heart, gastrointestinal tract, tumor growth and other diseases (HIV, thalassemia, thyroid acropachy, hyperparathyroidism) [71, 72].

Apparently, fibroblastic (FGF), PDGF and VEGF play a leading pathogenetic role in the development of osteoarthropathies in cyanotic CHD, which together with TGF-β, prostaglandins, bradykinin, serotonin, ferritin, etc., are synthesized in large quantities during inflammation (including autoimmune and peritumoral) and hypoxia (VEGF and PDGF are HIF targets, as mentioned above). These biologically active substances stimulate fibroblasts (connective tissue production), osteoclasts (acroosteolysis), osteoblasts (periostosis), angiogenesis, exudation.

The increased production of growth factors is complemented by their insufficient inactivation in the lungs due to venoarterial shunt, which can be observed in the following conditions [71, 72]:

- extrapulmonary bypass (CHDs with venoarterial shunting);
- intrapulmonary bypass at the level of large vessels (arteriovenous malformations);
- intrapulmonary bypass at the level of small vessels (lung diseases, systemic and splanchnic vasodilatation within liver diseases, hepatopulmonary syndrome, peritumoral angiogenesis).

In this case, the lungs cannot fully carry out their non-respiratory functions, which include megakaryocyte fragmentation, inactivation of prostaglandins, bradykinin, serotonin, ATP, CO and other biologically active substances.

According to the currently accepted hypothesis of Dickinson and Martin, it is megakaryocytes or their large fragments that reach systemic microcirculation and secrete PDGF and TGF-β (while the path from the heart to the fingers is shorter than to the feet, and the probability of fragmenting «along the way» is less) that play a crucial role in the pathogenesis of Hippocratic fingers (additional factors are probably necessary for the occurrence of other symptoms of hypertrophic osteoarthropathy). This assumption is supported by abnormal platelet morphology (macrothrombocytes, platelet distribution width), detection of megakaryocytes «stuck» in renal glomeruli, increased plasma concentration of von Willebrand factor antigen and other markers of endothelial and platelet hyperactivation in patients with cyanotic CHD [71–74].

Thus, venoarterial shunt compromises not only the respiratory functions of the lungs but also the non-respiratory function. At the same time, the nail clubbing symptom may be only the tip of the iceberg manifestation of this mechanism, which may play a role in the pathogenesis of target organ remodeling (PDGF- and TGF-β-dependent proliferation, inflammation, fibrosis), e.g., one of the two main types of glomerulopathy (non-vascular type) in patients with cyanotic CHD [75, 76]. Fragmentation of megakaryocytes in the systemic microcirculation (and not in the lungs) does not replenish the circulating pool of platelets and contributes to the pathogenesis of thrombocytopenia [43] (see above).

Another important non-respiratory function of the lungs is immune function. This includes the activity of alveolar macrophages. The blood flow shunting the pulmonary «filter», presumably, can contribute to bacteremia in the arterial system, which partly explains the increased risk of brain abscesses. This mechanism is complemented by a failure of microcirculation due to erythrocytosis and increased blood viscosity [30, 77].

References

1. Nedashkovski EV. Basic course of anesthesiologist. Arkhangelsk: North state medical university. 2010. 224 c.
2. Henig NR, Pierson DJ. Mechanisms of hypoxemia. Respir Care Clin N Am. 2000;6(4):501–21.
3. Langley R, Cunningham S. How should oxygen supplementation be guided by pulse oximetry in children: do we know the level? Front Pediatr. 2016;4:138.
4. Gutierrez JA., Theodorou AA. Oxygen delivery and oxygen consumption in pediatric critical care. In Pediatric critical care study guide. London: Springer; 2012. p. 19–38.
5. Vlasenko AV, Moroz VV, Yakovlev BN, Alekseev VG. Information content of oxygenation index when diagnosing acute respiratory distress syndrome. Intensive Care. 2009;5:54–62.
6. Elliott M, Tate R, Page K. Do clinicians know how to use pulse oximetry? A literature review and clinical implications. Aust Crit Care. 2006;19:139–44.
7. Sinha IP, Mayell SJ, Halfhide C. Pulse oximetry in children. Arch Dis Child-Educ Pract. 2014;99:117–8.
8. Ross PA, Newth CJ, Khemani RG. Accuracy of pulse oximetry in children. Pediatrics. 2014;133:22–9.
9. Hoffman JIE. False negative diagnoses of critical congenital heart disease with screening neonatal pulse oximetry. J Neonatal-Perinatal Med. 2019;13:1–5.
10. Schmitt HJ, Schuetz WH, Proeschel PA, Jaklin C. Accuracy of pulse oximetry in children with cyanotic congenital heart disease. J Cardiothorac Vasc Anesth. 1993;7:61–5.
11. Torres JA, Skender KM, Wohrley JD, Aldag JC, Raff GW, Bysani GK, Geiss DM. Pulse oximetry in children with congenital heart disease: effects of cardiopulmonary bypass and cyanosis. J Intensive Care Med. 2004;19:229–34.

12. Murphy D, Pak Y, Cleary JP. Pulse oximetry overestimates oxyhemoglobin in neonates with critical congenital heart disease. Neonatology. 2016;109:213–8.
13. Dennis M, Bowen WT., Cho L. Mechanisms of clinical signs (EPub3). Elsevier Health Sciences. 2016.
14. Barreto L., Amiel JB., Dugard A., Pichon N., Clavel M., François B., Vignon P. The rendu-osler-weber disease revealed by a refractory hypoxemia and severe cerebral fat embolism. Case Rep Crit Care. 2013:434965.
15. Zufall F., Munger SD. Chemosensory transduction: the detection of odors, tastes, and other chemostimuli. Academic Press. 2016.
16. Goodman LS, Hardman JG, Limbird LE. Goodman and gilman's the pharmacological basis of therapeutics. New York: McGraw-Hill; 2011.
17. Zipes DP., Libby P., Bonow RO., Mann DL, Tomaselli GF. Braunwald's heart disease e-book: a textbook of cardiovascular medicine. Elsevier Health Sciences. 2018.
18. Bockeria LA, Shatalov KV. Pediatric cardiac surgery. Moscow: Bakulev Scientific Center of Cardiovascular Surgery; 2016. p. 864.
19. Obacz J, Pastorekova S, Vojtesek B, Hrstka R. Cross-talk between HIF and p53 as mediators of molecular responses to physiological and genotoxic stresses. Mol Cancer. 2013;12:93.
20. Palazon A, Goldrath AW, Nizet V, Johnson RS. HIF transcription factors, inflammation, and immunity. Immunity. 2014;41:518–28.
21. Lee JW, Ko J, Ju C, Eltzschig HK. Hypoxia signaling in human diseases and therapeutic targets. Exp Mol Med. 2019;51:1–13.
22. Semenza GL. Pharmacologic targeting of hypoxia-inducible factors. Ann Rev Ppharmacology Toxicol. 2019;59:379–403.
23. Serocki M, Bartoszewska S, Janaszak-Jasiecka A, Ochocka RJ, Collawn JF, Bartoszewski R. MiRNAs regulate the HIF switch during hypoxia: a novel therapeutic target. Angiogenesis. 2018;21:183–202.
24. Soni S, Padwad YS. HIF-1 in cancer therapy: two-decade long story of a transcription factor. Acta Oncol. 2017;56:503–15.
25. Nam HJ, Baek SH. Epigenetic regulation of the hypoxic response. Curr Opin Physio. 2019;7:1–8.
26. Kumar V, Abbas AK, Fausto N, Aster JC. Robbins and Cotran pathologic basis of disease, professional edition e-book. Elsevier Health Sciences. 2014.
27. Hoffbrand AV, Higgs DR, Keeling DM, Mehta AB. Postgraduate haematology. Wiley; 2016.
28. Zabala LM, Guzzetta NA. Cyanotic congenital heart disease (CCHD): focus on hypoxemia, secondary erythrocytosis, and coagulation alterations. Pediatr Anesth. 2015;25:981–9.
29. Broberg CS, Jayaweera AR, Diller GP, Prasad SK, Thein SL, Bax BE, Burman J, Gatzoulis MA. Seeking optimal relation between oxygen saturation and hemoglobin concentration in adults with cyanosis from congenital heart disease. Am J Cardiol. 2011;107:595–9.
30. Gaeta SA, Ward C, Krasuski RA. Extra-cardiac manifestations of adult congenital heart disease. Trends Cardiovasc Med. 2016;26:627–36.
31. Planche V, Georgin-Lavialle S, Avillach P, Ranque B, Pavie J, Caruba T, Darnige L, Pouchot J. Etiologies and diagnostic work-up of extreme macrocytosis defined by an erythrocyte mean corpuscular volume over 130 fL: a study of 109 patients. Am J Hematol. 2014;89:665–6.
32. Green R, Dwyre DM. Evaluation of macrocytic anemias. Semin Hematol. 2015;52:279–86.
33. Saunders WB, Hoefer J, Streif W, Kilo J, Grimm M, Berger G, Velik-Salchner C. Surgery of a cyanotic heart defect in an 11-year-old boy with thrombocytopenic thrombocytopathy and severe anemia due to a GATA-1 defect: hemostatic therapy. Klin Padiatr. 2012;224:382–5.
34. Broberg CS. Challenges and management issues in adults with cyanotic congenital heart disease. Heart. 2016;102:720–5.
35. Ammash N, Warnes CA. Cerebrovascular events in adult patients with cyanotic congenital heart disease. J Am Coll Cardiol. 1996;28:768–72.
36. Heineke J, Kempf T, Bauersachs J. Inter-and intracellular mechanisms of cardiac remodeling, hypertrophy and dysfunction. In Heart failure. Cham: Springer; 2019. p. 39–56.

37. Kaemmerer H, Fratz S, Braun SL, Koelling K, Eicken A, Brodherr-Heberlein S, Pietrzik K, Hess J. Erythrocyte indexes, iron metabolism, and hyperhomocysteinemia in adults with cyanotic congenital cardiac disease. Am J Cardiol. 2004;94:825–8.
38. Nadeem O, Gui J, Ornstein DL. Prevalence of venous thromboembolisms in patients with secondary polycythemia. Clin Appl Thromb Hemost. 2013;19:363–6.
39. Perloff JK, Marelli AJ, Miner PD. Risk of stroke in adults with cyanotic congenital heart disease. Circulation. 1993;87:1954–9.
40. Patil S, Relan J, Hote M, Kothari SS. Severe thrombocytopenia in tetralogy of Fallot patients: a contraindication for corrective surgery? Ann Pediatr Cardiol. 2019;12:305–7.
41. Cullen WC, McDonald TP. Effects of isobaric hypoxia on murine medullary and splenic megakaryocytopoiesis. Exp Hematol. 1989;17:246–51.
42. McDonald TP, Cullen WC, Cottrell M, Clift R. Effects of hypoxia on the small acetylcholinesterase-positive megakaryocyte precursor in bone marrow of mice. Proc Soc Exp Biol Med. 1986;183:114–7.
43. Lill MC, Perloff JK, Child JS. Pathogenesis of thrombocytopenia in cyanotic congenital heart disease. Am J Cardiol. 2006;98:254–8.
44. Tempe DK, Virmani S. Coagulation abnormalities in patients with cyanotic congenital heart disease. J Cardiothorac Vasc Anesth. 2002;16:752–65.
45. Ekert H, Sheers M. Preoperative and postoperative platelet function in cyanotic congenital heart disease. Blood. 1976;55:216–23.
46. Cui Y, Hei F, Long C, Feng Z, Zhao J, Yan F, Liu J. Perioperative monitoring of thromboelastograph on blood protection and recovery for severely cyanotic patients undergoing complex cardiac surgery. Artif Organs. 2010;34:955–60.
47. Jensen AS, Johansson PI, Idorn L, Sørensen KE, Thilén U, Nagy E, Furenäs E, Søndergaard L. The haematocrit–an important factor causing impaired haemostasis in patients with cyanotic congenital heart disease. Int J Cardiol. 2013;167:1317–21.
48. Jensen AS, Johansson PI, Bochsen L, Idorn L, Sørensen KE, Thilén U, Nagy E, Furenäs E, Søndergaard L. Response letter to: "Hypocoagulable" thromboelastography profiles in patients with cyanotic congenital heart disease: Facts or technical artifacts? Int J Cardiol. 2013;168:4426.
49. Spiezia L, Campello E, Simioni P. "Hypocoagulable" thromboelastography profiles in patients with cyanotic congenital heart disease: facts or technical artifacts? Int J Cardiol. 2013;168:2914.
50. Zabolotskikh IB, Sinkov SV, Lebedinskii KM, Bulanov AY, Roytman EV. Perioperative care of patients with with abnormalities of hemostasis. Anesthesiol Intensive Care. 2018;1:58–81.
51. Yeh JT, Kavarana MN. Cardiopulmonary bypass and the coagulation system. Prog Pediatr Cardiol. 2005;21:87–115.
52. Averina TB. Cardio-pulmonary bypass. Ann Surg. 2013;2:5–12.
53. Hoffman JI. Normal and abnormal pulmonary arteriovenous shunting: occurrence and mechanisms. Cardiol Young. 2013;23:629–41.
54. De Smet F, Segura I, De Bock K, Hohensinner PJ, Carmeliet P. Mechanisms of vessel branching: filopodia on endothelial tip cells lead the way. Arterioscler Thromb Vasc Biol. 2009;29:639–49.
55. Herbert SP, Stainier DY. Molecular control of endothelial cell behaviour during blood vessel morphogenesis. Nat Rev Mol Cell Biol. 2011;12:551–64.
56. Carmeliet P, Jain RK. Molecular mechanisms and clinical applications of angiogenesis. Nature. 2011;473:298–307.
57. Fish JE, Wythe JD. The molecular regulation of arteriovenous specification and maintenance. Dev Dyn. 2015;244:391–409.
58. Kania A, Klein R. Mechanisms of ephrin–Eph signalling in development, physiology and disease. Nat Rev Mol Cell Biol. 2016;17:240–56.
59. Sandeep N, Uchida Y, Ratnayaka K, McCarter R, Hanumanthaiah S, Bangoura A, Zhao Z, Oliver-Danna J, Leatherbury L, Kanter J, Mukouyama YS. Characterizing the angiogenic activity of patients with single ventricle physiology and aortopulmonary collateral vessels. J Thorac Cardiovasc Surg. 2016;151:1126–35.

60. Liu ZL, Wu ZS, Hu JG, Yang YF, Chen Y, Gao H, Hu YR. Correlation of serum levels of VEGF and SDF-1 with the number and function of circulating EPCs in children with cyanotic congenital heart disease. Chin J Contemp Pediatr. 2009;11:267–72.
61. Ootaki Y, Yamaguchi M, Yoshimura N, Oka S, Yoshida M, Hasegawa T. Vascular endothelial growth factor in children with congenital heart disease. Ann Thorac Surg. 2003;75:1523–6.
62. Gogiraju R, Bochenek ML, Schäfer K. Angiogenic endothelial cell signaling in cardiac hypertrophy and heart failure. Front Cardiovasc Med. 2019;6:20.
63. Oldfield CJ, Duhamel TA, Dhalla NS. Mechanisms for the transition from physiological to pathological cardiac hypertrophy. Can J Physiol Pharmacol. 2020;98:74–84.
64. Oka T, Akazawa H, Naito AT, Komuro I. Angiogenesis and cardiac hypertrophy: maintenance of cardiac function and causative roles in heart failure. Circ Res. 2014;114:565–71.
65. Guan A, Gong H, Ye Y, Jia J, Zhang G, Li B, Ge J. Regulation of p53 by jagged1 contributes to angiotensin II-induced impairment of myocardial angiogenesis. PLoS ONE. 2013;8: e76529.
66. Yoshida Y, Shimizu I, Katsuumi G, Jiao S, Suda M, Hayashi Y, Minamino T. P53-Induced inflammation exacerbates cardiac dysfunction during pressure overload. J Mol Cell Cardiol. 2015;85:183–98.
67. Sermeus A, Michiels C. Reciprocal influence of the p53 and the hypoxic pathways. Cell Death Dis. 2011;2:e164–e164
68. Wang P, Guan D, Zhang XP, Liu F, Wang W. Modeling the regulation of p53 activation by HIF-1 upon hypoxia. FEBS Lett. 2019;593:2596–611.
69. Mak TW, Hauck L, Grothe D, Billia F. P53 regulates the cardiac transcriptome. Proc Natl Acad Sci. 2017;114:2331–6.
70. Kumar A, Kim CS, Hoffman TA, Naqvi A, DeRicco J, Jung SB, Lin Z, Jain MK, Irani K. P53 impairs endothelial function by transcriptionally repressing Kruppel-Like Factor 2. Arterioscler Thromb Vasc Biol. 2011;31:133–41.
71. Martinez-Lavin M. Hypertrophic osteoarthropathy. Best Pract Res Clin Rheumatol. 2020;34: 101507.
72. Dubrey S, Pal S, Singh S, Karagiannis G. Digital clubbing: forms, associations and pathophysiology. Br J Hosp Med. 2016;77:403–8.
73. Dickinson CJ, Martin JF. Megakaryocytes and platelet clumps as the cause of finger clubbing. The Lancet. 1987;330:1434–5.
74. Dickinson CJ. Etiology of clubbing and hypertrophic osteoarthropathy. Eur J Clin Invest. 1993;23:330–8.
75. Perloff JK, Latta H, Barsotti P. Pathogenesis of the glomerular abnormality in cyanotic congenital heart disease. Am J Cardiol. 2000;86:1198–204.
76. Morgan C, Al-Aklabi M, Guerra GG. Chronic kidney disease in congenital heart disease patients: a narrative review of evidence. Can J Kidney Health Dis. 2015;2:27.
77. Udayakumaran S, Onyia CU, Kumar RK. Forgotten? Not yet. Cardiogenic brain abscess in children: A case series–based review. World Neurosurg. 2017;107:124–129.

Myocardial Remodeling

A. K. Kade, P. P. Polyakov, S. A. Zanin, and Z. M. Dzhidzhikhiya

Abstract The presence of CHD influences on myocardial tissue through pressure and/or volume overload. Hemodynamic load along with arterial hypoxemia activate neurohumoral mechanisms which lead to pathological ventricular hypertrophy and partial or full adaptation. In turn, hypertrophy as a process of increase of myocardial mass as well as dilatation of cardiac chambers is responsible for myocardial remodeling. Though neurohumoral mechanisms serve for adaptative purpose, their hyperactivation has negative effects such as apoptosis, free radical damage and cytoplasmic calcium overload which are responsible for onset of fibrosis and eventually lead to heart failure.

Keywords Double-outlet right ventricle · Cyanotic congenital heart defects · Hypertrophy · Myocardial remodeling · Fibrosis

The term «remodeling», originally used to describe structural rearrangements of the heart—hypertrophy and dilatation, currently includes a wide range of changes at various morpho-functional levels (macrostructural, cellular, electrical), in particular [1]:

- hypertrophy and an increase in the mass of ventricular myocardium;
- change in the shape (dilation) and geometry of the ventricles (during systole, the ventricles take not an ellipsoid, but a spherical shape);
- replacement of a functioning myocardium with fibrous tissue;
- cardiomyocyte apoptosis;
- neurohormonal activation;
- development of systolic and diastolic myocardial dysfunction.

A. K. Kade · P. P. Polyakov (✉) · S. A. Zanin
Departement of Pathophisiology, Kuban State Medical University, Krasnodar, Russia
e-mail: palpal.p@yandex.ru

Z. M. Dzhidzhikhiya
Research Institute – Ochapovsky Regional Clinical Hospital №1, Krasnodar, Russia

K. V. Shatalov and K. M. Dzhidzhikhiya (eds.), *Double-Outlet Right Ventricle*,
https://doi.org/10.1007/978-3-031-49707-0_5

Myocardial remodeling is based on the process of its hypertrophy. In accordance with this, the classical stages of hypertrophy can describe the remodeling process itself [2]:

1. emergency stage—the impact of trigger factors;
2. the stage of completed hypertrophy and relatively stable hyperfunction is the reaction of the heart and the organism itself in the form of neurohormonal activation;
3. stage of exhaustion and fibrosis—development of fibrosis and heart failure.

1 Triggers of Myocardial Hypertrophy and Remodeling

The trigger factor for the development of hypertrophy in DORV is the load on the myocardium in the form of an excess volume of blood filling a ventricular chamber in diastole (preload), or excessive resistance to the cardiac output in systole (afterload).

Preload, or volume overload, is characterized by an increase in the filling of a ventricle in diastole, as a result of which its end-diastolic volume increases. Myocardial adaptation is provided by a heterometric mechanism (Frank–Starling phenomenon), i.e., increasing the size of sarcomeres. With this type of load, eccentric hypertrophy develops over time with thickening of the myocardial wall and an increased end-diastolic size of a ventricle.

An increased preload on the right ventricle in DORV occurs when there is pulmonary valve insufficiency after RVOT reconstruction. Increased preload on the left ventricle occurs in rare cases of aortic valve insufficiency in the long term after biventricular repair.

Afterload, or pressure overload, is characterized by an increased resistance to the output from a ventricle, which leads to increased stress to its walls. Myocardial adaptation to this type of overload is provided by a homeometric mechanism (Anrep phenomenon), i.e., an increased pressure of sarcomeres. In this case, concentric hypertrophy develops with thickening of the myocardial wall without increasing end-diastolic size of a ventricle.

An increase in the afterload of the right ventricle occurs in the presence of initial or residual (after correction) pulmonary artery stenosis, after pulmonary artery banding and in pulmonary hypertension. In addition, systemic systolic pressure from the left ventricle is directly transmitted to the right ventricle through VSD. For the left ventricle, an increased afterload may take place in restrictive nature of VSD, as well as initial or residual subaortic stenosis (obstruction of an intraventricular tunnel).

2 Mechanisms of Pathological Hypertrophy. The Role of Hemodynamic and Neurohumoral Factors

In DORV, pathological hypertrophy of ventricles is formed, which significantly differs from physiological one. The triggering factors of hypertrophy in DORV are severe hemodynamic overload of the heart chambers and arterial hypoxemia due to venoarterial shunt of blood (see Chap. 4).

2.1 *Primary Damage to Target Cells by Hemodynamic Overload*

Prolonged exposure to hemodynamic volume and pressure overload in DORV on the mechanosensitive structures of cardiomyocytes, vascular endothelium and endocardium, as well as fibroblasts, leads to a cascade of adverse intracellular events that cause the development of pathological hypertrophy and myocardial fibrosis [3, 4] (Fig. 1).

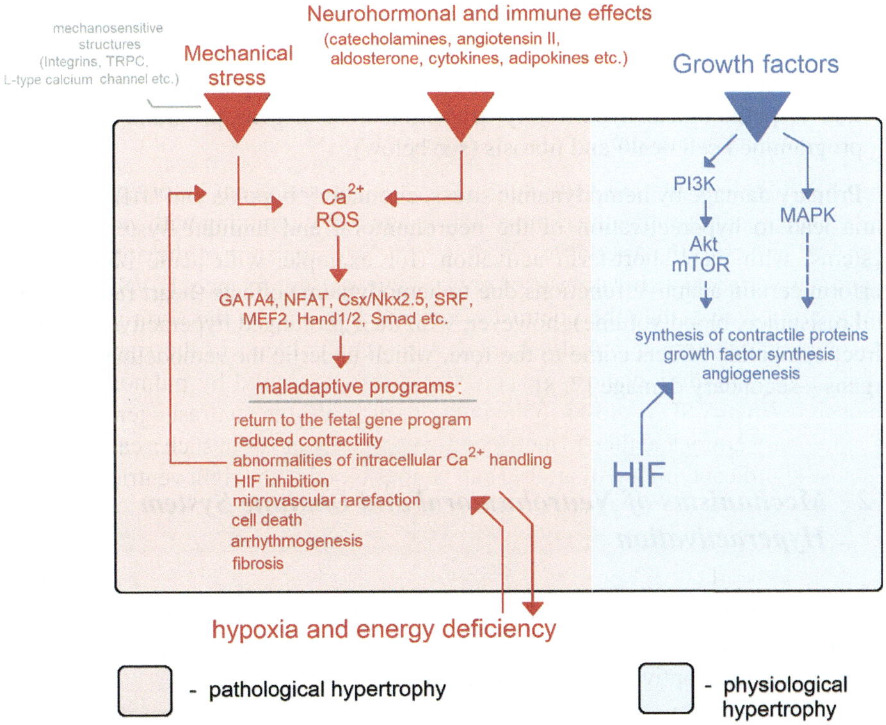

Fig. 1 Mechanisms of pathological hypertrophy and remodeling

Mechanosensitive Structures. The most important activated mechanosensitive cellular structures are as follows [4–6]:

- integrins on cell membranes that transmit a signal inside the cell using the enzyme focal adhesion kinase and other ways;
- cadherins as part of adherens junctions;
- dystroglycan complex;
- L-type calcium channels;
- cation channels TRPC, TRPM, TRPV, «letting in» Ca^{2+} inside the cell;
- STIM1 sensor molecule, store-operated calcium entry (SOCE) (activates with a lack of Ca^{2+} in sarcoplasmic reticulum);
- angiotensin (AT) II type 1 receptor (AT1R);
- intracellular proteins titin, LIM and others, coupled with contractile proteins and enzymes regulators of intracellular processes;
- extracellular matrix molecules.

A Cascade of Intracellular Events. The number and/or activity of mechanosensitive structures increases with chronic hemodynamic overload, which leads to:

- increase the cytoplasmic concentration of Ca^{2+} by elevated inflow into the cell (through L-type channels, TRPC, TRPV, TRPM) and exits from intracellular depot;
- increase the intracellular concentration of free radicals by enhancing activity of enzymes, for example, NADPH oxidases, producing superoxide radical;
- activation of intracellular signal transduction systems responsible for the formation of pathological hypertrophy, transition to fetal gene program, as well as programmed cell death and fibrosis (see below).

Primary damage by hemodynamic stress, circulatory hypoxia and arterial hypoxemia lead to hyperactivation of the neurohumoral and immune systems. These systems, with their short-term activation (for example, with acute blood loss), perform certain adaptive functions due to hemodynamic effects (heart rate, peripheral resistance, blood volume); however, with their prolonged hyperactivation, their direct cytopathic effects come to the fore, which underlie the remodeling of target organs—secondary damage [7, 8].

2.2 Mechanisms of Neurohumoral and Immune System Hyperactivation

Elevated hemodynamic stress and hypoxia cause hyperactivation of neurohumoral and immune systems, which, like hemodynamic overload, trigger intracellular programs of maladaptive hypertrophy and fibrosis.

Hypoxia and hypoxemia, for example, stimulate the chemoreceptors of the carotid sinuses and the aortic arch (see Chap. 4) and thus increase the activity of SNS and the concentration of its effector molecules: catecholamines and neuropeptide Y. Catecholamines stimulate the synthesis of prorenin and renin in the juxtaglomerular apparatus (through the stimulation of β1-adrenergic receptors), which hydrolyzes angiotensinogen to AT I. Angiotensin-converting enzyme, mainly in lungs, converts AT I to AT II—a component of renin–angiotensin system (RAS). AT II enhances the production of aldosterone by the activity of the enzymes StAR (transfers cholesterol to the mitochondria, providing the first stage of steroidogenesis) and aldosterone synthase (or CYP11B2) in the cells of the zona glomerulosa of the adrenal gland.

An important role is played by the activation of tissue RAS, for example, local renin production, enhanced uptake, expression of angiotensin-converting enzyme by cardiomyocytes, fibroblasts, endotheliocytes, conversion of angiotensinogen by cathepsin D, conversion of AT I by chymase, cathepsin G (mast cells), intracellular production of AT II (interacting with AT-receptor-like proteins, freely penetrating into the nucleus and inaccessible to existing medicines) [9–11].

Thus, the effect on target cells of catecholamines, AT II and aldosterone is enhanced.

Hemodynamic load on the endothelium leads to its dysfunction, which is manifested in the predominance of the following effects [12]:

- vasoconstrictor (production of endothelin-1, decline of NO production);
- proaggregant (exocytosis of Weibel–Palade bodies, von Willebrand factor, thromboxane A2, prostacyclin);
- procoagulant (tissue factor);
- antifibrinolytic (plasminogen activator inhibitor-1, TAFI—thrombin activatable fibrinolysis inhibitor);
- proinflammatory (adhesion molecules ICAM-1, VCAM-1, selectins, interleukins, chemokines);
- prooxidant (NADPH oxidases);
- mitogenic (vascular endothelial growth factor, fibroblast growth factor);
- profibrotic effects (TGF-β).

Secondary erythrocytosis is also a factor aggravating endothelial dysfunction and its consequences—pulmonary hypertension and remodeling of the heart. This is due to the binding and inactivation of NO by hemoglobin [13]. As a result, the effect of endothelin-1 and inflammatory mediators on blood vessels, heart and other target organs increases.

Hemodynamic load together with hypoxia also leads to activation and maintenance of the aseptic inflammatory process in several ways. Endothelial dysfunction includes endothelial production of cytokines, eicosanoids, platelet-activating factor, expression of adhesion molecules to which inflammatory cells «attach». Direct mechanical action on cardiomyocytes, fibroblasts, macrophages contributes to an increase in the number of non-specific receptors on their surface (scavenger receptors/CD36, toll-like receptors (TLR)), with the stimulation of which the inflammation process begins. The ligands for these receptors are endogenous molecules that are released from cells damaged due to mechanical stress and hypoxia. These molecules are called «damage-associated molecular patterns» (DAMP). Examples of such molecules are ATP (stimulates P2X7 receptors and potassium currents), chromatin-binding protein HMGB1 (stimulates TLR4), S100 proteins (stimulate TLR4, RAGE), mitochondrial DNA (unmethylated like bacterial, TLR9 is recognized), heat shock proteins (TLR2, 4), etc. Other important examples of DAMP are extracellular matrix molecules, (tenascin-C, biglycan, decorin, etc.). Hemodynamic load causes dysfunction of the extracellular matrix by directly transmitting mechanical stress or acting on the mechanosensitive molecules (see above) connecting cells to the extracellular matrix. Other ligands of non-specific receptors are exogenous microbial molecules called «pathogen-associated molecular pattern» (PAMP). Hypoxia contributes to an increase in their number in target organs, as it negatively affects the gut microbiome system—induces microbiome dysfunction and the movement of microbes, endotoxin and their waste products (trimethylamine N-oxide) into the bloodstream. Circulatory hypoxia and arterial hypoxemia also damage skeletal muscles, adipose tissue, spleen, which are the source of DAMP, proinflammatory monocytes (spleen), adipokines (adipose tissue). Stimulation of the above receptors by DAMP and PAMP molecules triggers early inflammatory events, for example, the assembly of a supramolecular complex called «inflammasome», which is involved in the synthesis of interleukin-1ß. Early inflammatory events (release of IL-1β, IL-6, TNFa, histamine) are followed by exudation, infiltration of tissue by immune cells, which synthesize even more inflammatory mediators [14–16].

As a result of the above-mentioned processes, the effect of cytokines on the damaged organ and the entire organism increases.

2.3 Adverse Effects of Neurohumoral and Immune System Activation

Hemodynamic load, hypoxia and hypoxemia contribute to an increased activity of catecholamines, prorenin, AT II, aldosterone, endothelin-1, cytokines, some adipokines (TNFa, IL-1β, IL-6, resistin, visfatin), whose effect on target organs (in particular, on the ventricular myocardium) is predominantly negative. On the contrary, natriuretic peptides (NP), apelin, CTRP (C1q/TNF-related proteins), CTRP-3, CTRP-6, CTRP-9, CTRP-15, omentin-1, some other adiponectins, NO, prostacyclin and counter-regulatory RAS (angiotensins 1-7, 1-9, alamandine, Mas receptors, MrgD) have rather an organoprotective effect. However, with cardiovascular diseases, their function may be reduced. For example, NP is inactivated when combined with «trap receptors», under the action of enzymes (for example, neprilysin), as well as during intracellular destruction of cGMP (a secondary messenger, which helps NP transmit information to protein kinase G and target molecules) by phosphodiesterase-5A and phosphodiesterase-9A [4, 17–19].

The specific effect of neurohumoral and immune system effector molecules is related to their distant (hormone-like), paracrine, autocrine and intracrine effects. The last three in the context of cardiovascular diseases play a more significant role, since it is these mechanisms that determine the direct cytopathic effect on target cells.

Distant effects. Some of the consequences of distant effects are as follows [9, 20]:

- increase in heart rate (β_1-adrenergic receptor inserted), peripheral resistance (α-adrenergic receptors, AT-1 receptor type), circulating blood volume, (mineralocorticoid receptors (MR));
- retention of Na^+ ions (AT receptors type 1 increase Na^+/H^+ exchanger loop of Henle, MR stimulate epithelial sodium channel (ENaC) of distal tubule), the loss of K^+ (MR stimulate the renal outer medullary potassium channel (ROMK)), chloride-resistant alkalosis (MR stimulate H^+-ATPase activity);
- secretion of antidiuretic hormone, adrenocorticotropic hormone (type 1 AT receptors);
- insulin resistance (type 1 AT receptors disrupt signal transmission from the insulin receptor);
- anemia of chronic disease (cytokines stimulate synthesis of hepcidin in liver, which disrupts the release of iron from storage).

Cytopathic Effects. Of the numerous cytopathic effects, the following most likely play a key role: 1) overload of cells with Ca^{2+}; 2) increased oxidative stress; 3) triggering apoptosis and activation of fibrosis (see below).

These processes are closely related to each other and, as mentioned above, are activated by hemodynamic stress (Fig. 1).

Calcium Overload. The mechanisms of cellular overload with Ca^{2+} when exposed to primary and secondary damaging factors include [9, 11, 21]:

- stimulation of Gq-coupled receptors (type 1 AT II receptor, α-adrenergic receptors, endothelin ETA receptors) increases inositol trisphosphate concentration in a cell, which stimulates the release of Ca^{2+} from sarcoplasmic reticulum;
- stimulation of Gs-coupled receptors (β1-adrenoreceptors, β2-adrenoreceptors; the latter "switches" to Gi during prolonged stimulation) increases intracellular concentration of cAMP, which activates protein kinase A, phosphorylates L-type calcium channels; β1-stimulation, however, enhances the reuptake of Ca^{2+} by the sarcoplasmic reticulum (with which positive lusitropic effect is associated), but this energy-dependent process is effective with sufficient oxygen supply;
- for the same reason, adrenergic desensitization in response to chronic catecholaminergic stimulation is related to decreased Ca^{2+} reuptake into the sarcoplasmic reticulum;
- in response to chronic exposure to catecholamines, it is associated with a decrease in the reverse transport of Ca^{2+} into sarcoplasmic reticulum;

- cAMP also activates EPAC-2 protein (exchange protein directly activated by cAMP), which stimulates the release of Ca^{2+} from sarcoplasmic reticulum;
- hypoxia and energy deficiency disrupt the functioning of Ca^{2+}-ATPase, which move Ca^{2+} ions into the extracellular environment, mitochondria, sarcoendoplasmic reticulum. Free radicals disrupt SERCA function by oxidative modifications;
- the effector molecules of the neurohumoral and immune systems launch transition to the fetal gene program (see below), one of the characteristics of which is inhibition of energy-dependent processes (energy saving in adverse conditions), including ATP-dependent transport of Ca^{2+} ions;
- Ca^{2+} ions, being second messengers, also trigger transition to the fetal gene program (Fig. 1).

As a result, the cytoplasmic concentration of Ca^{2+} ions increases due to its elevated inflow from extracellular space and intracellular depot. Cellular overload with Ca^{2+} entails a number of negative consequences:

- arrhythmogenesis, early afterdepolarization;
- Ca^{2+} ions, as secondary messengers, activate a number of enzymes (by binding directly, or with the help of calmodulins Ca^{2+}-binding proteins): calmodulin kinases, phosphatases (for example, calcineurin), proteases (for example, calpains). These enzymes, through phosphorylation (kinase), dephosphorylation (phosphatase) and proteolysis (protease), affect numerous transcription regulators (examples—NFAT, GATA4, MEF-2, SMAD, NF-KB), histone-modifying enzymes (histone deacetylases), histones themselves and other targets [22, 23]. As a result, transcription regulators NFAT, GATA4, MEF-2 trigger intracellular programs to return to the fetal phenotype, transcription factors SMAD activate fibrosis (see below), transcription factor NF-KB enhances cytokine synthesis and inflammation [24].

Ultimately, intracellular overload with Ca^{2+} can apoptosis or cause non-programmed cell death (manifested by necrosis at the tissue level). One of the mechanisms of launching of apoptosis is an increase in permeability of the mitochondrial membrane influenced by Ca^{2+}, release of cytochrome C into the cytoplasm, where it forms an apoptosome and activates proapoptotic enzymes (caspase-9 and caspase-3).

Non-programmed cell death during calcium overload is associated with activation of phospholipases (damage the plasma membrane and membrane organelles), proteases (damage integral membrane proteins, cytoskeleton), endonucleases (destroy nucleic acids, which is manifested by pyknosis, karyorrhexis and karyolysis) [3].

Oxidative Stress. Sources of reactive oxygen species (ROS) are as follows:

- in the mitochondria of the electron leak respiratory chain, the work of pyruvate decarboxylase complex, oxoglutarate dehydrogenase complex, glycerol-3-phosphate dehydrogenase, flavoprotein:ubiquinone oxidoreductase;
- peroxisomal β-oxidation;
- endoplasmic reticulum stress and unfolded protein response;

- microsomal oxidation;
- membrane-associated and cytoplasmic enzymes using oxygen, for example, NADPH oxidases, xanthine oxidases, cyclooxygenases;
- oxidation of the NO-synthase cofactor tetrahydrobiopterin (BH4) leads to the uncoupling of the enzyme, after which it produces a superoxide anion (O_2);
- non-enzymatic auto-oxidation of some molecules, for example, catecholamines to adrenochrome or oxymyoglobin to metmyoglobin with the formation of the same radical [21, 25–27].

These mechanisms are also closely related to each other. For example, radicals «produced» by NADPH oxidases induce mitochondrial dysfunction, endoplasmic reticulum stress (ROS-induced ROS release (RIRR)) and oxidize BH4 [27].

As a rule, the first of free radicals formed is a superoxide anion (except for some exceptions as the formation of a hydroxyl radical from water during water radiolysis), which by superoxide dismutase (SOD) is converted into hydrogen peroxide (H_2O_2). Unlike the superoxide anion, this molecule is stable, easily overcomes membranes by aquaporins. These properties allow it to perform the function of a secondary messenger by influencing SH-groups of redox-sensitive proteins. Fenton reaction occurs when hydroxyl radical is formed from H_2O_2 with the participation of iron or copper. In neutrophils, hydrogen peroxide myeloperoxidase is converted into hypochlorite (ClO^-). The superoxide anion and NO can form peroxynitrite ($ONOO^-$) [25].

When a heart is exposed to hemodynamic stress and neurohumoral factors, many of the above-mentioned mechanisms of ROS production are intensified. Thus, the activity of non-phagocytic NADPH oxidases and xanthine oxidase in cardiomyocytes, endothelium, fibroblasts and other cells increases by AT II (type 1 AT receptor), catecholamines (β2-adrenergic receptors), endothelin-1 (ETA receptors), cytokines (TNF receptor), PAMP and DAMP molecules (TLR, NLR, RLR receptors, etc.), aldosterone (nuclear receptor subfamily 3, group C, member 2, cell membrane-associated caveolin/striatin-associated MR, transactivation of type 1 AT receptor and growth factor receptors) [8, 15, 25, 28, 29].

Excessive amounts of free radicals contribute to the heart remodeling (as well as blood vessels, kidneys and other target organs) by the following mechanisms [7, 21, 23, 25]:

- activation of redox-sensitive signal transduction systems, for example, cascades of mitogen-activated protein kinase (ASK1, p38 MAPK, JNK), proinflammatory transcription factor NF-KB, etc.;
- damage to nucleic acids, resulting in the launch of complex processes of energy-dependent repair, induction of apoptosis with the participation of p53, including mitochondrial DNA;
- lipid peroxidation, leading to damage to the cytoplasmic membrane, mitochondria, endoplasmic reticulum and other structures;
- oxidative posttranslational protein modification (for example, SERCA exchangers, which leads to a weakening of Ca^{2+} reuptake into the sarcoplasmic reticulum);

- extracellular effects—activation of latent TGF-β, activation of matrix metalloproteinases, exposure of matricryptic sites (see below), etc.

The negative clinical consequences of the above-mentioned processes are as follows [23, 29–31]:

- overload of intracellular Ca^{2+} (because of the suppression of SERCA, Na^{+}/Ca^{2+}-exchangers);
- apoptosis: a) p53-dependent; b) associated with cytochrome C released from damaged mitochondria; c) associated with the effects of the enzyme p38 MAPK and JNK (including the stimulation of p53, inhibition of antiapoptotic proteins BCL-2 and BCL-XL); d) associated with endoplasmic reticulum stress, etc.;
- launching and propagation of fibrosis (hyperactivation of TGF-β, activation of fibroblasts);
- metabolic reprogramming (suppression of the proteins that regulate mitochondrial metabolism and biogenesis, for example, PGC1α);
- increased inflammation (damage to cells and extracellular matrix, release of DAMP, NF-KB-dependent synthesis of proinflammatory enzymes, cytokines);
- contractile dysfunction associated with the above-mentioned mechanisms—mitochondrial disorders, cell death, activation of p38 MAPK and JNK enzymes, impaired expression of functional proteins, fibrosis;
- severe irreversible damage to the cell, causing non-programmed death (at the tissue level manifested by necrosis).

2.4 Physiological and Pathological Hypertrophy. The Return to the Fetal Gene Program

The impact of primary (hemodynamic overload) and secondary (neurohumoral and immune) damaging factors on the heart contributes to the development of both pathological hypertrophy and subsequent remodeling of the myocardium. In addition to trigger factors, this type of hypertrophy in comparison with physiological one differs significantly.

In physiological hypertrophy, the ratio of end-diastolic diameter of a ventricle to wall thickness remains normal (proportional, adaptive dilatation), whereas in pathological hypertrophy this ratio is usually reduced—concentric hypertrophy, and then significantly increases at the terminal stage of compensation—maladaptive dilatation. In addition, pathological hypertrophy is accompanied by diastolic dysfunction and often heart failure with preserved ejection fraction, progression of hypoxia and energy deficiency, as well as further remodeling of the myocardium, fibrosis and ultimately the development of heart failure with reduced ejection fraction. The mentioned features of pathological hypertrophy determine its irreversible nature [7, 8].

The differences between the two types of hypertrophy and the mechanisms responsible for transformation from physiological to pathological hypertrophy are caused by launch of certain intracellular programs, i.e., activation of signal transduction systems, epigenetic, posttranscriptional, posttranslational modifications.

Intracellular programs implemented in physiological hypertrophy contribute to [32]:

- intensified angiogenesis and maintained capillary density adequate to the increased needs of cardiomyocytes, and other changes that increase energy supply of cells;
- optimization of energy consumption;
- cell proliferation and survival, which requires appropriate metabolic changes, control of apoptosis and autophagy;
- maintenance of contractile function of cardiomyocytes (for example, synthesis of contractile proteins, control of cytoplasmic concentration of Ca^{2+}, increased sensitivity to inotropic factors);
- inhibition of the negative effects of Ca^{2+} (for example, increased reuptake of Ca^{2+} into the sarcoplasmic reticulum);
- increased antioxidant potential of cells;
- adequate response to mechanical load;
- inhibition of processes observed in pathological hypertrophy (in many ways, the opposite of those listed above), including fibrosis, inflammation, cell death, β-adrenergic desensitization.

Sometimes, the main trend of molecular remodeling events is called the «return to the fetal gene program». This process, on the one hand, provides less energy consumption and therefore protects the cell from immediate death, but, on the other hand, makes it more vulnerable to long-term damage, for example, as some experiments show, it does not provide the phenomenon of preconditioning [33]. This duality is manifested by the hypofunction of the exchangers SERCA2a of the damaged heart, which helps to save energy, reduce contractility, but leads to an overload of the cytoplasm with Ca^{2+}. It is assumed that the transition to the fetal phenotype can prepare the heart for potential regeneration, which is preceded by dedifferentiation. However, under ongoing damage, the restoration of normal tissue does not occur [8].

The underlying changes in the expression of fetal genes and genes of the "adult" heart are regulated by transcription factors (GATA4, NFAT, Csx/Nkx2.5, SRF, MEF-2, Hand1/2, Smad, products of early response genes), prohypertrophic (microRNAs-21, −195, −199b, −208, −23, −499) and antihypertrophic microRNAs (−1, −133, −9), methyltransferases (G9a, SUV39H1), demethylases (Jumonji D1A, D2A, D2B), acetyltransferases (p300/CBP), deacetylases (I, IIa, III (sirtuins of sirtuins) classes, etc.), poly(ADP-ribose)-polymerase, chromatin remodeling complexes (SWI/SNF families), long non-coding RNAs (CHAER, CHAST, CHRF, H19, HOTAIR, MALAT1, MEG3, MHRT, etc.), etc. [24, 34, 35] Many of these transcription regulators, as mentioned above, are activated by Ca^{2+} and free radicals, which, in turn, transmit a signal from mechanosensitive structures, neurohumoral and immune effects (Fig. 1).

Such reprogramming has an impact on [8, 35, 36]:

- transdifferentiation of cells to myofibroblasts and fibrosis (expression of the transgelin-1 gene; see «Mechanisms of fibrosis»);
- structure of contractile apparatus (decrease in the α/β ratio of myosin heavy chain, change in isoform titin isoforms);
- HCN (hyperpolarization-activated cyclic nucleotide gated), normally expressed on pacemakers (HCN4), expression of T-type calcium channels;
- electromechanical coupling and control of intracellular Ca^{2+} concentration (T-type calcium channels, reduction of SERCA2/phospholamban ratio);
- arrhythmogenesis;
- reduction of contractility;
- humoral response to damage (ANP, BNP production); metabolism, etc.

Metabolic rearrangements of the damaged heart contribute to saving oxygen by using instead of fatty acids (105 ATP molecules from palmitic acid using 23 molecules, O_2 P/O = 2.3) substrates that are less "expensive" in this sense—glucose (31 ATP molecules from one glucose molecule using 6 O_2 molecules, P/O = 2.6), ketone bodies (P/O = 2.5), lactate utilization, branched-chain amino acid, strengthening anaplerotic reactions, etc. In other words, the Randle cycle is interrupted at the cardiomyocyte level (normally the heart captures fatty acids that inhibit glucose metabolism). The activity of key beta-oxidation regulators—intracellular receptors PPARα, ERRα and their coreceptor PGC1α (they are also the main regulators of mitochondrial functions)—decreases—the isoform composition of GLUT transporters changes: more GLUT-1 and 5 (fructose), less GLUT-4, and the activity of monocarboxylate transporters (MCT-1 and MCT-2) for capturing ketone bodies increases [37, 38].

However, these changes do not fully meet the energy needs. Glucose utilization under anaerobic conditions produces less ATP and decreases with the progression of the disease, and ketone bodies start to act relatively late, as some studies show. The biological activity of these substances and their metabolites also plays a positive or negative role: branched-chain amino acids aggravate mitochondrial dysfunction, leucine stimulates the mTOR signaling pathway, protein glycation (including transcription factors). β-Hydroxybutyrate inhibits lipolysis (via PUMA-G and GPR109A receptors), SNS activity (via GPR41 receptor), inflammasome assembly, inhibits class I histone deacetylase, oxidative stress, stimulates the synthesis of fibroblast growth factor-21 (cardioprotective effects) [37, 38]. Failure of ATP synthesis modifies the work of purinergic signaling (the release of ATP by pannexins, "transformation" into adenosine, interaction with receptors P1 (or A, four types), P2X (seven types), P2Y (eight types)), possibly having a cardioprotective function [37, 38].

It is these links of pathogenesis that remain the least accessible target of therapy so far, although neurohumoral inhibitors have pleiotropic and main metabolic effects (ranolazine and trimetazidine). Interestingly, the cardioprotective effect of sodium glucose co-transporter 2 (SGLT2) inhibitors may be associated not only with natriuresis, exposure to Na^+/H^+ exchangers, increased erythropoiesis, but also with hyperketonemia (increased glucagon/insulin ratio, stimulation of hepatic β-oxidation).

However, the protective effect of ketosis, not caused by SNS, remains a partially accepted hypothesis [38].

Thus, taking into account all the above, the molecular events of pathological hypertrophy and further remodeling can be described in a simplified way as follows: primary (hemodynamic) and secondary (neurohumoral and immune) damages contribute to an increase in the intracellular concentration of Ca^{2+} and free radicals, which, being second messengers, trigger the transition to the fetal gene program and other related maladaptive programs, including fibrosis.

3 Mechanisms of Fibrosis

Myocardial fibrosis is a morphological substrate of most severe heart diseases. It is found in children with «blue» heart defects, for example, by increasing the myocardial extracellular volume during MRI with cardiac magnetic resonance. At the same time, a feature of defects with insufficient filling of the left ventricle is a decrease in the mass of working cells. In arterial hypertension or aortic stenosis, on the contrary, there is a positive correlation between an increase in extracellular volume and the left ventricular mass index [39, 40].

Depending on the etiopathogenesis and localization, fibrosis variants can be divided into [40, 41]:

- reactive—connective tissue «between» working cells, the volume of which does not decrease at the initial stages. Develops in response to hemodynamic load, is critical for cardiomyocyte ischemia, hyperglycemia, in hypertrophic cardiomyopathy, sarcoidosis, chronic kidney disease or in the framework of degenerative changes during aging;
- replacement—after the death of cardiomyocytes (myocardial infarction, sarcoidosis, myocarditis, toxic/drug-induced damage, chronic kidney disease);
- infiltrative—amyloidosis, Anderson-Fabry disease and other infiltrative diseases;
- endomyocardial.

The main producers of excess connective tissue in the heart, as well as in other organs (in the liver with cirrhosis, in the kidneys with chronic diseases, in the gastrointestinal tract with inflammatory bowel disease) are myofibroblasts. These cells combine the properties of fibroblasts (for example, synthesis and secretion of certain markers: collagens of I and III types, periostin, fibronectin, tenascin-C) and smooth muscle alpha-actin (acta2, sma), transgelin (tagln, sm22). Myofibroblasts have an increased sensitivity to profibrogenic and proinflammatory mediators, including chemokines. In addition, they can produce many of mediators themselves (IL-1β, -6, -10, TNFa), mechanically affect the intercellular substance, for example, by means of fibronexus connecting the cytoskeleton with fibronectin, and developed focal adhesions [42]. When an organ is damaged, fibroblasts, epitheliocytes, pericytes, Ito cells, representatives of mononuclear phagocytes, bone marrow precursors and fibrocytes turn into myofibroblasts [41]. This transdifferentiation is the most important event of the «fibrosis program», which also includes hyperproduction of intercellular matrix components, violation of its degradation, changes in the function of leukocytes, epithelial cells, pericytes, cardiomyocytes and other cells.

The trigger factors that initiate the fibrosis program include:

- TGF-β, secreted by fibroblasts, macrophages, platelets, cardiomyocytes, vascular cells when exposed to mechanical overload, ATP II, aldosterone, cytokines;
- activation of already synthesized latent TGF-β bound to the extracellular matrix, which is produced by enzymes and free radicals;
- platelet growth factor-B (PDGFB), secreted by macrophages, platelets;
- hemodynamic overload, AT II and aldosterone. Cytokines also activate a number of mechanisms that are not directly related to TGF-β, among them increased synthesis of matricellular proteins (for example, connective tissue growth factor, CTGF or CCN2, tenascin-C), membrane proteoglycans (syndecans) lysyl oxidases, which have a profibrogenic effect.

As a result, there is excessive production of connective tissue by myofibroblasts, which replaces normal functional tissue, therefore, impairing the biomechanical properties of the heart, disrupting myocardial relaxation (diastolic dysfunction), reducing contractility (systolic dysfunction), aggravating circulatory hypoxia and also contributing to arrhythmogenesis (creating a morphological substrate for reentry arrhythmias) [43, 44].

References

1. Bockeria LA, Bockeria OL, Averina II. Electric remodeling in compensated hypertrophy of the heart. Annals of Arrythmol. 2010;3:5–15.
2. Meerson FZ. A mechanism of hypertrophy and wear of the myocardium. Am J Cardiol. 1965;15:755–60.
3. Kumar V, Abbas AK, Fausto N, Aster JC. Robbins and Cotran pathologic basis of disease, professional edition e-book. Elsevier Health Sciences; 2014.
4. Nakamura M, Sadoshima J. Mechanisms of physiological and pathological cardiac hypertrophy. Nat Rev Cardiol. 2018;15:387–407.
5. Lyon RC, Zanella F, Omens JH, Sheikh F. Mechanotransduction in cardiac hypertrophy and failure. Circ Res. 2015;116:1462–76.
6. Saucerman JJ, Tan PM, Buchholz KS, McCulloch AD, Omens JH. Mechanical regulation of gene expression in cardiac myocytes and fibroblasts. Nat Rev Cardiol. 2019;16:361–78.
7. Oldfield CJ, Duhamel TA, Dhalla NS. Mechanisms for the transition from physiological to pathological cardiac hypertrophy. Can J Physiol Pharmacol. 2020;98:74–84.
8. Cokkinos DV. Cardiac hypertrophy. Myocardial Preservation, Cham:Springer;2019. p. 63–86.
9. Forrester SJ, Booz GW, Sigmund CD, Coffman TM, Kawai T, Rizzo V, Scalia R, Eguchi S. Angiotensin II signal transduction: an update on mechanisms of physiology and pathophysiology. Physiol Rev. 2018;98:1627–738.
10. Lymperopoulos A, Rengo G, Zincarelli C, Kim J, Soltys S, Koch WJ. An adrenal β-arrestin 1-mediated signaling pathway underlies angiotensin II-induced aldosterone production in vitro and in vivo. Proc Natl Acad Sci. 2009;106:5825–30.
11. Franzoso M, Zaglia T, Mongillo M. Putting together the clues of the everlasting neuro-cardiac liaison. Biochimica et Biophysica Acta (BBA)-Molecul Cell Res. 2016;1863:1904–1915.

12. Vasina LV, Petrischev NN, Vlasov TD. Endothelial dysfunction and its main markers. Reg Circul Microcircul. 2017;16:4–15.
13. Cordina RL, Celermajer DS. Chronic cyanosis and vascular function: implications for patients with cyanotic congenital heart disease. Cardiol Young. 2010;20:242–53.
14. Zhang Y, Bauersachs J, Langer HF. Immune mechanisms in heart failure. Eur J Heart Fail. 2017;19:1379–89.
15. Murphy SP, Kakkar R, McCarthy CP, Januzzi JL Jr. Inflammation in heart failure: JACC state-of-the-art review. J Am Coll Cardiol. 2020;75:1324–40.
16. Van Linthout S, Tschöpe C. Inflammation–cause or consequence of heart failure or both? Curr Heart Fail Rep. 2017;14:251–65.
17. Paz OM, Riquelme JA, García L, Jalil JE, Chiong M, Santos RA, Lavandero S. Counter-regulatory renin–angiotensin system in cardiovascular disease. Nat Rev Cardiol. 2019;17:116–29.
18. Rubattu S, Volpe M. Natriuretic peptides in the cardiovascular system: multifaceted roles in physiology, pathology and therapeutics. Int J Mol Sci. 2019;20:3991.
19. Lau WB, Ohashi K, Wang Y, Ogawa H, Murohara T, Ma XL, Ouchi N. Role of adipokines in cardiovascular disease. Circ J. 2017;81:920–8.
20. Sztechman D, Czarzasta K, Cudnoch-Jedrzejewska A, Szczepanska-Sadowska E, Zera T. Aldosterone and mineralocorticoid receptors in regulation of the cardiovascular system and pathological remodelling of the heart and arteries. J Physiol Pharmacol. 2018;69:829–45.
21. Mann DL. Heart failure: a companion to Braunwald's heart disease E-book. Elsevier Health Sciences; 2010.
22. Bockeria LA, Glushko LA. Mechanisms of arrythmias. Annals of Arrythmol. 2010;7:69–79.
23. Silva JV, Freitas MJ, Fardilha M. Tissue-specific cell signaling. Springer Nature; 2020.
24. Dirkx E, da Costa Martins PA, De Windt LJ. Regulation of fetal gene expression in heart failure. Biochimica et Biophysica Acta (BBA)-Molecul Basis of Disease. 2013;12:2414–2424.
25. McCance KL, Huether SE. Pathophysiology-E-book: the biologic basis for disease in adults and children. Elsevier Health Sciences; 2018.
26. Holmström KM, Finkel T. Cellular mechanisms and physiological consequences of redox-dependent signalling. Nat Rev Mol Cell Biol. 2014;15:411–21.
27. Brito R, Castillo G, Gonzalez J, Valls N, Rodrigo R. Oxidative stress in hypertension: mechanisms and therapeutic opportunities. Exp Clin Endocrinol Diabetes. 2015;123:325–35.
28. Di Lisa F, Kaludercic N, Paolocci N. β2 Adrenoceptors, NADPH oxidase, ROS and p38 MAPK: another 'radical'road to heart failure? Br J Pharmacol. 2011;162:1009–11.
29. Touyz RM, Rios FJ, Alves-Lopes R, Neves KB, Camargo LL, Montezano AC. Oxidative stress—a unifying paradigm in hypertension. Can J Cardiol. 2020;36:659–70.
30. Turner NA, Blythe NM. Cardiac fibroblast p38 MAPK: a critical regulator of myocardial remodeling. J Cardiovascular Developm Disease. 2019;6:27.
31. Chen W, Frangogiannis NG. Fibroblasts in post-infarction inflammation and cardiac repair. Biochimica et Biophysica Acta (BBA)-Molecul Cell Res. 2013;4:945–953.
32. Schirone L, Forte M, Palmerio S, Yee D, Nocella C, Angelini F, Pagano F, Schiavon S, Bordin A, Carrizzo A, Vecchione C, Valenti V, Chimenti I, De Falco E, Sciarretta S, Frati GA. Review of the molecular mechanisms underlying the development and progression of cardiac remodeling. Oxid Med Cell Longev. 2017;2017:3920195.
33. Cokkinos DV, Pantos C. Myocardial remodeling, an overview. Heart Fail Rev. 2011;16:1–4.
34. Hobuß L, Bär C, Thum T. Long non-coding RNAs: at the heart of cardiac dysfunction? Frontiers in Fhysiol. 2019;10:30.
35. Nandi SS, Mishra PK. Harnessing fetal and adult genetic reprograming for therapy of heart disease. J Nat Sci. 2015;1: e71.
36. Aubert G, Vega RB, Kelly DP. Perturbations in the gene regulatory pathways controlling mitochondrial energy production in the failing heart. Biochimica Et Biophysica Acta (BBA)-Molecular Cell Res. 2013;4:840–847.
37. Taegtmeyer H, Sen S, Vela D. Return to the fetal gene program: a suggested metabolic link to gene expression in the heart. Ann NY Acad Sci. 2010;1188:191–8.

38. Selvaraj S, Kelly DP, Margulies KB. Implications of altered Ketone metabolism and therapeutic ketosis in heart failure. Circulation. 2020;141:1800–12.
39. Andrade AC, Jerosch-Herold M, Wegner P, Gabbert DD, Voges I, Pham M, Shah R, Hedderich J, Kramer HH, Rickers C. Determinants of left ventricular dysfunction and remodeling in patients with corrected tetralogy of Fallot. J Am Heart Assoc. 2019;8: e009618.
40. Tian J, An X, Niu L. Myocardial fibrosis in congenital and pediatric heart disease. Exp Ther Med. 2017;13:1660–4.
41. Liu T, Song D, Dong J, Zhu P, Liu J, Liu W, Ma X, Zhao L, Ling S. Current understanding of the pathophysiology of myocardial fibrosis and its quantitative assessment in heart failure. Front Physiol. 2017;8:238.
42. Fan D, Takawale A, Lee J, Kassiri Z. Cardiac fibroblasts, fibrosis and extracellular matrix remodeling in heart disease. Fibrogenesis and Tissue Repair. 2012;5:15.
43. Frangogiannis NG. Cardiac fibrosis: cell biological mechanisms, molecular pathways and therapeutic opportunities. Mol Aspects Med. 2019;65:70–99.
44. Nguyen MN, Kiriazis H, Gao XM, Du XJ. Cardiac fibrosis and arrhythmogenesis. Comprehens Physiol. 2017;7:1009–49.

Diagnostics

Echocardiography

I. Y. Baryshnikova

Abstract Echocardiography is a first-line diagnostic tool both for preoperative assessment of DORV anatomy and postoperative complications. The main goal of preoperative echocardiography in DORV is to evaluate VSD type, the presence of pulmonary artery stenosis and its nature, mitral–aortic continuity as well as relationship and course of the arterial trunks and associated cardiac anomalies. Evolving echocardiographic techniques such as speckle tracking method allows to obtain volumetric heart models and assess local abnormalities of myocardial performance, respectively. The great limitation of echocardiography is its subjectivity and low effectiveness in evaluation of extracardiac components of the disease. Overall, echocardiography is able to provide pivotal parameters for accurate surgical planning.

Keywords Double-outlet right ventricle · Diagnostics · Echocardiography

DORV is a complex conotruncal anomaly with a wide range of anatomical varieties. The difficulties of diagnosis of DORV on echocardiography (echo) arise already at the prenatal stage. In most fetuses, a conotruncal anomaly can be suspected as early as 11–14 weeks of gestation by echo, but it is difficult to distinguish whether a defect is tetralogy of Fallot or DORV, on the one hand, and TGA or DORV «TGA» type, on the other hand. This is not only due to the limited visualization of a fetal heart, but also due to the lack of universal echo criteria for DORV. As a rule, four-chamber view at the end of the first and second trimesters is visualized without any particularities; however, in five-chamber view, VSD and origin of the arterial trunks from the anterior chamber (right ventricle) are clearly visible [1, 2]. In postnatal period, echo can provide almost complete information for surgical planning [3].

Echo examination of DORV as well as all CHD should be performed in accordance with segmental approach with evaluation of each segmental level of a heart. Diagnosis of DORV by echo in some cases may be very complicated. Often, sonographers and

I. Y. Baryshnikova (✉)
Department of Ultrasound Investigations, A. N. Bakulev National Medical Investigation Center for Cardiovascular Surgery, Moscow, Russia
e-mail: jatropha@mail.ru

K. V. Shatalov and K. M. Dzhidzhikhiya (eds.), *Double-Outlet Right Ventricle*,
https://doi.org/10.1007/978-3-031-49707-0_6

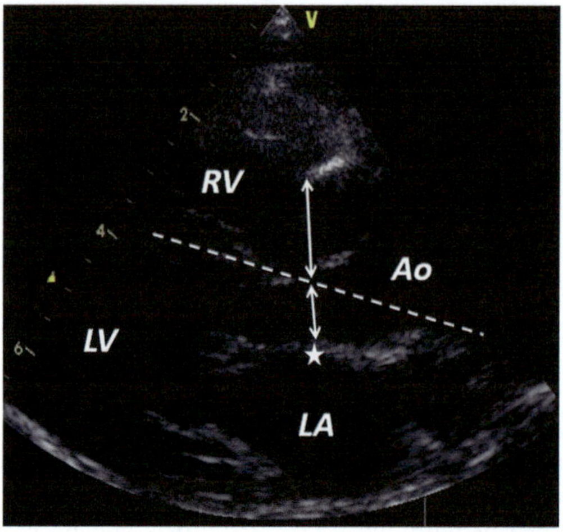

Fig. 1 The aorta more than 50% takes origin from the right ventricle (left parasternal long-axis view). The asterisk indicates mitral–aortic continuity. *Ao—aorta; RV—right ventricle; LV—left ventricle; LA—left atrium*

surgeons cannot come to an agreement regarding the degree of origin of the arterial trunks from the ventricles since this parameter is highly subjective and may be interpreted ambiguously depending on the plane of the ultrasound beam and cardiac phase. For example, from subxiphoid long-axis view aortic origin can be projected mainly from the right ventricle, whereas from the left parasternal long-axis view aorta predominantly origins from the left ventricle.

Some specialists in order to simplify the diagnostic of DORV consider the absence of mitral–aortic fibrous continuity as a direct sign of DORV. However, this approach can lead to an incorrect classification of ventriculoarterial connections, for example, when the aorta takes origin predominantly from the left ventricle and there is mitral–aortic muscular continuity (see "Transitional anatomical forms of DORV" in the Chap. 2). In this regard, many specialists use the "50% rule" for determining DORV when both aorta and pulmonary artery predominantly originate from the right ventricle (Fig. 1).

1 Preoperative Investigation

For correct preoperative surgical decision-making, echo protocol should include assessment of the following anatomical structures:

- VSD;
- morphology of mitral–aortic continuity;
- relationship and course of the arterial trunks;
- pulmonary artery stenosis;
- coronary artery anatomy;
- associated cardiac abnormalities.

1.1 VSD

Standard echo is a method of two-dimensional visualization. Sonographers virtually construct in a head a three-dimensional image of a whole heart based on the set of two-dimensional projections obtained during the investigation. By means of 3D echo, it is possible to obtain volumetric nonstandard cuts and provide additional information for careful surgical planning [4].

VSD location in DORV is determined depending on the projection obtained. On apical or subxiphoid four-chamber view, the inlet part of IVS is visualized (Fig. 2A), which helps in diagnosing non-committed VSD. In turn, to diagnose conoventricular VSD, the visualization of the outlet part of IVS is obtained by apical five-chamber or subxiphoid view, left parasternal long-axis view, or along the long axis of the right ventricle from the subxiphoid long-axis view (Fig. 2B–C).

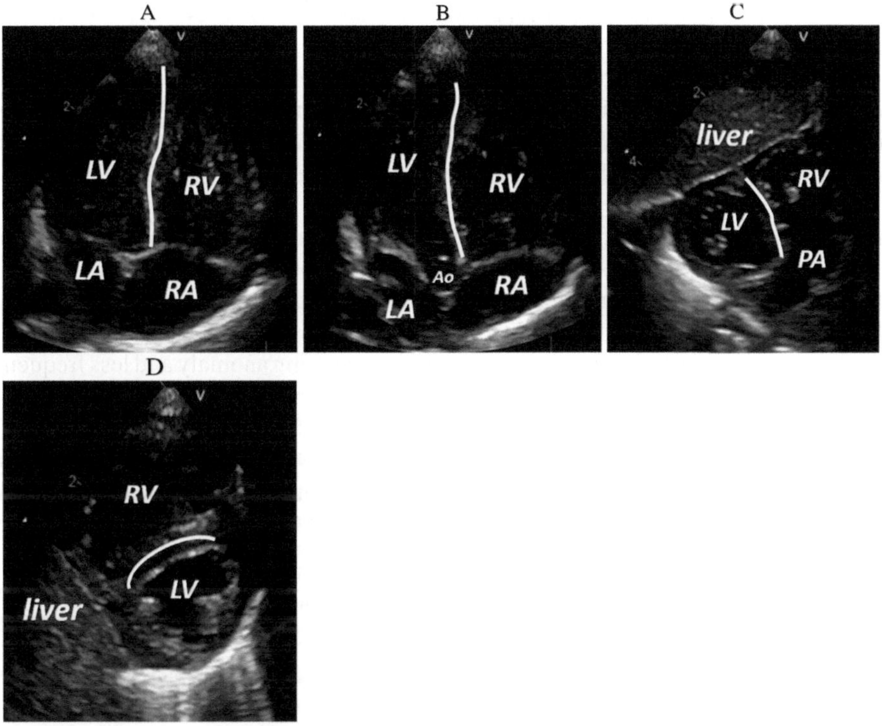

Fig. 2 Echo visualization of different parts of the IVS: **A**—four-chamber apical view. The line indicates the inlet part of IVS; **B**—five-chamber apical view. The line indicates the outlet IVS; **C**—subxiphoid short-axis view, cross section of the RVOT. The line indicates the outlet IVS; **D**—subxiphoid short-axis view, cross section at the level of the papillary muscles. The line indicates the IVS. *Ao—aorta; PA—pulmonary artery; RV—right ventricle; LV—left ventricle; RA—right atrium; LA—left atrium*

On echo cuts along the short axis of the left ventricle, the transverse size of VSD and its extension toward the basal, middle and apical segments are estimated (Fig. 2D).

When assessing conoventricular VSD from left parasternal short-axis view at the level of the aortic valve, the distance between the tricuspid and pulmonary valves is virtually divided into three equal parts. A tissue defect or blood shunting in the area of the nearest third to the tricuspid valve corresponds to the location of VSD in subaortic area. Similarly, when the same signs are detected in the middle or the closest third to the pulmonary valve, then subarterial and subpulmonary VSDs are determined, respectively. The projections for assessment different types of VSD in DORV are presented in Table 1.

In case of subaortic VSD, the area of potential tunneling is well visualized from subxiphoid view. It is important to determine the distance from the edge of VSD to the most distant point of the aortic valve as well as the risk of tunnel obstruction in case of prominent VIF which is typical for DORV with not directly committed subaortic VSD. Left parasternal long-axis view also allows to assess proximity of VSD to the arterial trunks.

In some cases, subaortic VSD is restrictive which may lead to subaortic obstruction after tunnel construction (Fig. 3E). To solve this problem, a ratio of VSD size to the aortic diameter has been proposed which if less than 4/5 indicates restrictive nature of VSD [5, 6].

There are also extremely rare forms of DORV with intact IVS characterized by hypoplasia of the left ventricle with the mitral valve atresia/hypoplasia [7]. In such cases, it is important to assess the presence and size of interatrial communication, intensity of left-to-right shunting and pressure gradient since the communication is the only outflow for the pulmonary veins.

Table 1 Echo projections for assessment of different types of VSD

<table>
<tr><th>VSD type</th><th>Description</th><th>Echo projection</th></tr>
<tr><td>Subaortic</td><td>Closer to the aortic valve (Fig. 3A)</td><td rowspan="3">– Left parasternal long-axis view and left parasternal short-axis view at the level of aortic valve
– Apical five-chamber view
– Subxiphoid long-axis and short-axis views</td></tr>
<tr><td>Subpulmonary</td><td>Closer to the pulmonary valve (Fig. 3B)</td></tr>
<tr><td>Subarterial</td><td>Usually very large and closely related to both arterial valves (Fig. 3C)</td></tr>
<tr><td>Noncommitted</td><td>Locates in the inlet IVS and is not related to either arterial valves (Fig. 3D)</td><td rowspan="2">– Left parasternal long-axis view
– Apical five-chamber view
– Individual views</td></tr>
<tr><td>Multiple VSDs</td><td>Multiple VSDs of various locations</td></tr>
</table>

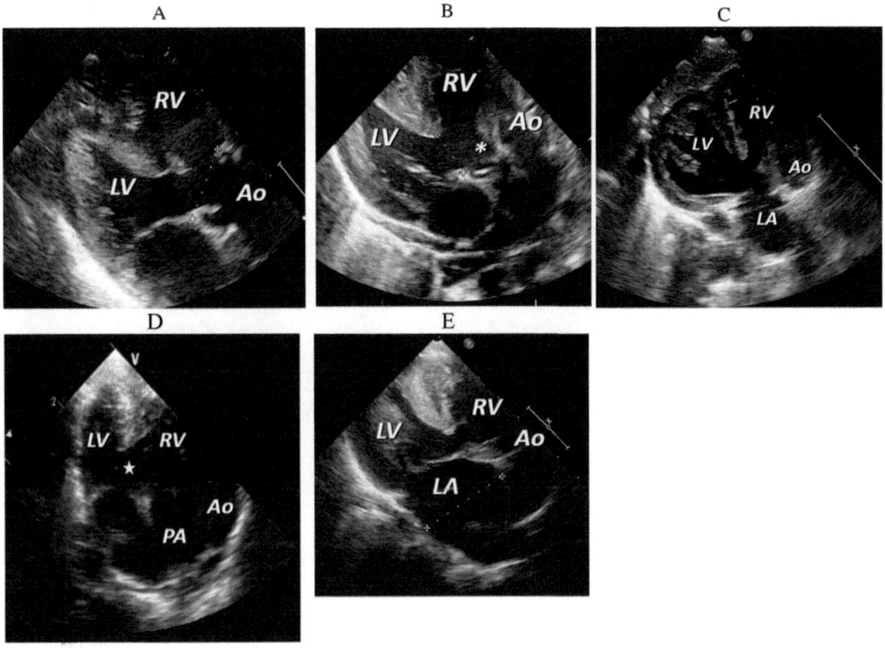

Fig. 3 Echo view of different types of VSD in DORV: **A**—subaortic VSD (left parasternal long-axis view). Despite mitral–aortic fibrous continuity, the aorta predominantly originates from the right ventricle; **B**—subpulmonary VSD (apical view, individual projection for visualization of the arterial trunks). The pulmonary artery (indicated by an asterisk) overrides the IVS; entrance to the aortic valve is separated from VSD by the OS; **C**—subarterial VSD (subxiphoid view, individual projection for visualization of the arterial trunks). In the plane of VSD both arterial valves are visualized; **D**—non-committed VSD located in the inlet IVS (apical view, individual projection for visualization of the arterial trunks); **E**—restrictive subaortic VSD (left parasternal long-axis view). *Ao—aorta; PA—pulmonary artery; RV—right ventricle; LV—left ventricle; LA—left atrium*

1.2 Morphology of Mitral–Aortic Continuity

The absence of mitral–aortic fibrous continuity is an important but not mandatory sign of DORV (according to the «50%» rule). The nature of mitral–aortic continuity can be easily visualized in left parasternal long-axis view (Fig. 3A).

1.3 Relationship and Course of the Arterial Trunks

The arterial trunks can have spiral course with the pulmonary artery twisting around the aorta (as it is in the normal heart) or parallel course (Fig. 4). Parallel course is visualized in LVOT view from the subxiphoid short-axis or left parasternal projections.

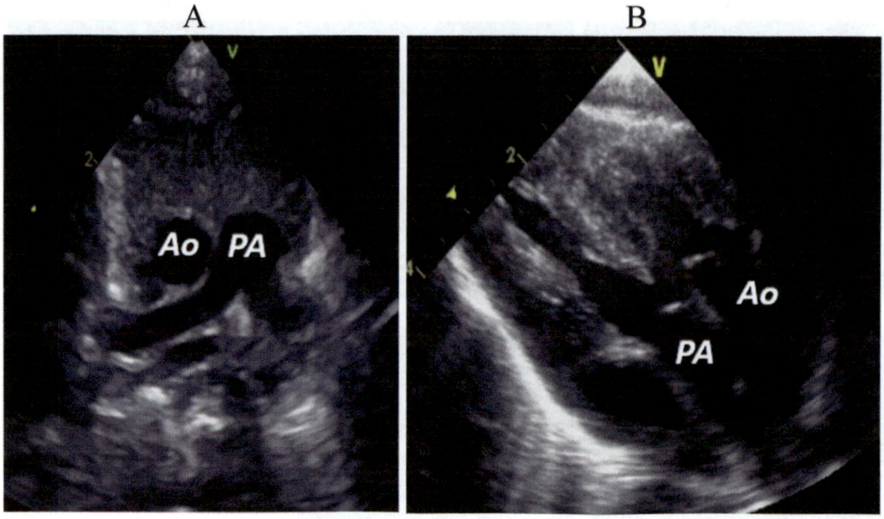

Fig. 4 Course of the arterial trunks in DORV: **A**—spiral course (normal). At the same echo projection, different planes of the arterial trunks are visualized: transverse axis of the ascending aorta and longitudinal axis of the pulmonary artery. This indicates a twisting of the trunks (left parasternal short-axis view with visualization of the pulmonary artery bifurcation); **B**—parallel course (Taussig-Bing anomaly). Longitudinal axes of both arterial trunks is visualized at the same projection; subpulmonary VSD is determined (subxiphoid long-axis view). *Ao—aorta; PA—pulmonary artery*

Relationship of the arterial valves is assessed in parasternal short-axis view at the level of the arterial valves (Fig. 5). To distinguish arterial trunks, it is necessary to visualize pulmonary artery bifurcation or coronary arteries ostia.

1.4 Pulmonary Artery Stenosis

Pulmonary artery stenosis is generally encountered in "tetralogy" type of DORV. It is preferable to assess pulmonary artery and RVOT obstruction from left parasternal or subxiphoid short-axis views at the level of the aortic valve or RVOT which allow to clearly visualize the level of obstruction and its morphological substrate. Thus, the cause of infundibular stenosis may be anterolateral deviation (to the right on echo) of the OS which in addition may be hypertrophied (Fig. 6) or anomalous muscle in the right ventricle (including the so-called double-chambered right ventricle).

The pulmonary valve is assessed mainly regarding morphology of the leaflets (thickening, fusion, quantity) and fibrous annulus diameter. Hypoplasia of the annulus, trunk and branches is evaluated according to the standardized Z-score scale. The values less than -2 are considered as hypoplasia. A thorough assessment of the anatomy and hemodynamics of the exit from the right ventricle is important for

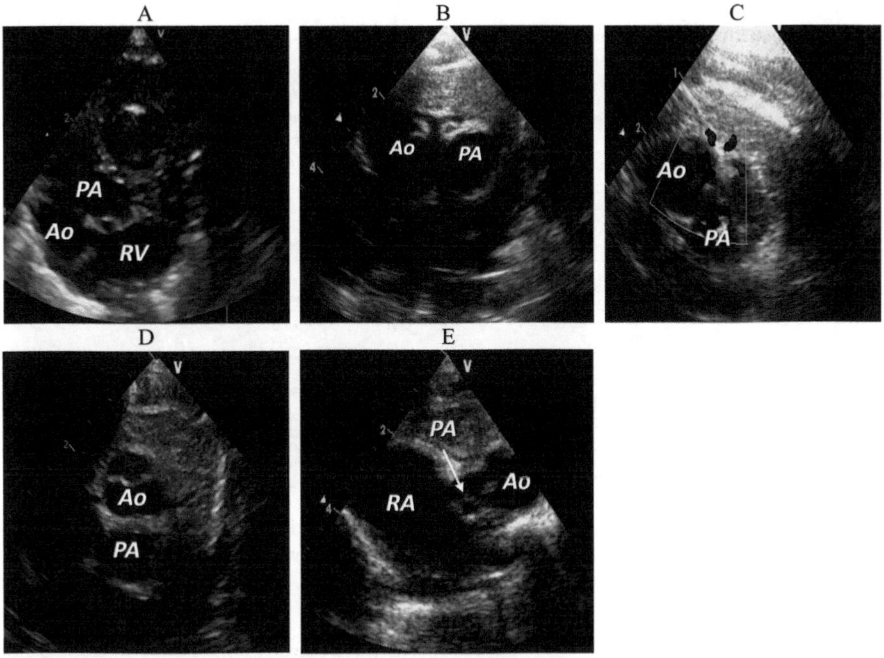

Fig. 5 Relationships of the arterial valves in DORV (high left parasternal short-axis view at the level of the aortic and the pulmonary valves): **A**—DP-aorta (normal relationship). The aorta is located right and posterior to the pulmonary artery; **B**—D-aorta. The aorta is right to the pulmonary artery ("side-by-side"); **C**—DA-aorta. The aorta is anterior and right to the pulmonary artery. The single left coronary artery: color Doppler mode shows trifurcation of the coronary artery; **D**—A-aorta. The aorta is in front of the pulmonary artery. Coronary arteries originate from the "facial" aortic sinuses; **E**—L-aorta. The aorta is in front and left to the pulmonary artery. *Ao—aorta; PA—pulmonary artery; RA—right atrium*

surgical planning. Echo has certain limitations in visualization of stenosis/hypoplasia of distal segments of the right and left pulmonary arteries (Fig. 7) [8, 9].

1.5 Coronary Artery Anatomy

Assessment of coronary artery anatomy is an important part of preoperative evaluation of patients with DORV. Detection of the coronary branches crossing RVOT can influence surgical treatment when transannular repair of RVOT is indicated (Fig. 8A).

High left parasternal short-axis view at the level of the aortic valve is used to visualize proximal segments of the coronary arteries. Sometimes in assessing coronary anatomy, left parasternal long-axis as well as apical or subxiphoid projection may be useful. Coronary arteries should originate from the facing sinuses. The absence of

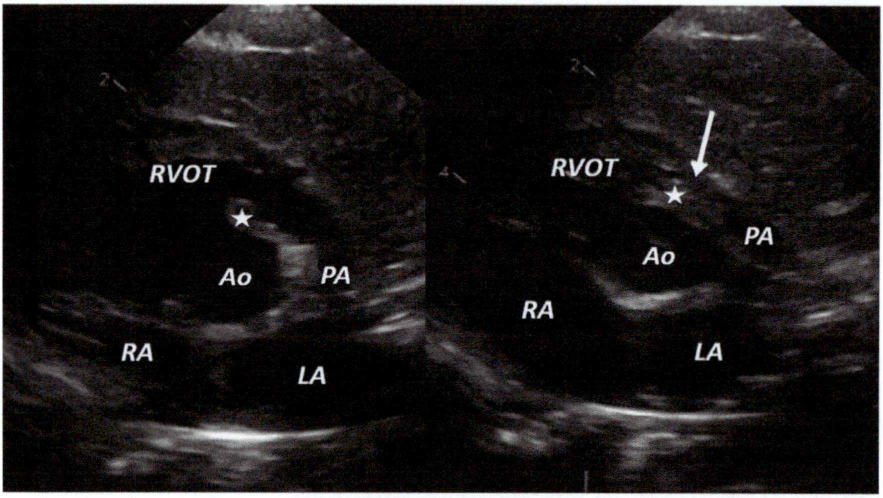

Fig. 6 Left parasternal short-axis view at the level of the aortic valve. The hypertrophied OS (asterisk) causes subpulmonary obstruction in systole (white arrow on the right panel). *Ao—aorta; RVOT—right ventricular outflow tract; PA—pulmonary artery; LA—left atrium; RA—right atrium*

Fig. 7 Hypoplasia of the right and dilation of the left pulmonary artery (left parasternal short-axis view at the level of the aortic valve with visualization of the pulmonary artery branches). *Ao—aorta; RVOT—right ventricular outflow tract; rPA—right pulmonary artery; lPA—left pulmonary artery*

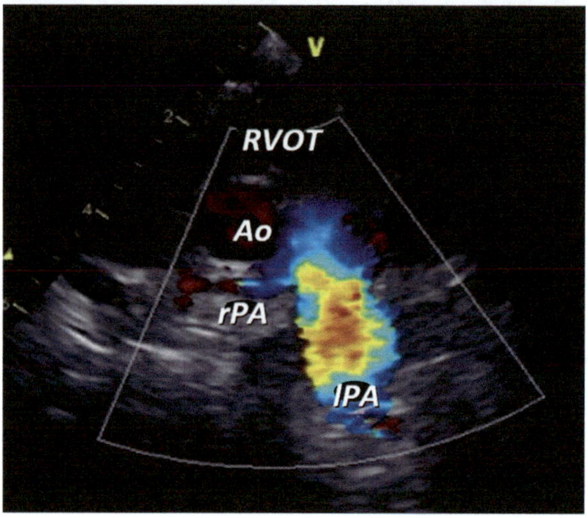

the left coronary artery bifurcation may indicate an anomalous origin of its branches, as well as possible intramural course [8, 9] (Fig. 8B).

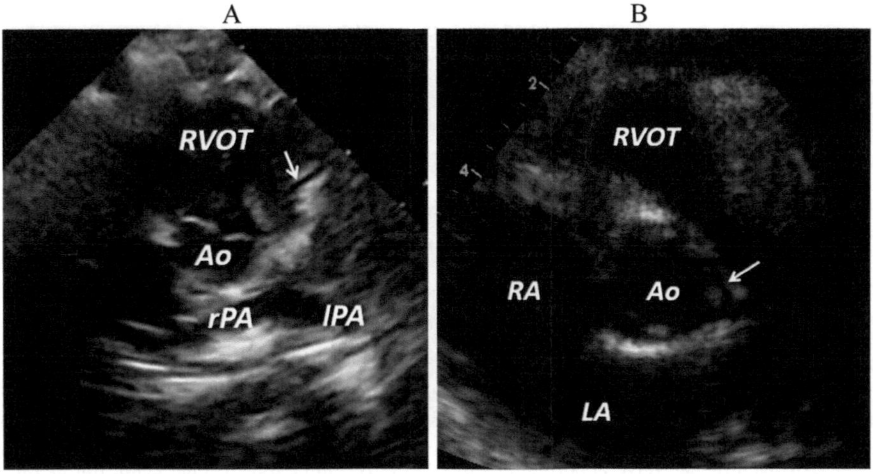

Fig. 8 Assessment of coronary artery anatomy by echo (left parasternal short-axis view at the level of aortic valve): **A**—coronary artery branch crossing RVOT (arrow); **B**—intramural course of the left coronary artery (arrow). *Ao—aorta; RVOT—right ventricular outflow tract; rPA—right pulmonary artery; lPA—left pulmonary artery; RA—right atrium; LA—left atrium*

1.6 Associated Cardiac Lesions

1.6.1 Atrioventricular Valve Anomalies

Mitral valve abnormalities in DORV are relatively common and usually are represented by the cleft of its anterior leaflet (Fig. 9A) or anomalous chordal attachment crossing left ventricular outflow tract (LVOT) which may potentially cause subsequent subaortic obstruction. Anatomy of the leaflets is evaluated from the left parasternal or subxiphoid short-axis view at the level of the mitral valve leaflets, and regurgitation area is determined using Doppler mode [8-11].

Straddling atrioventricular valve is visualized as an anomalous attachment of its chordae on both sides of the IVS or to papillary muscles of the contralateral ventricle. Four-chamber view from apical or subxiphoid approaches allow clearly identify the point of anomalous attachment (Fig. 9B).

One of the main signs of AVSD is a disproportion of the inlet and outlet components of the left ventricle due to the shortening of the former (see Fig. 2.17). Also, the location of the atrioventricular valves at the same level (apical four-chamber view) with a common fibrous annulus is a key diagnostic sign (Fig. 10). When evaluating DORV/AVSD, it is important to determine heart position in thorax, anatomy of common atrioventricular valve and its function, anatomy of subvalvular structures, degree of deficiency of the inlet part of IVS, RVOT and LVOT obstruction and size of the ventricles.

The definition of a balanced/unbalanced type of AVSD is based on the following echo parameters that allow biventricular repair:

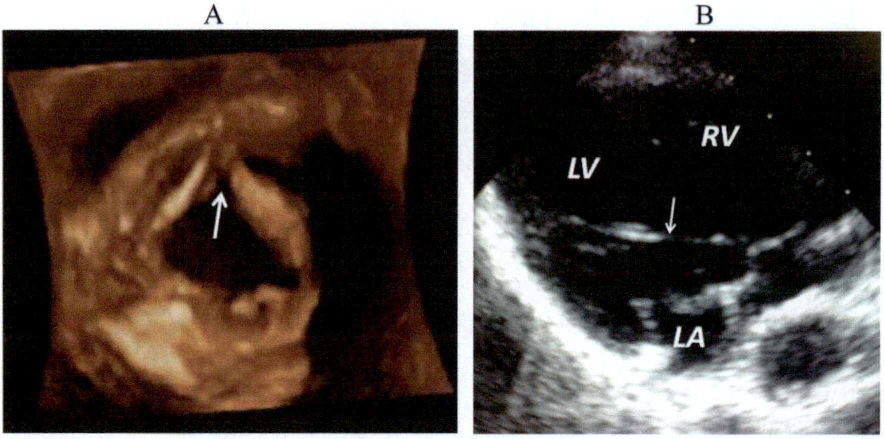

Fig. 9 Atrioventricular valve abnormalities in DORV: **A**—three-dimensional echo, mitral valve reconstruction, cleft of the anterior leaflet (arrow); **B**—anomalous chordal attachment of the tricuspid valve to the papillary muscle of the left ventricle—“straddling” type “C.” *RV—right ventricle; LV—left ventricle; LA—left atrium*

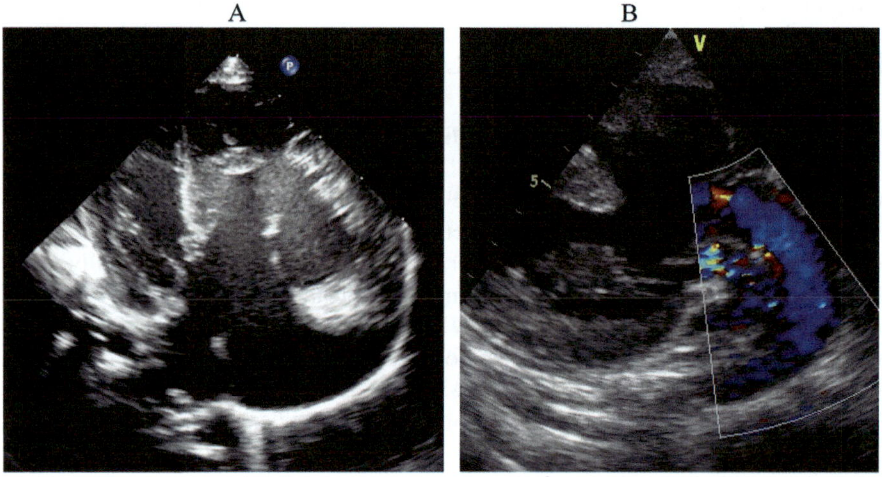

Fig. 10 DORV with AVSD: **A**—AVSD (apical four-chamber view); **B**—both arterial trunks originate from the right ventricle (subxiphoid long-axis view of RVOT)

- ratio of the left/right ventricles long axis > 0.65;
- ratio of the atrioventricular valves’ areas (smaller to larger). The edge of VSD serves as a point of separation. The ratio more than 0.67 indicates a balanced type, while less than < 0.3 determines an unbalanced type;

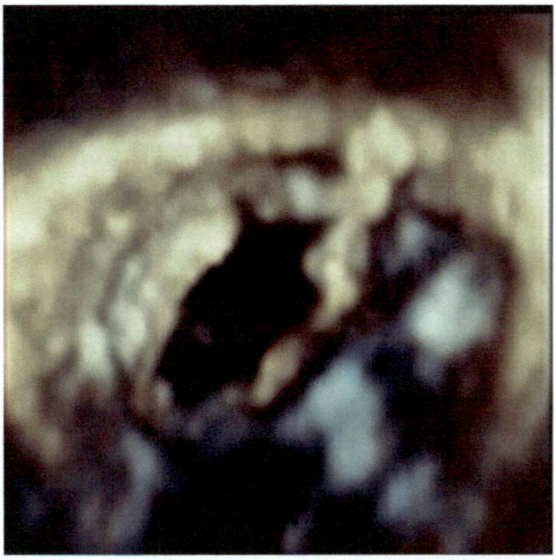

Fig. 11 Three-dimensional echo of the common atrioventricular valve in DORV

- modified valve area ratio index – the ratio of the area of the mitral component to common atrioventricular valve area (normal – 0.5; the value 0.19–0.39 is considered to be borderline) [8, 9].

Biventricular repair of DORV/AVSD depends on the ability of the left ventricle to support adequate systemic circulation after repair, which can be estimated by its myocardial mass, linear dimensions and volume of the left ventricle [12].

Clinical effectiveness of three-dimensional echo was first demonstrated in patients with AVSD, and today this method can be used routinely. Three-dimensional echo allows detailed assessment of anatomy and function of the common atrioventricular valve (Fig. 11) and subvalvular apparatus as well as to calculate the volumes and linear dimensions of the ventricles more accurately [11, 13, 14].

In a number of cases, DORV/AVSD is associated with heterotaxy syndrome with anomalous drainage of the systemic, pulmonary and hepatic veins. Subxiphoid projection may help in obtaining venous vessels draining into the common atrium (Fig. 12).

1.6.2 Aortic Arch Obstruction

Two-dimensional echo from suprasternal approach allows to evaluate the ascending aorta, aortic arch, isthmus and proximal thoracic aorta. During the investigation, the following parameters are to be estimated: aortic arch type (right/left), the presence of arch obstruction, area of the narrowing/interruption, type of coarctation, size, intensity and comparison of antegrade and retrograde blood flow patterns in pre- and poststenotic areas.

Using Doppler, acceleration and turbulent blood flow are assessed at the site of narrowing which allows to set the volume control more accurately to determine the peak systolic pressure gradient, indirectly reflecting the severity of coarctation.

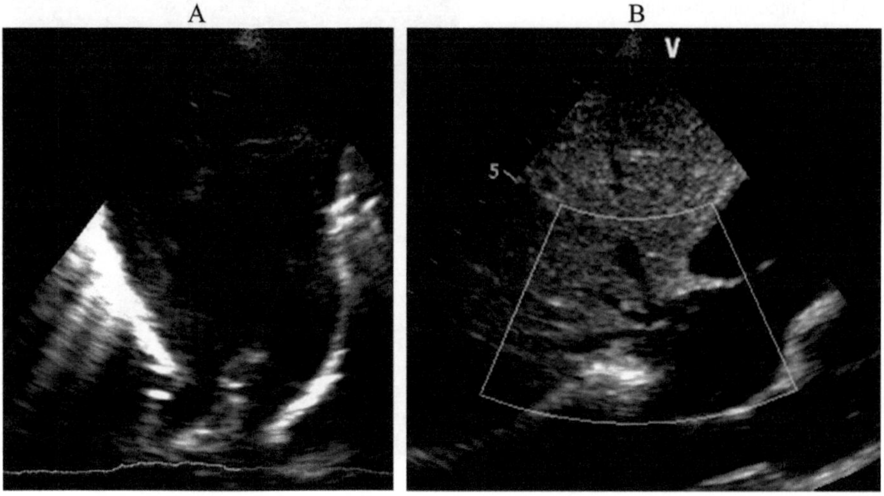

Fig. 12 Anomalous drainage of the systemic and hepatic veins into the common atrium in DORV associated with heterotaxy syndrome: **A**—left and right superior vena cava draining into the common atrium (subxiphoid projection, four-chamber view); **B**—hepatic veins draining directly into the right atrium, the absence of the hepatic segment of the inferior vena cava with azygos continuation (subxiphoid long-axis view of the inferior vena cava)

Due to decreased velocity and flow through the stenotic area, understated hemodynamic characteristics are possible in the presence of well-developed collateral arteries, patent ductus arteriosus, aortic arch hypoplasia, low ventricular performance, hemodynamically significant atrioventricular valve regurgitation. Overestimation of gradient is possible in the following circumstances: a) with a moderate increase in the flow in the descending aorta due to normal acceleration in the aortic arch after repair without signs of vessel narrowing, b) an increase in the systolic velocity of the flow and its turbulence due to the aortic rigidity in the repaired area in the absence of significant narrowing.

One of the typical signs of arch obstruction is a diastolic flow in abdominal aorta (collateral blood flow) and/or retrograde blood flow during diastole when ductus arteriosus is patent (Fig. 13). To diagnose coarctation, it is necessary to take into account the combination of hemodynamic parameters (peak systolic pressure gradient in a narrowing area, blood flow velocity and flow spectrum in abdominal aorta) and anatomical features of the aorta [8, 9].

Aortic arch hypoplasia is diagnosed when diameter ratio of the ascending aorta to the proximal arch is less than 60%, to the distal arch is less than 50% and to the isthmus is less than 40% [15]. For practical convenience, a formula of normal diameter of the aortic isthmus in a newborn was developed, according to which the minimal size of the isthmus should be equal to "body weight + 1 mm." [16] Z-score < -2 and diameter of the aortic isthmus less than 50% of the abdominal aorta are also criteria in favor of hypoplasia of the arch and the aortic isthmus [17, 18].

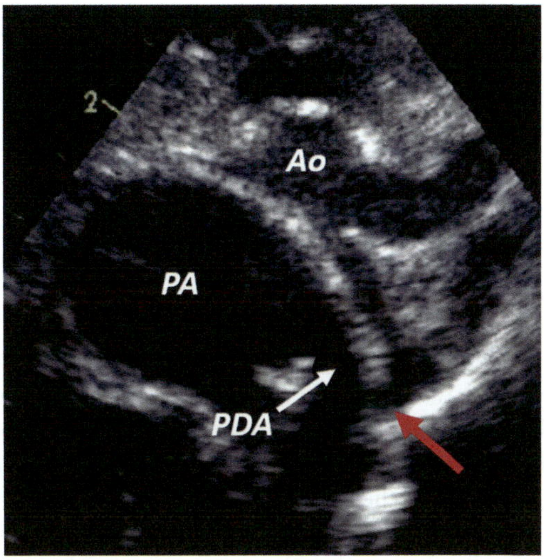

Fig. 13 Juvenile type of coarctation, arch hypoplasia, narrowing of the isthmus (red arrow). Suprasternal long-axis view. *Ao—aorta; PA—pulmonary artery; PDA—patent ductus arteriosus*

In fact, echo being a method of two-dimensional visualization has certain limitations in evaluation of extracardiac structures. Thus, interrupted aortic arch type B with aberrant right subclavian artery can be confused with type C. In case of large patent ductus arteriosus, assessment of the aortic arch distally to the left subclavian artery may be complicated. Analysis of flow patterns as well as evaluation of pressure gradients helps to verify the diagnosis [8, 9]. The final verification of the anatomy in some cases is possible only by means of CT/MRI or ACG.

2 Postoperative Investigation

Echo protocol after anatomical repair of DORV both in early and late postoperative periods should include the assessment of the following main complications:

- residual VSD;
- residual RVOT obstruction;
- pulmonary valve insufficiency;
- tricuspid valve insufficiency;
- subaortic obstruction;
- myocardial contractility.

2.1 Residual VSD

Residual blood shunting at the level of intraventricular patch is determined using color Doppler. Shunting can be determined at the any level of a patch but most often in its upper. It is necessary to evaluate the IVS in complex intraventricular tunnels appropriately [9, 17, 19].

2.2 *Residual RVOT Obstruction*

When assessing residual RVOT obstruction, it is important to determine the level of stenosis using a combination of ultrasound methods – color, impulse-wave and continuous-wave Doppler. Often after repair of DORV «tetralogy» type, a multilevel residual obstruction takes place. Following ASO, the presence of pulmonary artery stenosis is the most common complication due to the tension of pulmonary artery branches after the Lecompte maneuver in patients with Taussig-Bing anomaly. Left and right parasternal, suprasternal and subxiphoid projections are routinely used to visualize the pulmonary arteries. Diameter of the pulmonary trunk should be measured in its mid-third during the systolic phase. In the presence of supravalvular stenosis, the smallest diameter of the trunk should be measured. Diameter of the right and left pulmonary arteries is measured at the area of their origin if good visualization is achieved. Doppler allows to identify stenotic areas at the sites before the division of pulmonary arteries into the lobar branches. Distal segment of the left pulmonary artery is more difficult to visualize than that of the right one.

Flow spectrum in RVOT can help in differentiation between the dynamic obstruction in the right ventricle and residual valvular or supravalvular stenosis: In the former, there is a late peak of the Doppler signal while the latter is characterized by a mid-systolic peak (Fig. 14).

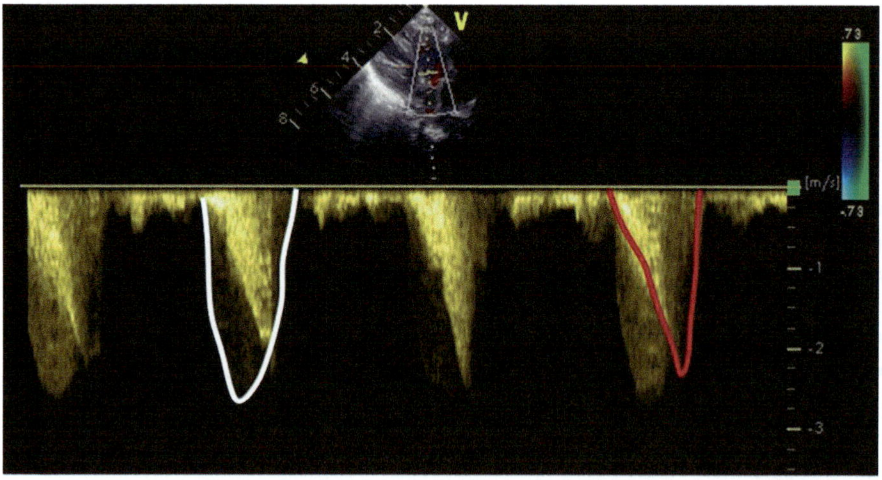

Fig. 14 Flow spectrum in RVOT obtained by continuous-wave Doppler. Dynamic obstruction in the right ventricle—red contour; residual valvular stenosis—white contour

The degree of obstruction is determined by peak systolic pressure gradient [17, 20]:

- severe (> 64 mmHg);
- moderate (36–64 mmHg);
- mild (< 36 mmHg).

According to some authors, RVOT obstruction is diagnosed when systolic pressure gradient exceeds 30 mmHg. For asymptomatic patients reintervention is indicated when peak systolic pressure gradient is more than 64 mmHg or right ventricle systolic pressure is more than 2/3 of the systemic pressure [17, 20, 21].

Multilevel obstruction of RVOT and pulmonary arteries represents a specific problem in terms of contribution of each stenotic level in right ventricle afterload especially when stenotic areas are close to each other [20].

2.3 *Pulmonary Valve Insufficiency*

Pulmonary valve insufficiency is an important factor initiating the pathophysiological cascade which leads to impairment of systolic and diastolic function of the right ventricular and, as a result, decreased exercise tolerance, risk of atrial and ventricular tachycardia as well as sudden death [20].

Evaluation of pulmonary regurgitation is an important component of echo examination. In a large study, it was revealed that predictors of severe pulmonary regurgitation are [20]as follows:

- ratio of the regurgitant jet width to the diameter of pulmonary annulus more than 0.5–0.7 (Fig. 15);
- ratio of the duration of the pulmonary regurgitation signal to the period of diastole in the spectral Doppler mode of less than 0.77;
- pressure half-time less than 100 ms (but unreliable with high end-diastolic pressure of the right ventricle).

Postoperative RVOT aneurysm is assessed by short-axis projection at the level of the aortic valve or long-axis projection of RVOT (Fig. 16).

2.4 *Tricuspid Valve Insufficiency*

After biventricular repair, tricuspid valve regurgitation may develop due to straddling valve, diastasis between the septal and anterior leaflets, dilation of the tricuspid annulus, etc. The valve function is assessed from apical view in four- or five-chamber projections, left parasternal short-axis view at the level of the aortic valve and from the same positions of subxiphoid view, as well as projections of individual scanning [10].

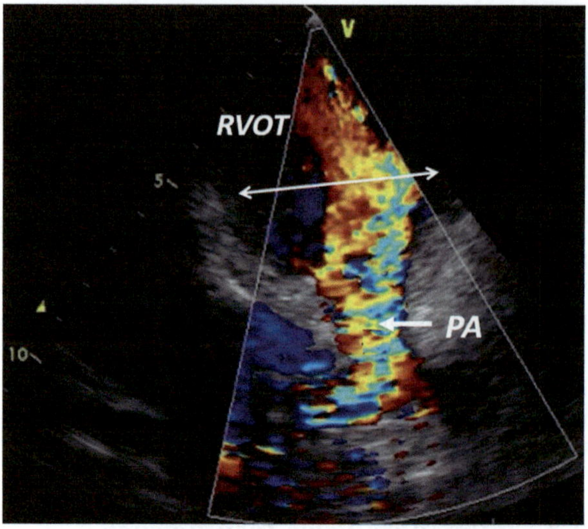

Fig. 15 Left parasternal long-axis view of RVOT, color Doppler mode. The double-headed arrow indicates RVOT aneurysm. Turbulent orange blood flow occupies the entire diameter of the pulmonary valve annulus—severe pulmonary regurgitation. *RVOT—right ventricular outflow tract; PA—pulmonary artery*

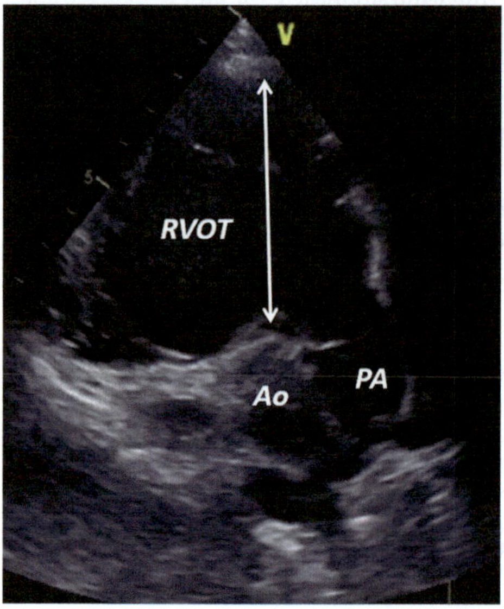

Fig. 16 RVOT aneurism (indicated by the arrow) (left parasternal short-axis view at the level of the aortic valve). *Ao—aorta; PA—pulmonary artery; RVOT—right ventricular outflow tract*

For extended assessment of tricuspid valve anatomy and function, it is advisable to use a two- or three-dimensional image in combination with color Doppler. Visualization through atrial and/or ventricular sections can be especially informative with a high-quality "live" image of the atrioventricular valves [10, 11].

Quantitative assessment of tricuspid regurgitation is limited compared to mitral regurgitation. The ratio of the regurgitant jet area to the atrium area in the color Doppler mode is a universal method for assessing its severity. The width of *vena contracta* and the intensity of the regurgitation flow reflect the degree of valve insufficiency [10, 20].

It is important to note that with the dilation of the tricuspid annulus regurgitation must be visualized from several echo approaches to minimize underestimation of its degree. In practice, the width of *vena contracta* is the most reliable parameter for quantifying tricuspid regurgitation. Width of *vena contracta* more than 0.7 cm in adults indicates a severe valve insufficiency [10].

In addition to assessing the regurgitant jet and *vena contracta,* it is necessary to measure the diameter of the inferior vena cava, hepatic veins and right atrium size. Reverse venous blood flow in inferior vena cava and hepatic veins is used as a marker of severe tricuspid regurgitation. However, these indirect signs are also influenced by other factors such as right ventricular stiffness, right ventricular preload and atrial tachyarrhythmia [8, 9, 20].

2.5 Subaortic Obstruction

Subaortic obstruction should always be excluded during the echo examination in repaired DORV. In color Doppler mode, turbulent blood flow in LVOT indicates an increased flow in the intracardiac tunnel. In case of univentricular palliation, it is useful to assess "late" LVOT restriction due to the myocardial hypertrophy and progressive volumetric hypoplasia of the left ventricle [23]. Using continuous-wave Doppler, subaortic obstruction is quantitatively measured in accordance with the following scale (Fig. 17) [17, 22]:

- mild (<30 mmHg);
- moderate (30–50 mmHg);

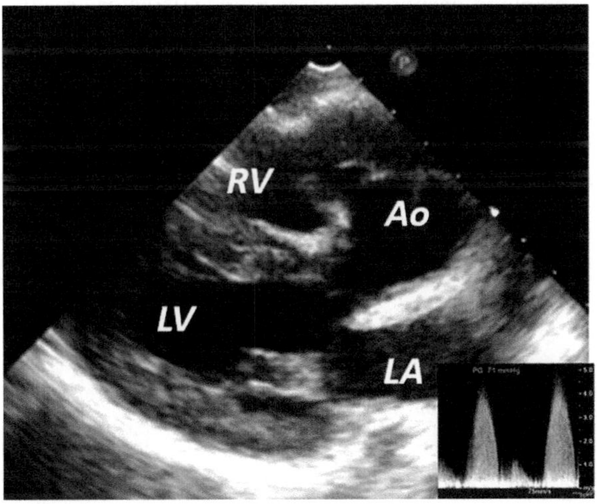

Fig. 17 Subaortic obstruction after repair of DORV with noncommitted VSD and systolic pressure gradient 71 mmHg (left parasternal long-axis view). *Ao—aorta; RV—right ventricle; LV—left ventricle; LA—left atrium*

– severe (>50 mmHg).

In asymptomatic patients, reoperation is indicated if systolic pressure gradient is more than 50 mmHg at rest [17, 22].

2.6 Myocardial Contractility

Long-term adequate myocardial contractility of both ventricles is one of the most topical subjects in pediatric cardiology, in particular in patients with repaired DORV. The measurement of myocardial deformity and its velocity obtained by tissue Doppler and two-dimensional speckle tracking method have recently appeared as tools for detecting subclinical myocardial dysfunction, as well as for patients with normal ventricular function (ejection fraction, shortening fraction) [8, 9, 24]. An increasing number of investigations confirm the high diagnostic value of two-dimensional speckle tracking and recommend this method as the main for the quantitative assessment of myocardial deformity in various clinical situations including patients after surgical repair of CHD, especially after DORV.

Nowadays, the assessment of myocardial function should include the use of tissue Doppler and speckle tracking pre- and postoperatively [8, 9, 25]. It is especially important to use new echo techniques in cases of repaired DORV with long intraventricular tunnel, IVS resection and operations with coronary artery reimplantation (Fig. 18). It is also of great clinical importance to determine the function of the right ventricle in patients with "tetralogy" type of DORV, as well as after univentricular palliation with a dominant right ventricle. The main goals for surgeons and cardiologists are to prevent pulmonary regurgitation after repair and thus progressive right ventricular dilation. To date, the optimal time for reintervention in such patients is widely discussed and still remains unsolved. A number of clinics adhere to the principle of early reoperation with satisfactory results [8, 20, 22].

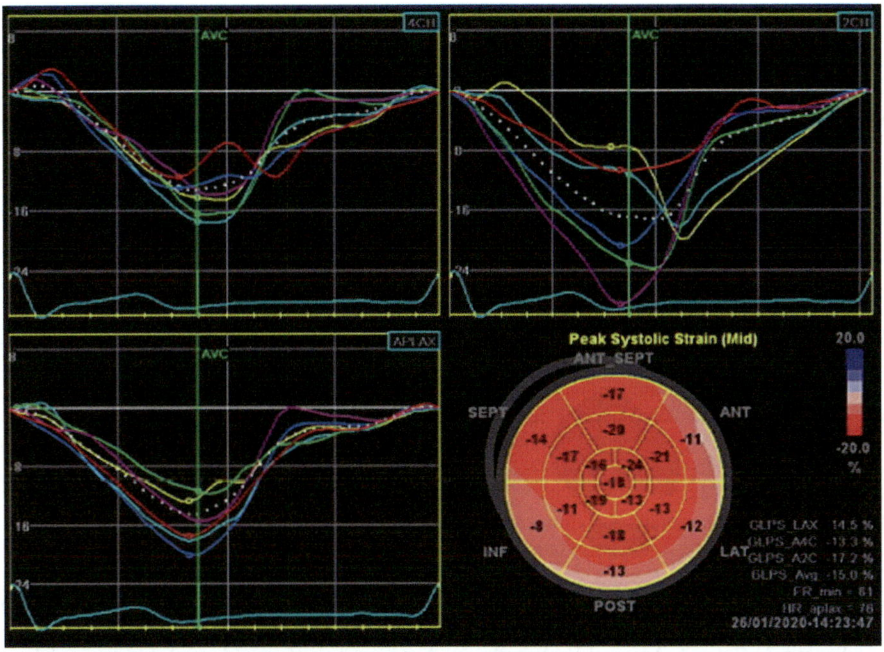

Fig. 18 Speckle tracking method after ASO in a patient with repaired Taussig-Bing anomaly. There is a slight decrease (to −15%) in global deformity of the left ventricular myocardium (normal = −19%)

References

1. Smith RS, Comstock CH, Kirk JS, Lee W, Riggs T, Weinhouse E. Double-outlet right ventricle: an antenatal diagnostic dilemma. Ultrasound Obstet Gynecol. 1999;14:315–9.
2. Abuhamad A, Chaoui R. A practical guide to fetal echocardiography. 2010.
3. Macartney FJ, Rigby ML, Anderson RH, Stark J, Silverman NH. Double outlet right ventricle. Cross sectional echocardiographic findings, their anatomical explanation, and surgical relevance. British Heart J. 1984;52:164–77.
4. Simpson JM, Miller O. Three-dimensional echocardiography in congenital heart disease. Arch Cardiovasc Dis. 2011;104:45–56.
5. Rychik J, Jacobs ML, Norwood WI. Early changes in ventricular geometry and ventricular septal defect size following Rastelli operation or intraventricular baffle repair for conotruncal anomaly. A cause for development of subaortic stenosis. Circulation. 1994;90:II13–19.
6. Mahle WT, Martinez R, Silverman N, Cohen MS, Anderson RH. Anatomy, echocardiography, and surgical approach to double outlet right ventricle. Cardiol Young. 2008;18(Suppl. 3):39–51.
7. Zamora R, Moller JH, Edwards JE. Double-outlet right ventricle. Anatomic types and associated anomalies. Chest. 1975;68:672–677.
8. Lai WW, Mertens LL, Cohen MS, Geva T. Echocardiography in pediatric and congenital heart disease. From fetus to adult. 2nd edn. Wiley Blackwell; 2016.
9. Anderson RH, Baker EJ, Penny DJ, Redington AN, Rigby ML, Wernovsky G. Paediatric cardiology. 3rd edn. Elsevier;2009.
10. Zoghbi WA, Adams D, Bonow RO, Enriquez-Sarano M, Foster E, Grayburn PA, Hahn RT, Han Y, Hung J, Lang RM, Little SH, Shah DJ, Shernan S, Thavendiranathan P, Thoman JD,

Weissman NJ. Recommendations for noninvasive evaluation of native valvular regurgitation: a report from the American society of echocardiography developed in collaboration with the Society for cardiovascular magnetic resonance. J Amer Soc Echocardiography. 2017;30:303–71.
11. Simpson J, Lopez L, Acar P, Friedberg MK, Khoo NS, Ko HH, Marek J, Marx G, McGhie JS, Meijboom F, Van den Bosch A, Miller O, Shirali G. Three-dimensional echocardiography in congenital heart disease: an expert consensus document from the European association of cardiovascular imaging and the American society of echocardiography. J Amer Soc Echocardiography. 2017;30:1–27.
12. Phoon CK, Silverman NH. Conditions with right ventricular pressure and volume overload, and a small left ventricle: "“hypoplastic”" left ventricle or simply a squashed ventricle? J Amer College of Cardiol. 1997;30:1547–53.
13. Espinola-Zavaleta N, Vargas-Barron J, Keirns C, Rivera G, Romero-Cardenas A, Roldan J, Attie F. Three-dimensional echocardiography in congenital malformations of the mitral valve. J Amer Soc Echocardiography. 2002;15:468–72.
14. Prakash A, Lacro RV, Sleeper LA, Minich LL, Colan SD, McCrindle B, Covitz W, Golding F, Hlavacek AM, Levine JC, Cohen MS. Challenges in echocardiographic assessment of mitral regurgitation in children after repair of atrioventricular septal defect. Pediatr Cardiol. 2012;33:205–14.
15. Backer CL, Mavroudis C. Congenital heart surgery nomenclature and database project: patent ductus arteriosus, coarctation of the aorta, interrupted aortic arch. Ann Thorac Surg. 2000;69:S298-307.
16. Moulaert AJ, Bruins CC, Oppenheimer-Dekker A. Anomalies of the aortic arch and ventricular septal defects. Circulation. 1976;53:1011–5.
17. Saxena A, Relan J, Agarwal R, Awasthy N, Azad S, Chakrabarty M, et al. Indian guidelines for indications and timing of intervention for common congenital heart diseases: revised and updated consensus statement of the working group on management of congenital heart diseases. Ann Pediatr Cardiol. 2019;12:254–86.
18. Karl TR, Sano S, Brawn W, Mee RB. Repair of hypoplastic or interrupted aortic arch via sternotomy. J Thorac Cardiovasc Surg. 1992;104:688–95.
19. Pang KJ, Meng H, Hu SS, Wang H, Hsi D, Hua ZD, Pan XB, Li SJ. Echocardiographic classification and surgical approaches to double-outlet right ventricle for great arteries arising almost exclusively from the right ventricle. Tex Heart Inst J. 2017;44:245–51.
20. Valente AM, Cook S, Festa P, Ko HH, Krishnamurthy R, Taylor AM, Warnes CA, Kreutzer J, Geva T. Multimodality imaging guidelines for patients with repaired tetralogy of Fallot: a report from the American Society of Echocardiography developed in collaboration with the society for cardiovascular magnetic resonance and the society for pediatric radiology. J Amer Soc Echocardiography. 2014;27:111–41.
21. Rao V, Kadletz M, Hornberger LK, Freedom RM, Black MD. Preservation of the pulmonary valve complex in tetralogy of Fallot: how small is too small? Ann Thorac Surg. 2000;69:176–80.
22. Stout KK, Daniels CJ, Aboulhosn JA, et al. 2018 AHA/ACC guideline for the management of adults with congenital heart disease: a report of the American college of cardiology/American heart association task force on clinical practice guidelines. J Amer College of Cardiol. 2019;73:e81–192.
23. Meadows J, Pigula F, Lock J, Marshall AJ. Transcatheter creation and enlargement of ventricular septal defects for relief of ventricular hypertension. Thoracic and Cardiovascular Surgery. 2007;133:912–8.

24. Mor-Avi V, Lang RM, Badano LP, Belohlavek M, Cardim NM, Derumeaux G, Galderisi M, Marwick T, Nagueh SF, Sengupta PP, Sicari R, Smiseth OA, Smulevitz B, Takeuchi M, Thomas JD, Vannan M, Voigt JU, Zamorano JL. Current and evolving echocardiographic techniques for the quantitative evaluation of cardiac mechanics: ASE/EAE consensus statement on methodology and indications endorsed by the Japanese society of echocardiography. J Amer Soc Echocardiography. 2011;24:277–313.
25. Black D, Vettukattil J. Advanced echocardiographic imaging of the congenitally malformed heart. Curr Cardiol Rev. 2013;9:241–52.

Angiocardiography

M. G. Pursanov and K. M. Dzhidzhikhiya

Abstract Angiocardiographic (ACG) investigation is a second-line diagnostic tool after echo in assessment DORV. The development of X-ray equipment paved the way to modern state of investigation when specialists can get detailed images of a heart and great vessels simultaneously in two planes. This made it possible to conduct intracardiac examinations more safely and efficiently and to improve the diagnosis of CHDs. Heart catheterization and ACG are necessary for accurate analysis of intracardiac hemodynamics, anatomy of the pulmonary arteries, major aortopulmonary collateral arteries, coronary arteries and associated cardiac lesions. In patients with DORV, the main anatomical structures to be assessed by ACG are VSD location and size, relationship and course of the arterial trunks, pulmonary artery stenosis, aortic arch obstruction, size and orientation of the OS, AVSD and size of ventricles.

Keywords Double-outlet right ventricle · Diagnostics · Angiocardiography

To date, echo provides almost all the necessary information for appropriate understanding of intracardiac anatomy and surgical decision-making in patients with DORV [1–6]. CT angiography and ACG are used when echo data are insufficient or ambiguous and at the same time play a key role in assessment of extracardiac components of the malformation. Computer diagnostic methods develop rapidly and are promising for a detailed assessment of intracardiac anatomy and surgical planning since obtained 3D images of a heart can be printed to convey an objective anatomy [7–12].

ACG plays an important role in assessment of complex malformations, in particular DORV, and remains the final diagnostic method in most cases [13–17].

M. G. Pursanov
Departement of Emergency Cardiac Surgery and Interventional Cardiology, Morozov Children's Clinical Hospital, Moscow, Russia

K. M. Dzhidzhikhiya (✉)
Departement of Emergency Surgery of Congenital Heart Diseases, A. N. Bakulev National Medical Investigation Center for Cardiovascular Surgery, Moscow, Russia
e-mail: d.m.konstantine@mail.ru

K. V. Shatalov and K. M. Dzhidzhikhiya (eds.), *Double-Outlet Right Ventricle*,
https://doi.org/10.1007/978-3-031-49707-0_7

The development of X-ray equipment paved the way to modern state of investigation when specialists can get detailed images of a heart and great vessels simultaneously in two planes (biplane ACG). This made it possible to conduct intracardiac examinations more safely and efficiently and to improve the diagnosis of diseases. Modern ACG equipment should allow performing biplane investigation of patients with complex CHDs. The use of angular projections and the emergence of the concept of axial angiography have solved many problems and limitations associated with superimposition and/or overlapping, inherent in the standard technique of visualization.

Heart axis is oriented obliquely with the left ventricle apex oriented to the left and anterior. The IVS is a complex «S-shaped» structure. The IVS bends at an angle of 100–120° in cranio-caudal direction. To visualize such a complex configuration, as well as to identify the composite features of DORV, modern ACG equipment allows to obtain a wide range of projections using cranial and caudal angulations in order to identify all the necessary heart structures and great vessels. Axial angiography establishing an accurate diagnosis and identifying many associate anomalies is a step to the new era of ACG examination.

For diagnosing DORV, the use of axial projections is mandatory. Biplane ACG is more suitable for the diagnosis of complex CHDs since one injection of contrast agent allows to get almost full information of a heart anatomy in two mutually opposite planes. In addition, the method allows to reduce the amount of contrast agent and declines the radiation impact on both patient and medical staff. The use of angular projections and the emergence of axial ACG allowed specialists to solve the number of widespread problems that arise with conventional heart visualization techniques—skew, superpose and overlay of images.

Catheterization and ACG are necessary for accurate analysis of intracardiac hemodynamics, anatomy of the pulmonary arteries, major aortopulmonary collateral arteries, coronary arteries and associated cardiac lesions.

ACG protocol depends on the specific CHD. The main anatomical components of DORV and ACG projections for their assessment are presented in Table 1.

The examination begins with measurement of pressure in the right and the left cardiac chambers and in the arterial trunks. This allows to determine severity of pulmonary hypertension, measure pulmonary and systemic vascular resistance, as well as to evaluate the entire intracardiac hemodynamics. In some patients with pulmonary hypertension, catheterization may be needed to assess vascular reactivity in response to injection of vasodilators.

When performing right and left ventriculography from different projections, it is necessary to estimate the following components of DORV:

- VSD location and size;
- relationship and course of the arterial trunks;
- pulmonary artery stenosis;
- aortic arch obstruction;
- OS;
- AVSD and size of ventricles.

Table 1 ACG projections used to assess different anatomical components of DORV [13]

Anatomical structure		ACG projection
Size of the right ventricle		Anterior and lateral projections with cranial angulation
Arterial trunks relationship		
LVOT/RVOT obstruction		Anterior projection and right anterior oblique projection, right ventriculography
Subarterial infundibulums and the OS	parallel course	Anterior projection, right ventriculography
	spiral course	Right/left anterior oblique projections with cranial angulation, right ventriculography
Location and size of VSD		Left anterior oblique projection, left ventriculography
Size of the left ventricle		
LVOTO		
AVSD or noncommitted (inlet) VSD		Hepatoclavicular position (four-chamber)
Coronary arteries		«Laid-back» projection, aortography
Pulmonary arteries		Anterior projection and anterior left oblique projection with cranial angulation, pulmonary artery arteriography
Aortic arch obstruction		Left anterior oblique projection, aortography

1 Preoperative Investigation

1.1 DORV «Tetralogy» and «VSD» Types

ACG assessment protocol:

- VSD location;
- relationship and course of the arterial trunks;
- pulmonary artery stenosis;
- atrioventricular valve anatomy;
- coronary artery anatomy.

VSD Location. VSD is typically subaortic or subarterial, and the arterial trunks are spiraling. On left ventriculography the contrast agent from the left ventricle through subaortic VSD first appears in the ascending aorta and after this in the pulmonary artery (Fig. 1A). Egress from the left ventricle to the ascending aorta on the left anterior oblique projection is characterized by Z-shape. On right ventriculography, the opposite scenario is observed because noncontrast blood from the left ventricles washes away the contrast agent from subaortic area; therefore, the pulmonary artery is visualized first followed by the ascending aorta (Fig. 1B).

As a rule, subarterial VSD is usually associated with hypoplasia/absence of the OS as a muscular structure and is a rarest form of DORV. The main ACG feature in favor of subarterial VSD is simultaneous opacification of the aorta and the pulmonary

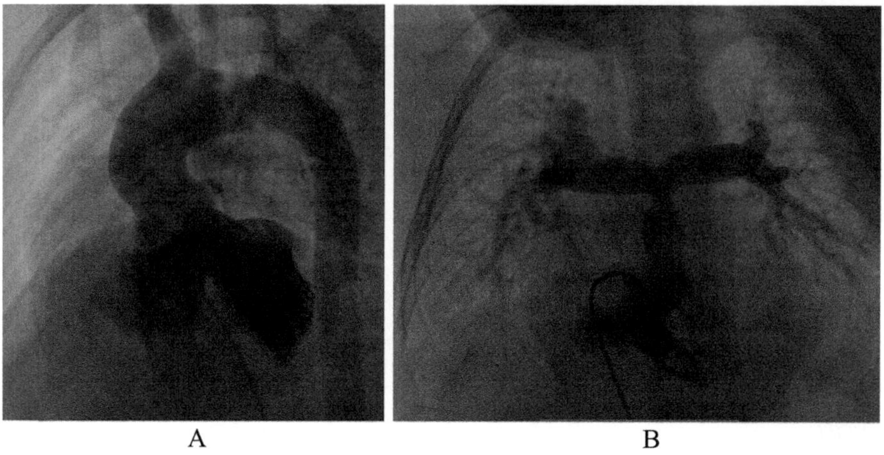

Fig. 1 DORV with subaortic VSD: **A**—left ventriculography, left anterior oblique projection, opacification of the ascending aorta. The aortic valve overrides the IVS and predominantly takes origin from the right ventricle; **B**—right ventriculography, frontal projection. Opacification of the pulmonary arteries

artery on left ventriculography, as well as almost complete absence of the shadow of the OS both in frontal and lateral projections (Fig. 2). As it was mentioned in Chap. 2, there is also an atypical form of DORV with subarterial VSD but with the prominent OS, when simultaneous opacification of the aorta and the pulmonary artery also takes place. In this case, on left ventriculography, shadow of the OS between the aorta and the pulmonary artery is clearly visualized. In addition, the arterial trunks have a parallel course. These two ACG signs are the distinctive for DORV with atypical subarterial VSD with the OS (Fig. 3).

Additional VSDs as well as their size and location are visualized on left ventriculography in left anterior oblique projection (Figs. 4, 5).

Relationship and Course of the Arterial Trunks. «Tetralogy» and «VSD» types of DORV are characterized by spiral course of the arterial trunks (Fig. 6A). If left ventriculography shows subaortic location of VSD but the aorta and the pulmonary artery have parallel course, then subaortic not directly committed VSD should be suspected. Parallel course of the trunks in this case is explained by the elongated subaortic infundibulum (i.e., the prominent VIF between the mitral and the aortic valves), which causes anterior shifting of the aortic valve and eventually leads to the "unspiraling" of the arterial trunks. Along with this, reorientation of the OS takes place and it becomes visible in frontal projection (Fig. 6B–C).

Pulmonary Artery Stenosis. In «tetralogy» type, pulmonary artery stenosis is usually represented by a combination of subvalvular (infundibular) and valvular stenosis which are well visualized on right ventriculography (Fig. 7A). Stenosis of the right and/or left pulmonary artery can be represented by local or diffuse variants, and

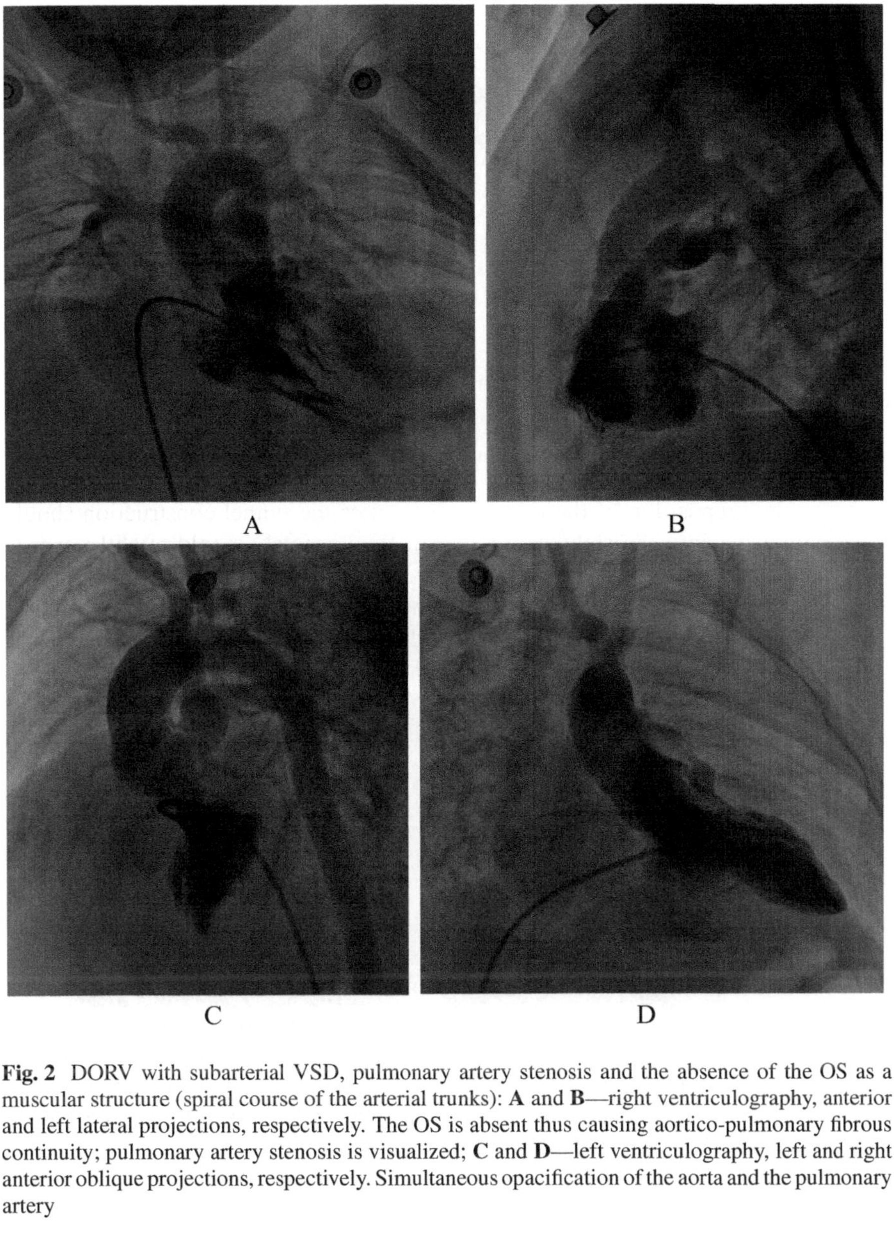

Fig. 2 DORV with subarterial VSD, pulmonary artery stenosis and the absence of the OS as a muscular structure (spiral course of the arterial trunks): **A** and **B**—right ventriculography, anterior and left lateral projections, respectively. The OS is absent thus causing aortico-pulmonary fibrous continuity; pulmonary artery stenosis is visualized; **C** and **D**—left ventriculography, left and right anterior oblique projections, respectively. Simultaneous opacification of the aorta and the pulmonary artery

their preoperative detection is an important part of surgical decision-making (Fig. 7B–D). In some cases, obstructive lesions can be represented by unilateral absence of pulmonary artery, which may be suspected by contrast interruption between the pulmonary trunk and the distal segment of an absent artery (so-called hilar artery) (Fig. 8). Since in this case, blood supply to hilar artery is provided by ipsilateral

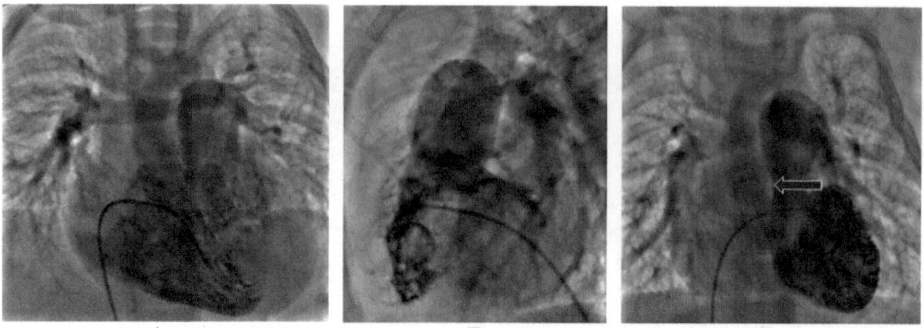

A B C

Fig. 3 DORV with subarterial VSD and the OS (parallel course of the arterial trunks): **A** and **B**—right ventriculography, anterior and left lateral projections, respectively. The aorta and the pulmonary artery are separated by the OS and originate predominantly from the right ventricle; **C**—left ventriculography, anterior projection. Simultaneous opacification of the aorta and the pulmonary artery (the arrow points at the OS)

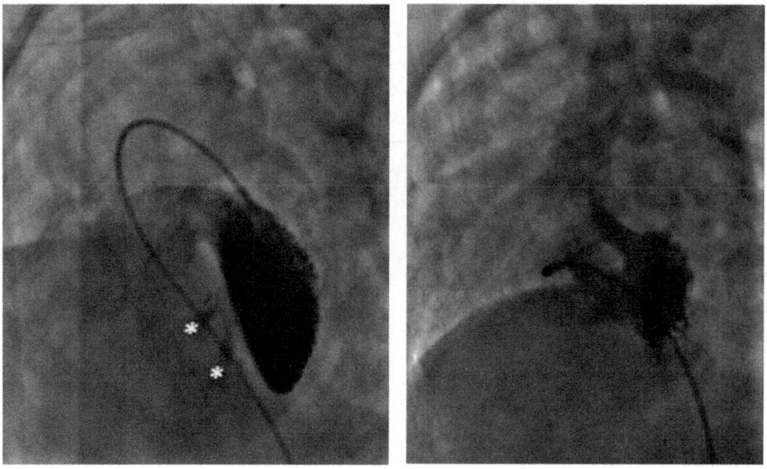

A B

Fig. 4 DORV with multiple VSDs: **A**—left ventriculography, left anterior oblique projection. Subaortic VSD and two additional trabecular VSDs (asterisks); **B**—left ventriculography, left anterior oblique projection. Large trabecular and restrictive subaortic VSDs are visualized

patent ductus arteriosus, it is necessary to additionally perform aortography in order to assess anatomy of distal vascular bed.

If on right ventriculography the aorta is contrasted first, then severe stenosis or pulmonary artery atresia should be suspected. To confirm the diagnosis, it is necessary to assess a lateral projection on which the contrast interruption between the right ventricle and the pulmonary artery is visualized (Fig. 9).

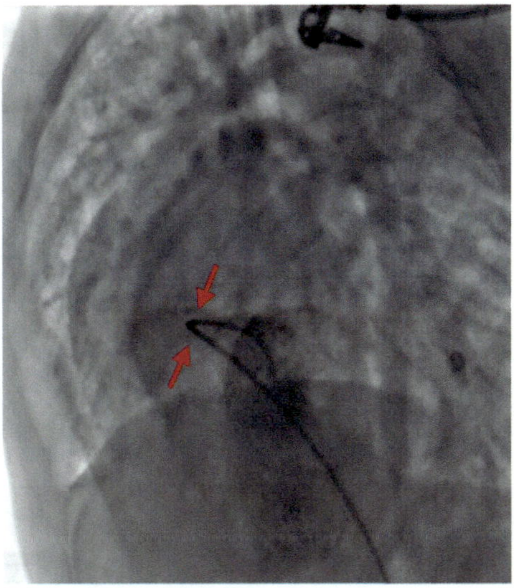

Fig. 5 Restrictive subaortic VSD (the boundaries of the VSD are indicated by arrows) (left ventriculography, left anterior oblique projection)

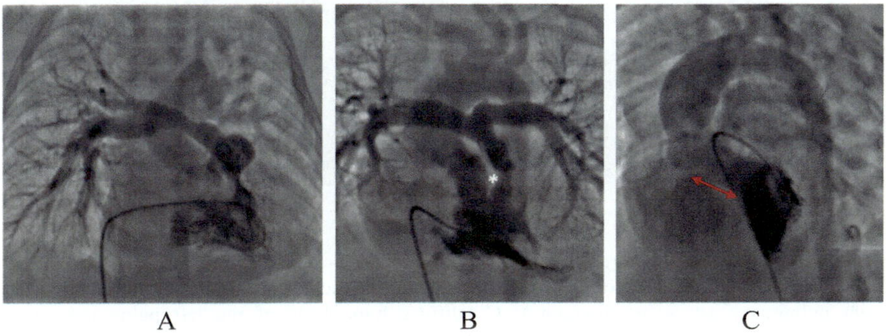

Fig. 6 DORV with subaortic VSD: **A**—«tetralogy» type (right ventriculography, anterior projection). Spiral course of the arterial trunks, shadow of the OS is not visualized; **B**—not directly committed subaortic VSD (right ventriculography, anterior projection). Parallel course of the arterial trunks, shadow of the OS is well seen (asterisk); **C**—not directly committed subaortic VSD (left ventriculography, left anterior oblique projection). Elongated subaortic conus that remotes the aortic valve from VSD

If pulmonary artery banding was done previously, right ventriculography clearly shows the level of a band (Fig. 7D). At the same time, if a band dislocated distally toward the pulmonary bifurcation, then proximal stenosis of both pulmonary arteries often develops as a complication. To assess severity of pulmonary hypertension and risk of biventricular repair, it is necessary to measure systolic, diastolic and mean pressure in the right and/or left pulmonary artery, as well as peak systolic

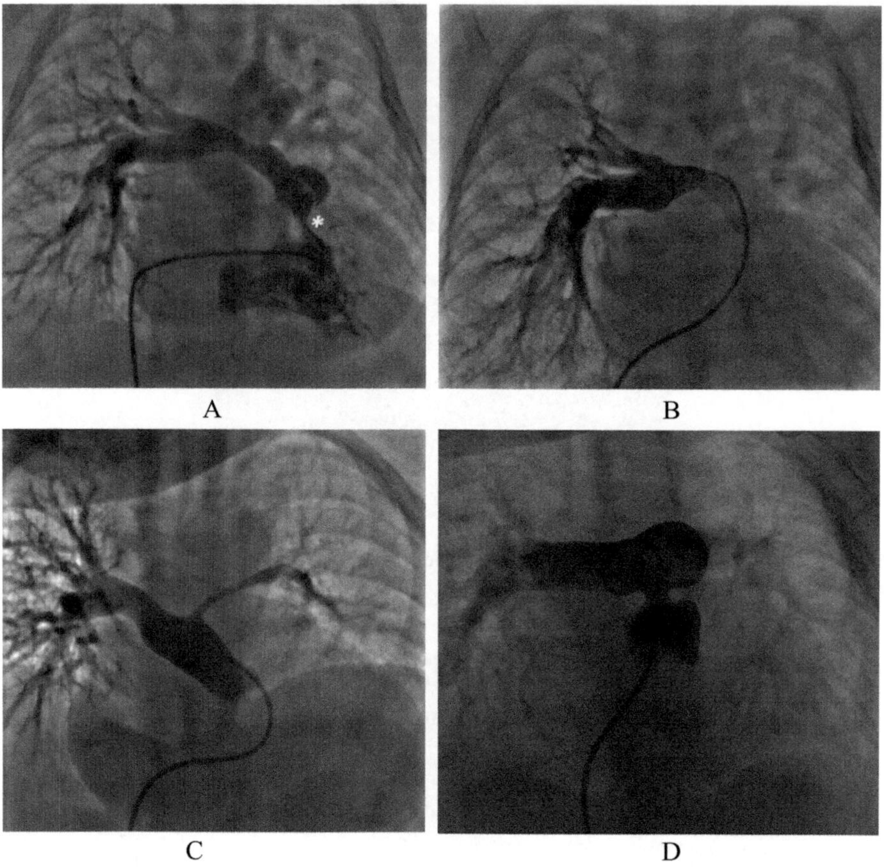

Fig. 7 Pulmonary artery obstructive lesions in DORV: **A**—severe infundibular stenosis (asterisk) (right ventriculography, anterior projection); **B**—proximal stenosis of the right pulmonary artery (right pulmonary artery arteriography); **C**—diffuse hypoplasia of the left pulmonary artery (pulmonary artery arteriography); **D**—site of the band after pulmonary artery banding operation (pulmonary artery arteriography)

pressure gradient on a band. Isolated high systolic pressure distally to a band indicates insufficient banding of the pulmonary artery, while in the presence of pulmonary hypertension, diastolic and mean pressure increase accordingly.

Atrioventricular Valve Anatomy. Echo may provide detailed assessment of anatomy and function of both atrioventricular valves, whereas ACG in most cases allows to detect only the presence of AVSD. Despite common atrioventricular valve, AVSD is characterized by shortening of the inlet and relative elongation of the outlet part of the IVS (see Fig. 2.17 in Chap. 2), which may be seen on ACG as a «goose neck» sign (Fig. 10).

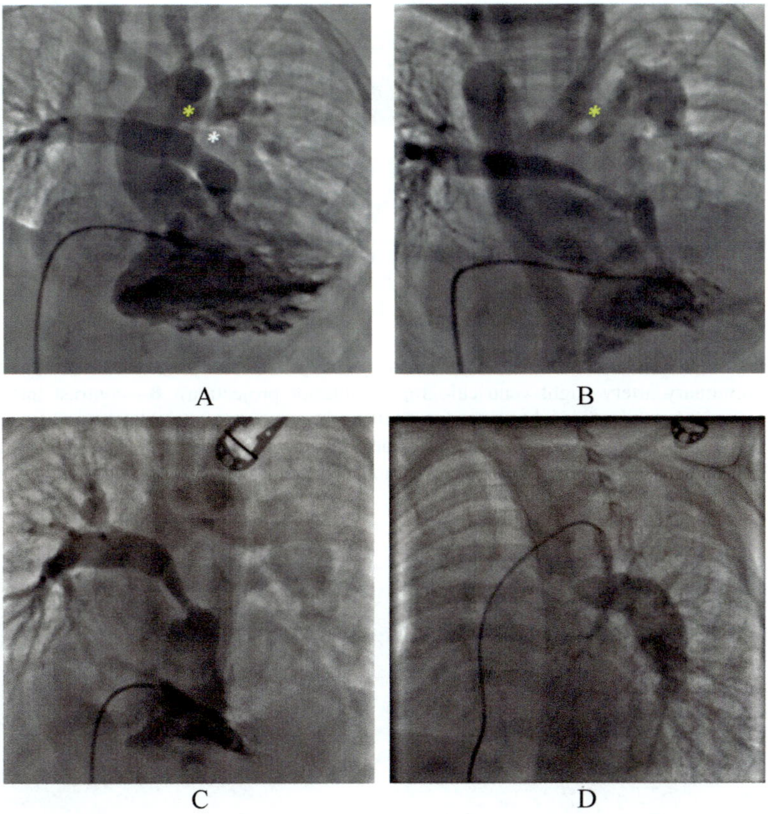

Fig. 8 DORV «tetralogy» type with unilateral absence of the left pulmonary artery: **A**—no opacification (white asterisk) between the pulmonary trunk and the hilar artery which receives blood through the patent ductus arteriosus (yellow asterisk) (right ventriculography, anterior projection); **B**—a similar situation as in the panel A but with right aortic arch and mirror-imaged branching of brachiocephalic arteries; the hilar artery receives blood from the patent ductus arteriosus (yellow asterisk) arising from the brachiocephalic trunk (right ventriculography, anterior projection); **C**—no opacification of the left pulmonary artery (right ventriculography, anterior projection); **D**—blood supply to the hilar artery is provided by the systemic-to-pulmonary shunt

Coronary Artery Anatomy. Due to spiral course and normal relationship of the arterial trunks, in most cases, anatomy of the coronary arteries remains normal. It is of practical importance for these types of DORV to determine the presence and size of infundibular branch of the right coronary artery crossing RVOT as it may preclude transannular repair if nedeed.

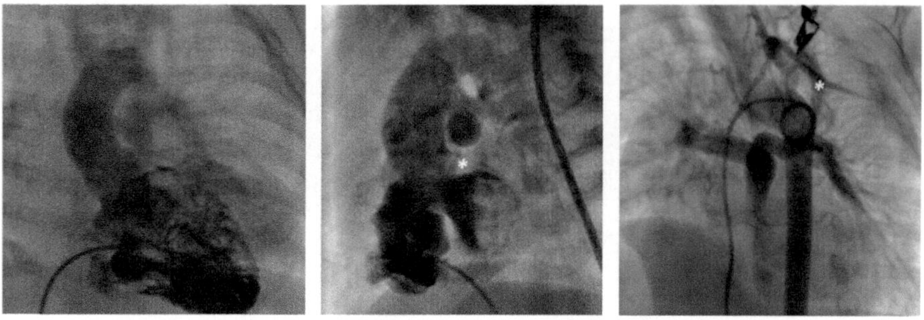
A B C

Fig. 9 DORV with subaortic VSD and pulmonary artery atresia: **A**—no antegrade opacification of the pulmonary artery (right ventriculography, anterior projection); **B**—contrast interruption (white asterisk) between the right ventricle and the pulmonary artery (right ventriculography, left lateral projection); **C**—the pulmonary arteries are opacified through the systemic-to-pulmonary shunt (yellow asterisk); the stump of the pulmonary trunk is visualized (aortography, anterior projection)

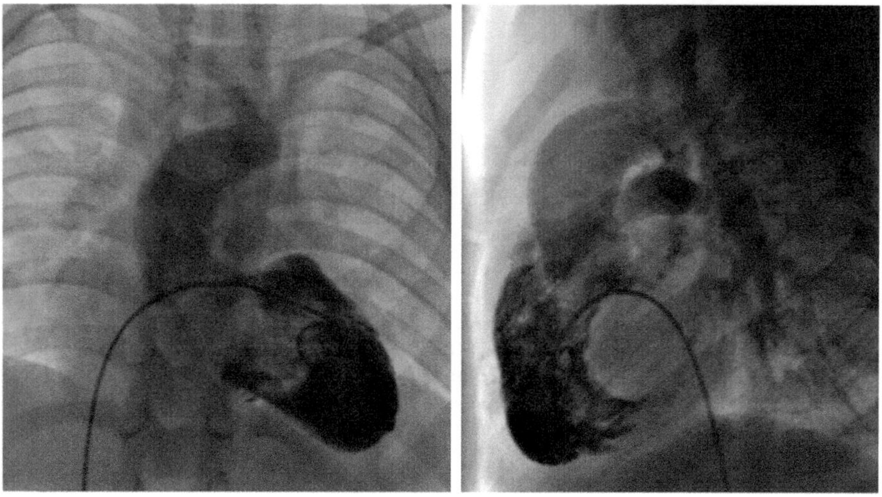
A B

Fig. 10 DORV/AVSD and pulmonary artery stenosis: **A** and **B**—left ventriculography, anterior and left lateral projections, respectively. A typical ACG sign of AVSD is a «goose neck» due to shortening of the inlet part and relative elongation of the outlet part of the IVS

1.2 DORV «TGA» Type

ACG assessment protocol:

- VSD location;

- relationship and course of the arterial trunks;
- orientation of the OS;
- subaortic obstruction;
- aortic arch obstruction;
- pulmonary artery anatomy;
- coronary artery anatomy.

VSD Location. On left ventriculography, opacification of the pulmonary artery is visualized first due to its proximity to VSD (Fig. 11A). Because of the aorta locates right/right anterior to the pulmonary artery and is separated from it and VSD by the OS, opacification of the ascending aorta occurs after the pulmonary artery. The degree of pulmonary artery overriding depends on size of the VIF interposed between the mitral and the pulmonary artery valves: the smaller the VIF the more the pulmonary valve is displaced toward the left ventricle and vice versa.

Relationship and Course of the Arterial Trunks. In the vast majority of cases, the aorta locates right (D-aorta) or right anterior (DA-aorta) to the pulmonary artery (Fig. 11B). In rare cases, anteroposterior relationship of the arterial trunks (A-aorta) can be observed, so that only the ascending aorta is visualized in anterior projection, while in lateral projection both trunks with the OS between them are well recognized. In subpulmonary VSD spiral twisting of the aorta and the pulmonary artery is never observed, so the course of the arterial trunks in DORV «TGA» type is always parallel.

Orientation of the OS. Assessment of the OS orientation is an important part of examination due to its possible deviation with corresponding consequences. Rightward deviation of the OS causes not only subaortic stenosis but in some cases also leads to different types of aortic arch obstructions due to limitation of blood flow

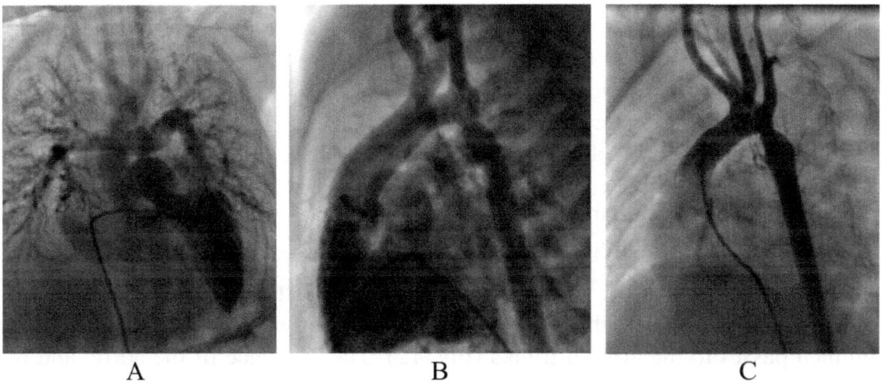

Fig. 11 DORV «TGA» type after palliative pulmonary artery banding and coarctation repair: **A** and **B**—VSD locates in subpulmonary area, both arterial trunks predominantly originate from the right ventricle, the aorta locates to the right and anterior to the pulmonary artery, the OS separates subarterial infundibulums (left ventriculography, anterior and left lateral projections, respectively); **C**—narrowing of the aortic isthmus with aberrant right subclavian artery (*arteria lusoria*) (aortography)

into the ascending aorta. In turn, leftward deviation of the OS leads to formation of subpulmonary stenosis.

Subaortic Obstruction. The morphological substrate of subaortic obstruction is represented by the VIF and the OS deviated to the right which is relatively frequent in Taussig-Bing hearts.

Aortic Arch Obstruction. One of the mechanisms of aortic arch obstruction is insufficient hemodynamic load, which in Taussig-Bing anomaly occurs due to rightward deviation of the OS and thus limited blood flow into the ascending aorta. Morphologically arch obstruction may be represented by coarctation with or without arch hypoplasia, or different types of interrupted aortic arch (Fig. 7.11C).

Pulmonary Artery Anatomy. One of the main signs of Taussig-Bing anomaly is a large pulmonary artery which can sometimes be twice the diameter of the ascending aorta. Concomitant stenosis of the pulmonary arteries is detected when the OS is deviated to subpulmonary area.

Coronary Artery Anatomy. Assessment of the coronary arteries is one of the main parts of preoperative evaluation of DORV «TGA» type regarding ASO as well as other alternative surgical techniques requiring coronary artery reimplantation (see Chap. 10). Detection of looping and intramural course of the coronary arteries is critically important. In some cases of pulmonary artery stenosis when aortic tunneling along with RVOT reconstruction is planned, it is important to evaluate the presence and size of an infundibular branch of the right coronary artery potentially impeding transannular repair.

1.3 DORV with Non-committed VSD

ACG assessment protocol:

- VSD location;
- OS;
- subaortic obstruction;
- aortic arch obstruction;
- pulmonary artery anatomy;
- coronary artery anatomy.

VSD Location. On left ventriculography the contrast agent before passing into the ascending aorta enters the right ventricle significantly mixing with venous blood and then passes to the arterial trunks (Fig. 12). The sequence of the aortic and the pulmonary artery opacification is of great diagnostic importance. If VSD is closer to the aortic valve, then the contrast agent will first pass to the aorta and then to the pulmonary artery minimally mixing with venous blood in the right ventricle which results in mild cyanosis (except if cyanosis is caused by pulmonary artery stenosis). When VSD is closer to the pulmonary valve, the contrast agent goes first to pulmonary artery and then to the ascending aorta. Cyanosis in such a case is severe because significant mixing of arterial and venous blood in the right ventricle. If VSD

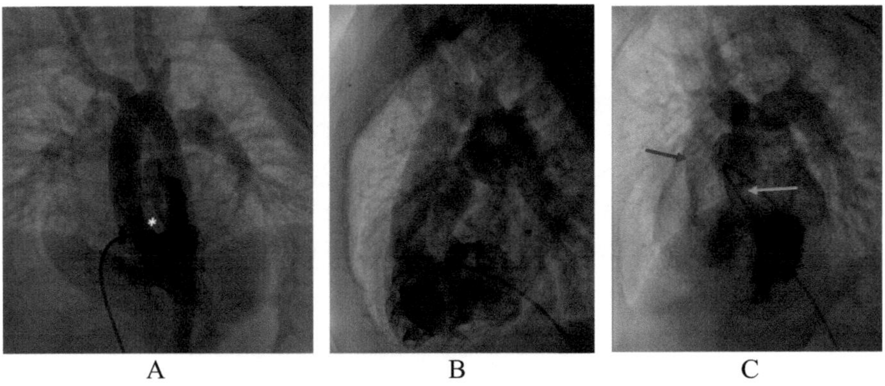

Fig. 12 DORV with non-committed (inlet) VSD after palliative pulmonary artery banding: **A** and **B**—hypertrophy of the OS (asterisk) causing subaortic obstruction, aorta is right and anterior to the pulmonary artery (right ventriculography, anterior and left lateral projections, respectively); **C**—VSD locates in the inlet IVS and is remote from both arterial valves (red and blue arrows point at the aortic and the pulmonary valves, respectively) (left ventriculography, left anterior oblique projection)

is equally distant from both arterial valves, then both arterial trunks are opacified simultaneously.

One of the main characteristics of «non-committed» type of DORV is high position of the aortic valve above the right ventricle due to prominent subaortic infundibulum, which lifts the aortic valve and makes it remote from inlet VSD. This anatomical feature can indirectly serve as a differential criterion with subaortic VSD. In addition, delayed opacification of the arterial trunks on left ventriculography, severe hypertrophy of the OS and the VIF, more frequent subaortic stenosis, as well as aortic arch obstruction are the supportive signs in favor of non-committed VSD.

OS. In this type of DORV, the OS is usually severely hypertrophied which may cause subaortic and subpulmonary obstruction (Fig. 13).

Subaortic Obstruction. The morphological substrate of subaortic obstruction is mainly represented by the hypertrophied VIF and the OS.

Aortic Arch Obstruction. See DORV «TGA» type.

Pulmonary Artery Anatomy. See DORV «tetralogy» and «VSD» types.

Coronary Artery Anatomy. See DORV «TGA» type.

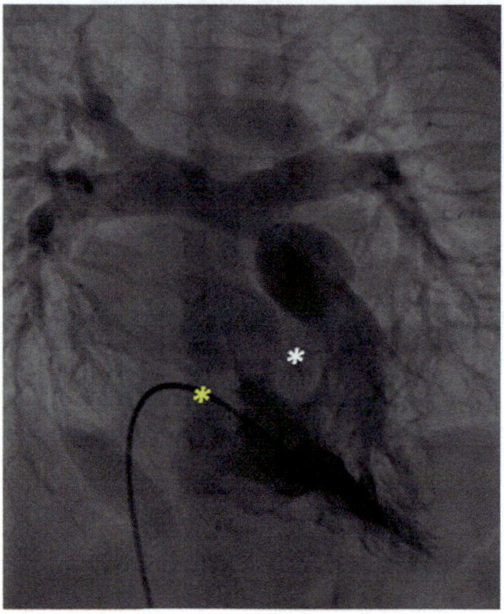

Fig. 13 DORV with non-committed (inlet) VSD after palliative pulmonary artery banding. Malposed arterial trunks (D-aorta). «Drop»-shaped hypertrophied OS is clearly visualized (white asterisk) which in couple with the VIF (yellow asterisk) causes subaortic obstruction

1.4 DORV with L-Aorta

Although DORV with L-aorta may be associated with any type of VSD, mostly the defect locates in subaortic area (see Chap. 2). The main ACG sign of the malformation is that the aorta is positioned anterior and left to the pulmonary artery (Fig. 14).

2 Postoperative Investigation

The main and most common complications after biventricular repair of DORV include:

- residual VSD;
- RVOT aneurism;
- RVOT and pulmonary artery stenosis;
- LVOT obstruction.

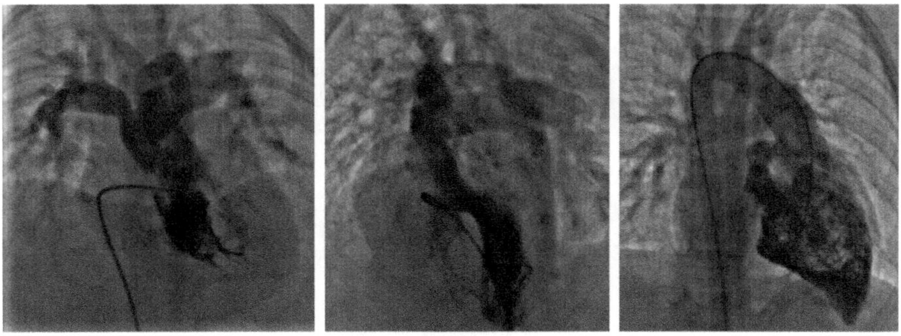

Fig. 14 DORV with L-aorta and subpulmonary VSD: **A**—right ventriculography, anterior projection. Both arterial trunks originate from the right ventricle, the aorta locates anterior and left to the pulmonary artery (L-malposition). Subvalvular pulmonary artery stenosis; **B**—left ventriculography, left anterior oblique projection. Additional trabecular apical VSD is seen; **C**—right ventriculography, anterior projection

2.1 Residual VSD

Residual VSD is one of the most frequent complications in patients with repaired DORV and may occur both in early and late postoperative periods. Usually, residual shunting occurs on the suture line, especially at the sites of the resected myocardium which were not reinforced by pledgeted sutures (Fig. 15). Sometimes, shunting may be caused by so-called intramural VSD as a result of applying a patch to a trabecula of the right ventricle instead of the rims of VSD (see DORV «tetralogy» and «TGA» types in Chap. 10).

2.2 RVOT Aneurism

RVOT aneurism is usually formed late after surgery and can develop both after patch reconstruction and an extracardiac biological conduit implantation. Aneurism itself is asymptomatic and in most cases leads to right ventricle overload (Fig. 16). Also, aneurism sac tightly adheres to the sternum, and its preoperative detection is extremely important for safe repeat sternotomy.

2.3 RVOT and Pulmonary Artery Stenosis

Residual obstructive lesions of RVOT and pulmonary arteries can manifest as infundibular stenosis and pulmonary artery stenosis of various location and severity.

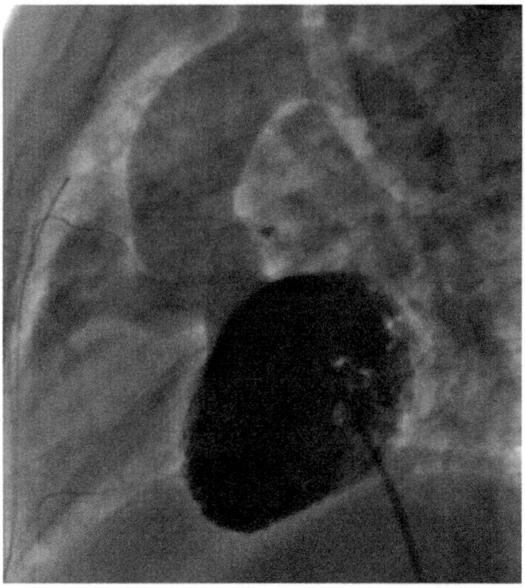

Fig. 15 Residual left to right shunting after repair of DORV «tetralogy» type

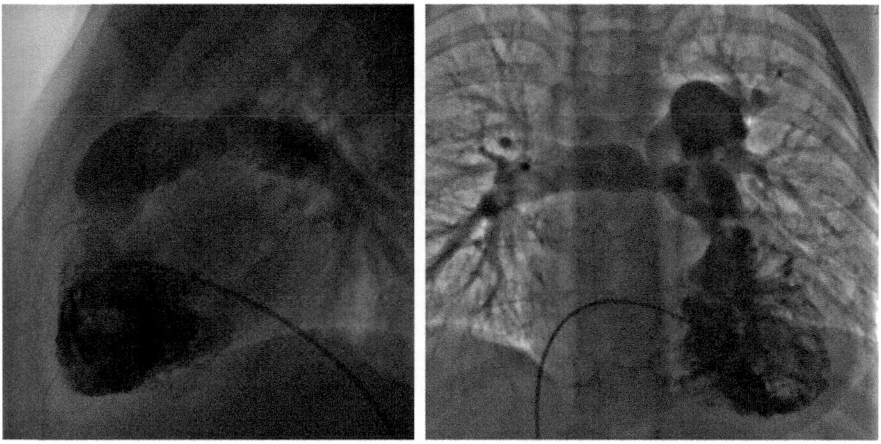

A B

Fig. 16 RVOT aneurism: **A**—patch aneurism after repair of DORV «tetralogy» type; **B** – aneurism of an extracardiac xenograft

As a rule, residual infundibular stenosis occurs due to incomplete resection of muscle structures contributing to initial subvalvular stenosis (Fig. 17A). In addition, ongoing right ventricular hypertrophy due to residual afterload and preload may significantly progress stenosis.

Residual pulmonary artery stenosis usually develops in combination with infundibular stenosis and most often locates at the site of bifurcation (Fig. 17B).

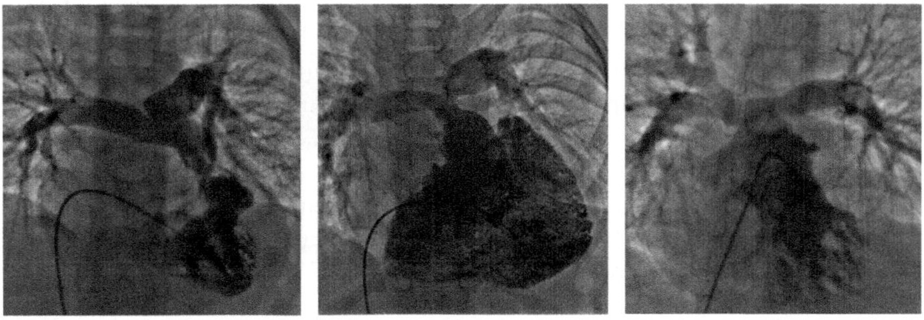

A B C

Fig. 17 Residual right-sided obstruction after anatomical repair of DORV: **A**—infundibular stenosis; **B**—left pulmonary artery stenosis; **C**—stenosis at the bifurcation site due to the Lecompte maneuver after ASO (Taussig-Bing anomaly)

Sometimes, stenosis may develop at the site of systemic-to-pulmonary shunt. After ASO branch pulmonary artery stenosis develops due to the Lecompte maneuver (Fig. 17C).

2.4 LVOT Obstruction

Intraventricular tunnel obstruction is the most serious complication after biventricular repair of DORV which finally leads to the necessity of reoperation. Hemodynamically significant stenosis should be considered when peak systolic pressure gradient exceeds 40–50 mmHg.

In the presence of local narrowing, usually located just under the aortic valve, balloon angioplasty in most cases is inefficient and can only lead to a temporary decrease in pressure gradient and systolic load on the left ventricle, and therefore, reintervention is required. Diffuse obstruction is usually caused by hypertrophied muscular elements of the OS, muscular rims of VSD involved in a tunnel, as well as the VIF between the mitral and the aortic valves limiting the egress from the left ventricle (Fig. 18).

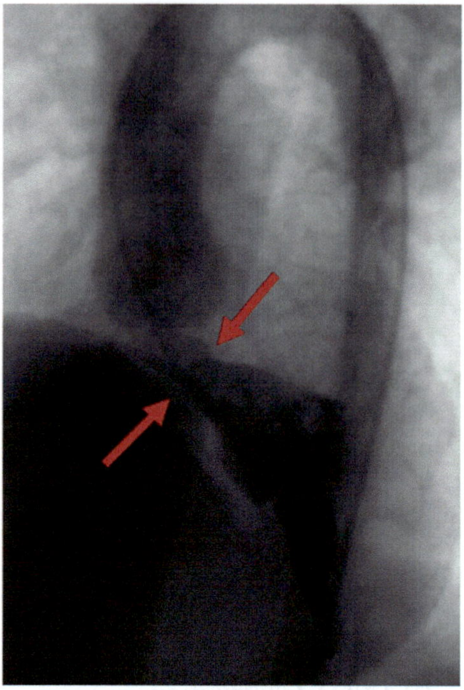

Fig. 18 Intraventricular tunnel obstruction after the aortic tunneling to the left ventricle (red arrows)

References

1. Pang KJ, Meng H, Hu SS, Wang H, Hsi D, Hua ZD, Pan XB, Li SJ. Echocardiographic classification and surgical approaches to double-outlet right ventricle for great arteries arising almost exclusively from the right ventricle. Tex Heart Inst J. 2017;44:245–51.
2. Pushparajah K, Anna BA, Hons BA, Tran V, Miller OI, Zidere V, Vaidyanathan B, Simpson JMA. Systematic three-dimensional echocardiographic approach to assist surgical planning in double outlet right ventricle. Echocardiography. 2013;30:234–8.
3. Mahle WT, Martinez R, Silverman N, Cohen MS, Anderson RH. Anatomy, echocardiography, and surgical approach to double outlet right ventricle. Cardiol Young. 2008;18:S39-51.
4. Smallhorn JF. Double-outlet right ventricle: an echocardiographic approach. Pediatric Cardiac Surgery Annual of the Seminars in Thoracic and Cardiovascular Surgery. 2000;3:20–33.
5. Macartney FJ, Rigby ML, Anderson RH, Stark J, Silverman NH. Double outlet right ventricle. Cross sectional echocardiographic findings, their anatomical explanation, and surgical relevance. British Heart J. 1984;52:164–177.
6. Martinez OA, Casado JA, de la Cruz MV, Diaz F, Cubero O. Double outlet right ventricle—an echocardiographic study. Cardiol Young. 1993;3:124–31.
7. Yoo S, Spray T, Austin EH, Yun T, Van Arsdell GS. Hands-on surgical training of congenital heart surgery using 3-dimensional print models. J Thorac Cardiovasc Surg. 2017;153:1530–40.
8. Xu J, Luo Y, Wang J, Xu W, Shi Z, Fu J, Shu Q. Patient-specific three-dimensional printed heart models benefit preoperative planning for complex congenital heart disease. World J Pediatrics. 2019. https://doi.org/10.1007/s12519-019-00228-4.
9. Meier LM, Meineri M, Hiansen JQ, Horlick EM. Structural and congenital heart disease interventions: the role of three-dimensional printing. Neth Hear J. 2017;25:65–75.

10. Vettukattil JJ, Nijres BM, Gosnell JM, Samuel BP, Haw MP. Three-dimensional printing for surgical planning in complex congenital heart disease. J Cardiac Surgery. 2019;1–7. https://doi.org/10.1111/ocs.14180
11. Samuel BP, Pinto C, Pietila T, Vetukattil JJ. Ultrasound three-dimensional printing in congenital heart disease. J Digit Imaging. 2015;28:459–61.
12. Sun Z, Lau I, Wong YH, Yeong CH. Personalized three-dimensional printed models in congenital heart disease. J Clin Med. 2019. https://doi.org/10.3390/jcm8040522.
13. Freedom RM, Yoo SL. Double-outlet right ventricle: pathology and angiocardiography. Pediatric Cardiac Surgery Annual of Seminars in Thoracic and Cardiovascular Surgery. 2000;3:3–19.
14. *Baron M.G.* Angiographic differentiation between tetralogy of Fallot and double-outlet right ventricle. Relationship of the mitral and aortic valves. *Circulation.* 1971.43:451–455
15. Hallerman FJ, Kincaid OW, Ritter DG, Titus JL Mitral-semilunar valve relationships in the angiography of cardiac malformations. Radiology. 1970;94:63–68.
16. Hallerman FJ, Kincaid OW, Ritter DG, Ongley PA, Titus JL. Angiocardiographic and anatomic findings in origin of both great arteries from the right ventricle. Am J Roentgenol Radium Ther Nucl Med. 1970;109:51–66.
17. Coelho E, Paiva E, Nunes A, Amram SS. Origin of both great vessels from the right ventricle with pulmonary stenosis. Am Heart J. 1963;65:766–73.

Computed Tomography

K. M. Dzhidzhikhiya

Abstract Echo being a first-line diagnostic tool allows quickly and easily evaluate intracardiac anatomy of DORV. However, in some cases, when there is a need of precise assessment of intra- and extracardiac anatomy computer tomography (CT) may be necessary. In compared to ACG, CT appears as a less invasive procedure and allows to accurately assess any area of interest from different projections simultaneously. In this regard, multiplanar reconstruction serves as a method of advanced evaluation of anatomy but requires certain manual skills in deriving individual projections from different planes and appropriate knowledge of complex anatomy of DORV. By CT a set of three-dimensional high-resolution images can be obtained in an extremely short scanning period, which makes it a valuable diagnostic tool for newborns and young children. Ultimately, the goal of CT when diagnosing DORV is to analyze anatomical components of the malformation that are necessary for the surgeon to make a correct preoperative decision-making among which the most important ones are VSD type, the presence of pulmonary artery stenosis and tricuspid-to-pulmonary valve distance.

Keywords Double-outlet right ventricle · Diagnostics · Computer tomography

Echo being a first-line diagnostic tool allows quickly and easily evaluate intracardiac anatomy of DORV. However, in some cases, when there is a need to obtain additional data about extracardiac components of the disease (aortic arch obstruction, insufficient visualization of the pulmonary arteries, major aortopulmonary collateral arteries, pulmonary veins anomalies, anomalous drainage of the systemic, pulmonary and hepatic veins) CT-angiography or MRI may be necessary [1–11].

CT-angiography has a higher resolution compared to echo and does not depend on the subjective judgment of the specialist. In turn, diagnostic value of ACG may be limited by poor opacification of heart chambers, erroneous interpretation due to

K. M. Dzhidzhikhiya (✉)
Department of Emergency Surgery of Congenital Heart Diseases, A. N. Bakulev National Medical Investigation Center for Cardiovascular Surgery, Moscow, Russia
e-mail: d.m.konstantine@mail.ru

K. V. Shatalov and K. M. Dzhidzhikhiya (eds.), *Double-Outlet Right Ventricle*,
https://doi.org/10.1007/978-3-031-49707-0_8

overlapping of cardiac structures as well as difficulties in catheterization of femoral vessels in a number of cases [5]. CT-angiography in DORV appears as a less invasive procedure, and allows to accurately assess any area of interest from different projections simultaneously. In this regard, multiplanar mode allows obtaining almost complete information about intracardiac details but requires certain skills in deriving individual projections from different planes and appropriate knowledge of complex anatomy of DORV.

CT also allows to obtain a set of three-dimensional high-resolution images in an extremely short scanning period, which makes it a valuable diagnostic tool for newborns and young children, as general sedation is not needed. One of the main related problems is radiation load, which correlates with image quality, especially with ECG-synchronization. Despite technological progress and development of CT scans that provide low radiation load, frequent use of the method in a same patient should be limited, especially in young children, as X-rays have an impact on a genetic apparatus. CT-angiography is a method of choice when MRI cannot provide necessary data for decision-making, for example, when evaluating anatomy of respiratory tract and lungs, pulmonary veins, major aortopulmonary collateral arteries (their number and diameter), in the presence of metal implants, as well as when MRI is contraindicated.

The appearance of method of 3D computer reconstruction has revolutionized and significantly simplified the diagnosis of complex forms of DORV due to its ability to assess anatomy of the disease taking into account relationships of all intracardiac and extracardiac structures, which is a significant limitation for two-dimensional models. The method of 3D reconstruction is the result of postprocessing of primary data and allows specialists to visualize an area of interest from an arbitrary angle [12–15]. Also, this method gives clear picture of location of anatomical structures and allows their accurate and detailed assessment, which makes it useful for preoperative planning. At the same time, structures with high density can hide other structures with equal or lower density. This problem can be solved by manual or automatic removal of outer layers with a higher density, which allows to obtain reconstruction of an area of interest with different degrees of transparency.

Ultimately, the goal of CT-angiography when diagnosing DORV is to analyze anatomical components of the malformation that are necessary for the surgeon to make a correct preoperative decision-making.

Anatomical correction of DORV involves tunneling of the aorta or the pulmonary artery to the left ventricle, which depends on VSD location and its proximity to the arterial valves. When tunneling aorta in order to create a nonobstructive tunnel, it is necessary to estimate tricuspid-to-pulmonary valve distance, which should be greater than the aortic valve diameter. In turn, the type of anatomical correction primarily depends on the presence of pulmonary artery stenosis. In this regard, when analyzing CT images, it is of primary goal to first clearly determine:

- VSD type;
- tricuspid-to-pulmonary valve distance;
- pulmonary artery stenosis.

1 VSD Type

Since VSD is a key characteristic of DORV, determination of its type, size and commitment to the arterial valves is a primary diagnostic task. Committed VSDs on CT-angiography are presented by contrasting of the outlet IVS due to left to right shunting, while the inlet IVS is intact (Fig. 1B). Non-committed VSDs own to their location are characterized by contrasting of the inlet IVS.

When committed VSD is detected, the next stage is to access its proximity to the arterial valves. For this, the angle of a particular plane should be changed so as to find the point «left ventricle-VSD-arterial valve», on which direct flow of contrasted blood from the left ventricle to the aorta/pulmonary artery can be clearly visualized (Figs. 1, 2, 3, 4, 5, and 6).

In some cases, it is difficult to visualize the IVS especially with poor opacification. So, it can be difficult to distinguish subaortic VSD (especially not directly committed) from non-committed VSD. Differential diagnostic signs in favor of non-committed VSD can be a high position of the aortic valve above the right ventricle and severe hypertrophy of the OS, which serves as a morphological substrate of subaortic stenosis, as well as obstructive lesions of the aortic arch, which is not typical for subaortic VSD.

VSD size must be determined in at least two mutually perpendicular projections due to its oval shape in most cases.

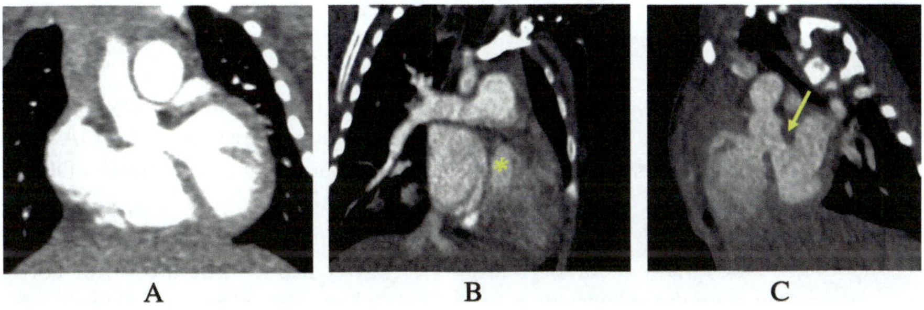

Fig. 1 DORV with subaortic VSD: **A**—the aorta overrides the IVS; subpulmonary infundibulum is not seen; transverse axis of the pulmonary artery and longitudinal axis of the ascending aorta are visualized in the same plain, which indicates their spiral course; **B**—VSD locates in the outlet IVS (asterisk) while the inlet component is intact; **C**—straight exit from the left ventricle to the ascending aorta; mitral-aortic muscular continuity is seen (arrow) (see Fig. 2 in Chapter 9)

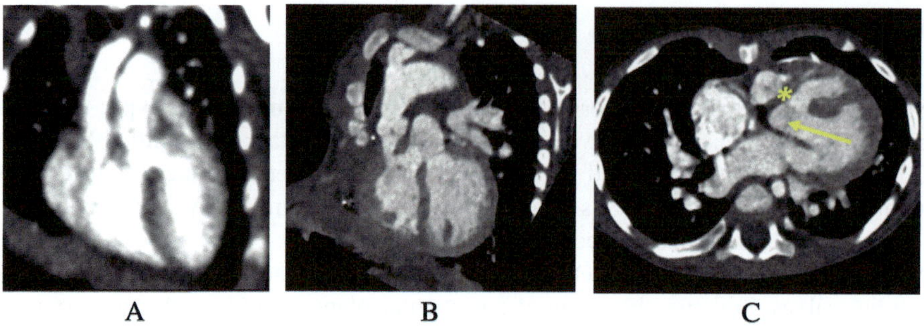

Fig. 2 DORV with subpulmonary VSD and subaortic obstruction: **A**—the pulmonary artery overrides the IVS; the aorta is right and anterior to the pulmonary artery and significantly remote from the VSD; longitudinal axes of the arterial trunks are visualized in the same plane—parallel course of the trunks; **B**—the pulmonary artery seems to be predominantly (≈60%/40%) originating from the left ventricle—anatomically transitional form with TGA; the OS is deviated to the right and anterior causing subaortic obstruction; **C**—straight exit from the left ventricle to the pulmonary artery (arrow); subaortic infundibulum is completely separated from the VSD by the OS (asterisk) (see Fig. 4 in Chapter 9)

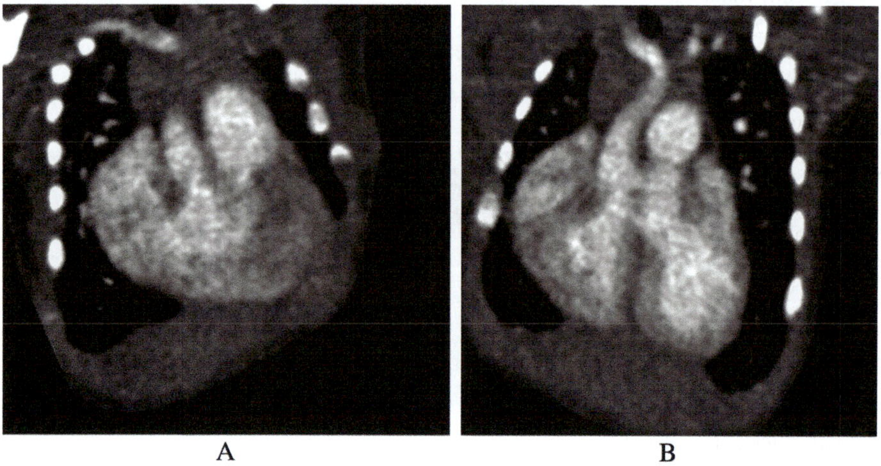

Fig. 3 DORV with subarterial VSD and the OS: **A**—aorta and pulmonary artery are separated by the OS and originate from the right ventricle (parallel course of the trunks); **B**—straight exit from the left ventricle to the both arterial trunks through the VSD (see Fig. 5 in Chapter 9)

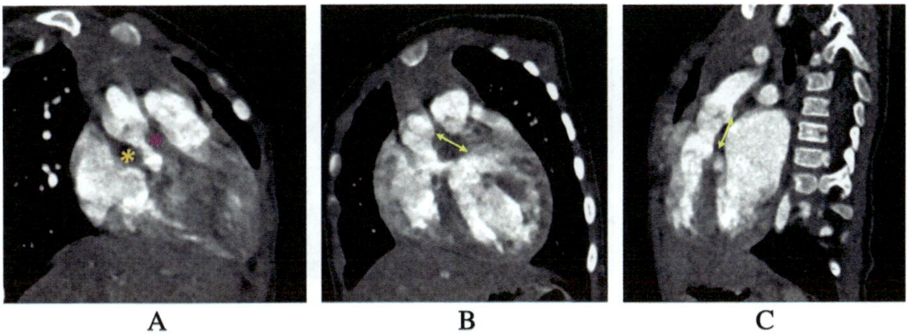

Fig. 4 DORV with not directly committed restrictive subaortic VSD: **A**—the VSD locates in subaortic area in the outlet IVS; hypertrophy of the OS (violet asterisk) and the VIF (orange asterisk) is clearly visualized, which serve as substrates of subaortic obstruction (parallel course of the trunks); **B**—elongated subaortic conus (mitral-aortic muscular continuity) which remotes the aortic valve from the VSD (arrow); there is a direct communication between the left ventricle and the ascending aorta; subpulmonary infundibulum is separated from the VSD by the OS; **C**—elongated subaortic conus (arrow) causing in couple with the IVS restrictive nature of the VSD (see Fig. 3 in Chapter 9)

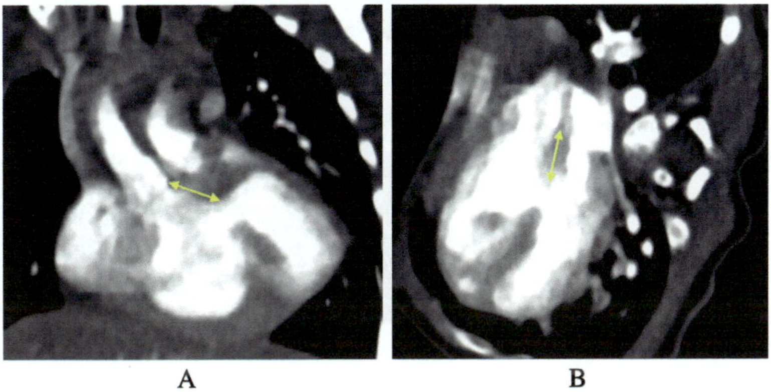

Fig. 5 DORV with non-committed VSD: **A**—the VSD locates in the inlet IVS. The distance between the VSD and the arterial valves (arrow) exceeds the diameter of the aortic valve; **B**—elongated subaortic conus (arrow) (see Fig. 6 in Chapter 9)

2 Tricuspid-to-Pulmonary Valve Distance

When planning biventricular repair with aortic tunneling to the left ventricle, tricuspid-to-pulmonary valve distance is a reliable indicator of nonobstructive intraventricular tunnel since this dimension determines its width. The distance can be estimated from individual «tricuspid valve-pulmonary valve» projection, and, if possible, it is important to conduct a cut through the middle of the aortic valve (Fig. 7).

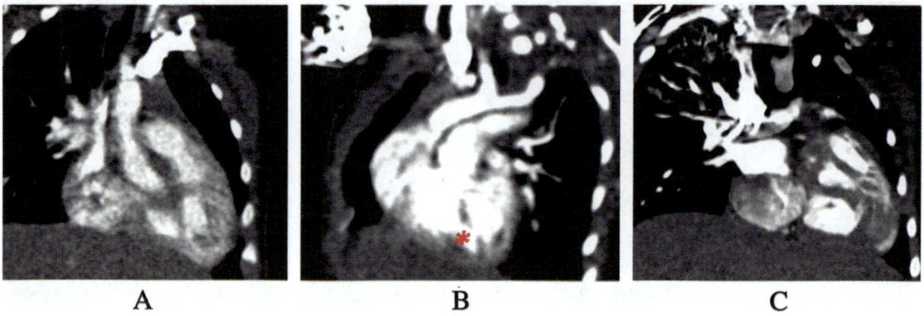

Fig. 6 DORV with multiple VSDs: **A**—the both arterial trunks originate from the right ventricle; two VSDs located in the inlet and trabecular IVS are visualized; **B**—the pulmonary artery predominantly originates from the right ventricle and overrides one of the VSDs; additional VSD locates in the inlet IVS (asterisk); **C**—three large VSDs in different parts of the IVS are visualized—functionally univentricular heart

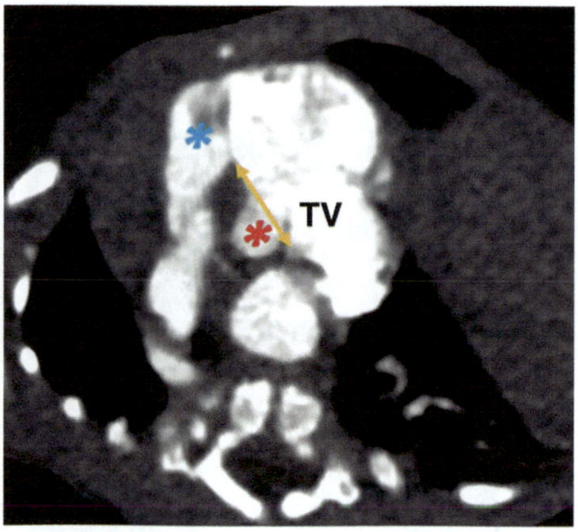

Fig. 7 DORV with subaortic VSD. Tricuspid-to-pulmonary valve distance (arrow) measured between the tricuspid septal leaflet and subpulmonary conus (blue asterisk) exceeds the diameter of the aortic valve (red asterisk). *TV – tricuspid valve*

Within the usual relationship of the arterial trunks (DP-aorta) or as long as the aorta locates behind or to the right to the pulmonary artery (D-aorta) tricuspid-to-pulmonary valve distance is usually sufficient to create a wide tunnel (see Fig. 4 in Chapter 10). If the aorta locates in front and to the right to the pulmonary artery (DA-aorta), then specialist should proceed with assessment of tricuspid-to-pulmonary valve distance, because interposition of the pulmonary artery in the tunnel projection is likely to occur, that may complicate tunnel construction.

3 Pulmonary Artery Stenosis

Pulmonary artery obstructive lesions are relatively frequent in DORV and most often found in patients with «tetralogy» type (Fig. 8). Preoperative evaluation of pulmonary arteries is of exceptional importance for surgical decision-making. Assessment of infundibular stenosis is best achieved by echo. In this regard, the main task of CT-angiography is to evaluate pulmonary artery branches, especially their distal segments.

Obstructive lesions of pulmonary arteries can be represented by local and diffuse variants. Assessment of confluence of pulmonary arteries is especially important. In case of pulmonary valve atresia, it is necessary to assess major aortopulmonary collateral arteries, which can also complicate early postoperative course due to pulmonary overcirculation and resulting respiratory disorders.

Another extremely rare variant of nonconfluent pulmonary circulation is unilateral absence of pulmonary artery. Blood supply to ipsilateral lung in this case is provided

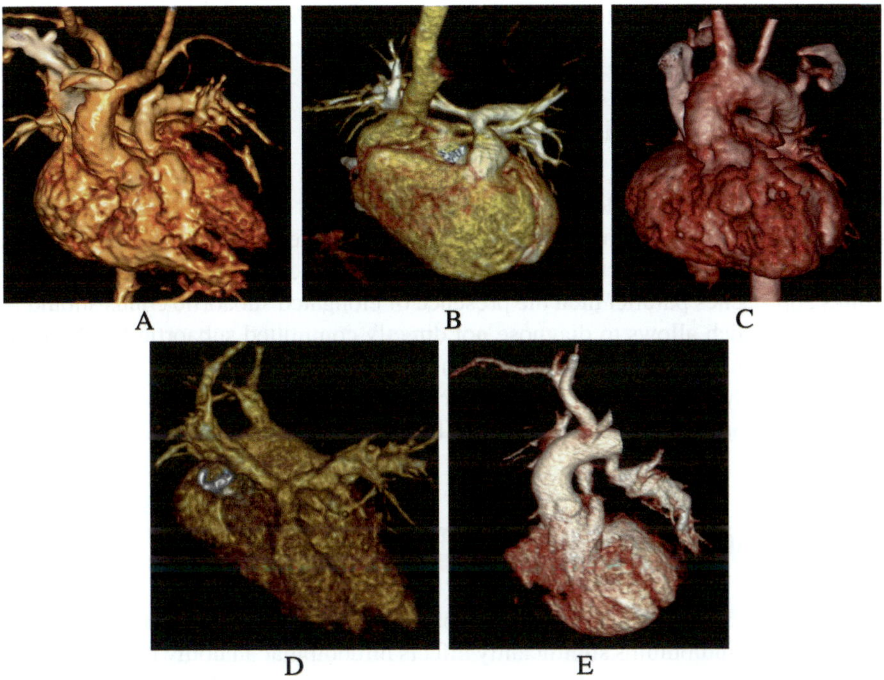

Fig. 8 Pulmonary artery obstructive lesions in DORV (3D reconstructions): **A**—pulmonary valvular stenosis; **B**—diffuse hypoplasia of the right pulmonary artery; **C**—pulmonary artery atresia (type I); contrast interruption between the right ventricle and the pulmonary artery; **D**—hypoplasia of the pulmonary artery system; **E**—unilateral absence of the left pulmonary artery; contrast interruption between the pulmonary trunk and the left hilar artery; blood supply is provided through the patent ductus arteriosus

either through patent ductus arteriosus or systematic-to-pulmonary shunt [16]. If there is no alternative blood flow in distal part of an absent pulmonary artery (so-called hilar artery), then ipsilateral lung should be evaluated for its hypoplasia or fibrosis as well as anatomy of compromised bronchi and vessels [17].

4 Arterial Valves Relationship

Relationship of the arterial valves is assessed on the axial plane as an angle between their axis (a line drawn through the centers of the arterial valves) and frontal plane. This angle is determined by degree of conotruncal rotation in embryonic period. In DORV «tetralogy» and «VSD» types course of the arterial trunks is usually spiral and angle of rightward rotation of the conotruncus is approximately 30–40° (Fig. 9A). In all other types of DORV, parallel course of the trunks with different degrees of rotation is seen (Fig. 9B, C). In Taussig-Bing anomaly with DA-aorta leftward rotation of the conotruncus takes place, and therefore, the axis of the arterial valves is oriented mirror-imaged compared to DORV «tetralogy» type (Fig. 9D).

5 Course of the Arterial Trunks

In the vast majority DORV «tetralogy» and «VSD» types are characterized by spiral course of the arterial trunks with the aorta located right and posterior to the pulmonary artery (DP-aorta) (Fig. 10A). If in subaortic VSD course of the arterial trunks approaches parallel then the presence of elongated subaortic conus should be suspected, which allows to diagnose not directly committed subaortic VSD, and in this case it is useful to measure the length of the conus.

All other types of DORV are characterized by parallel course of the trunks regardless of arterial valves relationship (Fig. 10B–E).

6 Orientation, Deviation and Size of the OS

The OS being an anatomical structure separating the arterial valves and accordingly subarterial infundibulums significantly affects infundibular anatomy if it is deviated. So, separating subarterial infundibulums the OS is perpendicular to the axis of the arterial valves. Thus, based on the OS orientation, it is possible to determine the axis of the arterial valves and vice versa.

The final position of the OS is the result of rotation of the conotruncus during embryogenesis, on which arterial valves relationship depends. On CT-angiography orientation of the OS is easily assessed on a cross-section at the level of the arterial valves. If the OS is oriented in sagittal plane and axis of the arterial valves is oriented

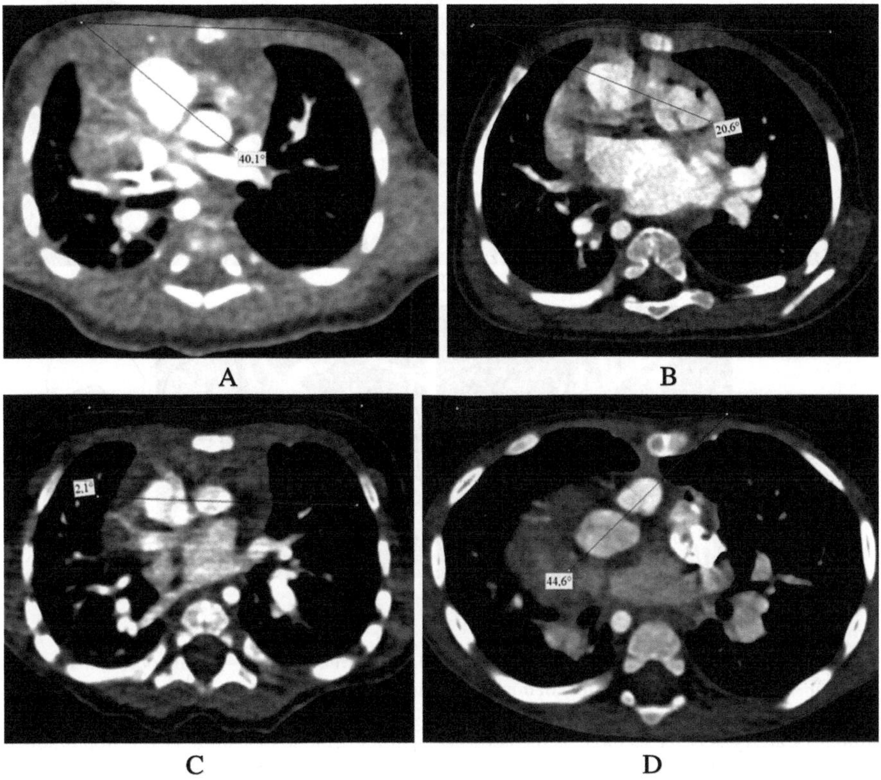

Fig. 9 Arterial valves relationship (i.e. angle of conotruncal rotation) in different types of DORV seen on the axial scans (view from above): **A**—«VSD» type; **B**—not directly committed subaortic VSD; **C**—non-committed type; **D**—Taussig-Bing anomaly with anterior and right aorta (conotruncal rotation to the left)

in frontal plane, then this indicates parallel course of the arterial trunks (Fig. 9C). If the arterial valves axis rotated to the right and oriented at an angle closer to 30°–40° relative to the frontal plane, then the course of the arterial trunks will be spiral, which indicates rightward rotation of the conotruncus and corresponding reorientation of the OS (Fig. 9A–B). Leftward rotation of the axis of the arterial valves also indicates corresponding conotruncal rotation and reorientation of the OS, which is typical for DORV with subpulmonary VSD with DA-aorta (Fig. 9D).

Deviation of the OS towards any subarterial infundibulums leads to either subaortic or subpulmonary stenosis. An anterolateral deviation of the OS in DORV with subaortic VSD leads to subvalvular pulmonary artery stenosis as it occurs in tetralogy of Fallot—«tetralogy» type of DORV. Thus, with spiral course of the arterial trunks, the OS can deviate to subpulmonary infundibulum. On the other hand, with parallel course of the trunks, the OS can deviate both to subpulmonary and subaortic infundibulums. The latter is common for Taussig-Bing anomaly with aortic arch obstruction (Fig. 2B).

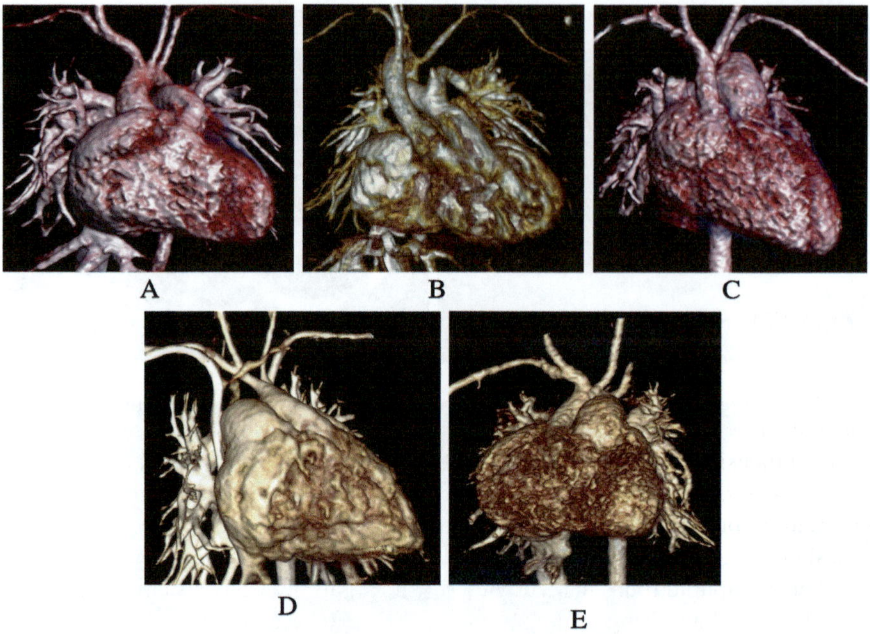

Fig. 10 Course of the arterial trunks in DORV (3D reconstruction): **A**—spiral course in subaortic VSD (DP-aorta); **B**—parallel course in non-committed VSD (D-aorta); the aorta and the pulmonary artery are almost of the same size; **C**—parallel course in subpulmonary VSD (D-aorta); the pulmonary artery is twice as large as the aorta; **D**—parallel course in L-aorta (with subpulmonary VSD in this case); **E**—parallel course in subarterial VSD with the OS (D-aorta)

The OS hypertrophy is most often seen in non-committed VSD. The OS in couple with the VIF squeeze aortic valve thus causing subaortic obstruction (Fig. 11). This scenario is similar to DORV with subarterial VSD and the prominent OS, when subaortic obstruction can develop by the same mechanism (see Fig. 8 in Chapter 2).

7 Aortic Arch Obstruction

Aortic arch obstruction is observed mainly in Taussig-Bing anomaly and less frequent in non-committed VSD. The mechanism of obstruction is based on insufficient hemodynamic load caused by limited blood flow to the ascending aorta. In case of Taussig-Bing anomaly it is due to deviation of the OS to subaortic area, while in case of non-committed VSD it is caused by hypertrophy of the OS and the VIF. In this regard, if aortic arch obstruction is diagnosed by CT, the next step is to determine the morphology and severity of subaortic stenosis and vice versa. Anatomically obstructive component may be represented by aortic coarctation (including arch hypoplasia) as well as different types of arch interruption (Fig. 12).

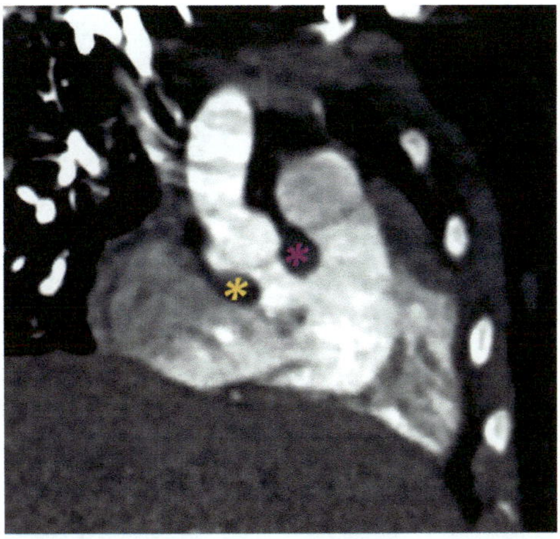

Fig. 11 DORV with non-committed VSD. The aorta and the pulmonary artery «200%» originate from the right ventricle. Subaortic obstruction due to hypertrophy of the OS (purple asterisk) and the VIF (orange asterisk) is clearly visualized

8 Coronary Artery Anatomy

Anatomy of the coronary arteries in DORV mainly depends on relationship of the arterial valves rather than on morphological type of DORV. When the aorta is right and posterior to the pulmonary artery (DP-aorta) then the coronary pattern is as in a normal heart. With side-by-side arterial trunks coronary artery abnormalities are found more frequently. It is of great practical importance to determine looping and intramural coronary arteries as well as their very proximal course to the aortic/pulmonary annulus for preoperative planning of operation requiring coronary artery reimplantation (see Chapter 10). When the aorta is right and anterior to pulmonary artery (DA-aorta), the left coronary artery, as a rule, crosses pulmonary trunk in front of it and thus precludes transannular repair of RVOT if necessary (Fig. 13).

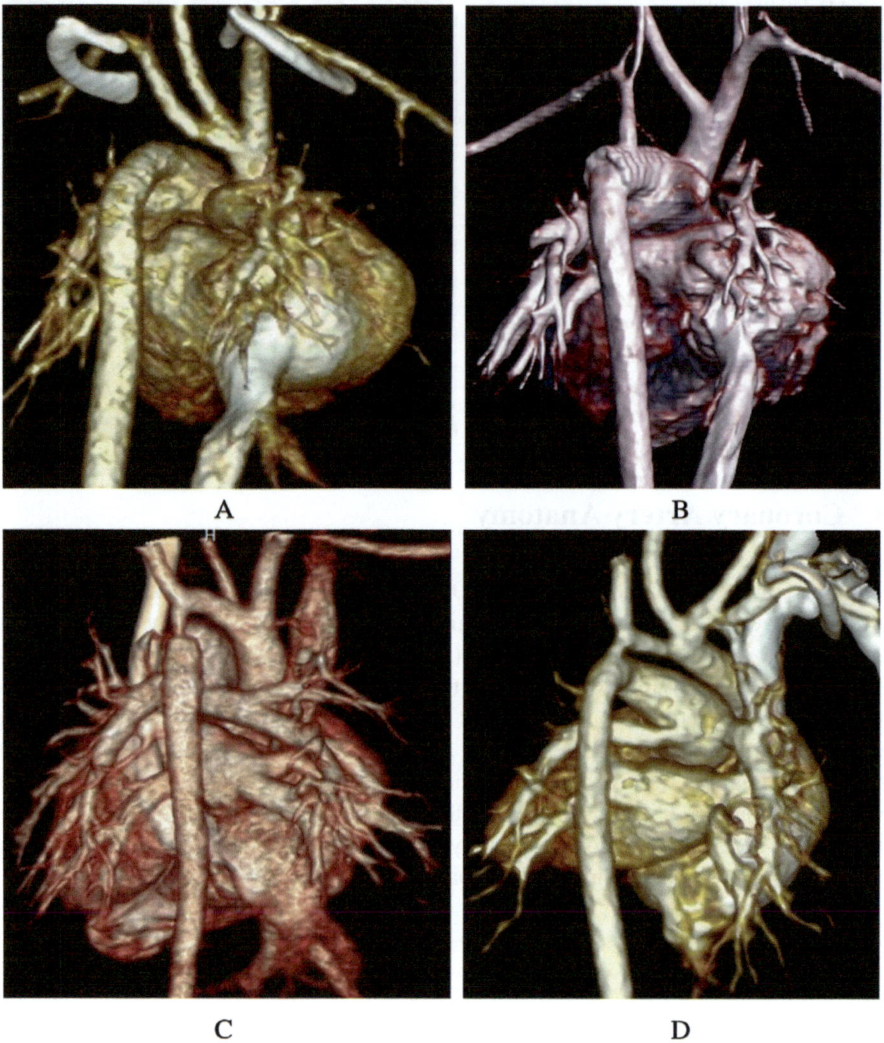

Fig. 12 Types of aortic arch obstruction (3D reconstructions): **A**—interrupted aortic arch type «A»; **B**—interrupted aortic arch type «B» (stented patent ductus arteriosus); **C**—aortic coarctation; **D**—aortic coarctation with arch hypoplasia

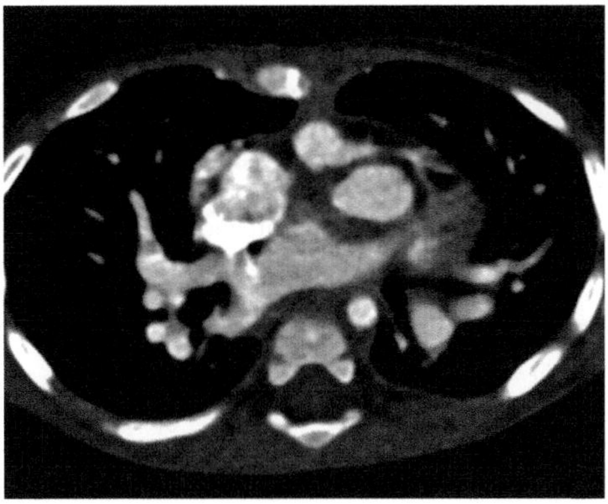

Fig. 13 DORV with subpulmonary VSD (with the right and anterior aorta). The left coronary artery crosses the pulmonary artery anteriorly

References

1. Chung KJ, Simpson IA, Newman R, Sahn DJ, Sherman FS, Hesselink JR. Cine magnetic resonance imaging for evaluation of congenital heart disease: role in pediatric cardiology compared with echocardiography and angiography. J Pediatr. 1988;6:1028–35.
2. Shi K, Yang Z, Chen J, Zhang G, Xu H, Guo Y. Assessment of double outlet right ventricle associated with multiple malformations in pediatric patients using retrospective ECG-gated dual-source computed tomography. PLOS ONE. 10(6):e0130987. doi:https://doi.org/10.1371/journal.pone.01309.
3. Uehara M, Funabashi N, Ogawa Y, Minamino T, Komuro I. Double outlet right ventricle demonstrated by multislice computed tomography. Int J Cardiol. 2007;121:218–20.
4. Ntsinjana HN, Hughes ML, Taylor AM. The role of cardiovascular magnetic resonance in pediatric congenital heart disease. J Cardiovasc Magn Reson. 2011;13:51.
5. Chen S, Lin M, Liu K, Chang C, Chen H, Wang J, Lee W, Tsang Y, Li1Y. Usefulness of 3D reconstructed computed tomography imaging for double outlet right ventricle. J Formosan Med Assoc. 2008;107:371–80.
6. Beekman RP, Roest AAW, Helbing WA, Hazekamp MG, Schoof PH, Bartelings MM, Sobotka MA, de Roos A, Ottenkamp J. Spin echo MRI in the evaluation of hearts with a double outlet right ventricle: usefulness and limitations. Magn Reson Imag. 2000;18:245–53.
7. Niezen RA, Beekman RP, Helbing WA, van der Wall EE, de Roos A. Double outlet right ventricle assessed with magnetic resonance imaging. Int J Card Imag. 1999;15:323–9.
8. Yoo S, Ho SY, Kilner PJ, Seo J, Anderson RH. Sectional anatomy of the ventricular septal defect in double outlet right ventricle—correlation of magnetic resonance images from autopsied hearts with anatomic sections. Cardiol Young. 1993;3:118–23.
9. Akins EW, Martin TD, Alexander JA, Knauf DG, Victorica BE. MR imaging of double-outlet right ventricle. Am J Roentgenol. 1989;152:128–30.
10. Parsons JM, Baker EJ, Anderson RH, Ladusans EJ, Hayes A, Fagg N, Cook A, Qureshi SA, Deverall PB, Maisey MN, Tynan M. Double-outlet right ventricle: morphologic demonstration using nuclear magnetic resonance imaging. J Am Coll Cardiol. 1991;18:168–78.
11. Yoo S, Lim TH, Park I, Hong CY, Song MG, Kim SH, Lee HJ. MR anatomy of ventricular septal defect in double-outlet right ventricle with situs solitus and atrioventricular corcondance. Radiology. 1991;181:501–5.
12. Prakash A, Powell AJ, Geva T. Multimodality noninvasive imaging for assessment of congenital heart disease. Circul Cardiovascul Imag. 2010;3:112–125.
13. Rajiah P, Schoenhagen P. The role of computed tomography in pre-procedural planning of cardiovascular surgery and intervention. Insights Imag. 2013;4:671–89.

14. Young C, Xie C, Owens CM. Pediatric multi-detector row chest CT: what you really need to know. Insights Imag. 2012;3:229–46.
15. Dillman JR, Hernandez RJ. Role of CT in the evaluation of congenital cardiovascular disease in children. Am J Roentgenol. 2009;192:1219–31.
16. Aposopolopoulou SC, Kelekis NL, Brountzos EN, Rammos S, Kelekis DA. «Absent» pulmonary artery in one adult and five pediatric patients: imaging, embryology, and therapeutic implication. Am J Roentgenol. 2002;179:1253–60.
17. Welch K, Hanley F, Johnston T, Cailes C, Shah MJ. Isolated unilateral absence of right proximal pulmonary artery: surgical repair and follow-up. Ann Thorac Surg. 2005;79:1399–402.

3D Printing

K. M. Dzhidzhikhiya

Abstract Two-dimensional methods of visualization are essential part of preoperative diagnostics of CHDs. Because of biplanar nature of obtained screens they need appropriate interpretation especially in cases of complex CHDs and require specific skills and experience which is a great limitation of such diagnostic tools. 3D printing is continuously evolving diagnostic tool in the field of congenital heart surgery, mainly in cases of DORV due to its extreme anatomical variability and thus complicated preoperative diagnostics. Already at a preprinting stage 3D computer reconstructed heart models may provide pivotal details of intracardiac anatomy which in many cases have vital role regarding surgical options.

Keywords Double-outlet right ventricle · Diagnostics · 3D-printing · 3D reconstruction

The main goal of all diagnostic tools is to provide a surgeon data necessary for accurate preoperative planning. Knowledge of precise anatomy of a CHD simplifies intracardiac revision during the operation. The development of 3D methods (3D echo, CT/MRI, rotational angiography) paved the way to taking a step forward to 3D volumetric heart models as close as possible to the real anatomy. Moreover, the implementation of 3D printing has brought cardiac surgery very close to solving the problem of underdiagnosis of CHDs.

Since 2000, the 3D printing method has been gradually introduced into the clinical practice of cardiac surgeons and today is gaining more and more popularity among specialists due to the ability of 3D heart models to convey real intracardiac anatomy [1–17].

K. M. Dzhidzhikhiya (✉)
Department of Emergency Surgery of Congenital Heart Diseases, A. N. Bakulev National Medical Investigation Center for Cardiovascular Surgery, Moscow, Russia
e-mail: d.m.konstantine@mail.ru

K. V. Shatalov and K. M. Dzhidzhikhiya (eds.), *Double-Outlet Right Ventricle*,
https://doi.org/10.1007/978-3-031-49707-0_9

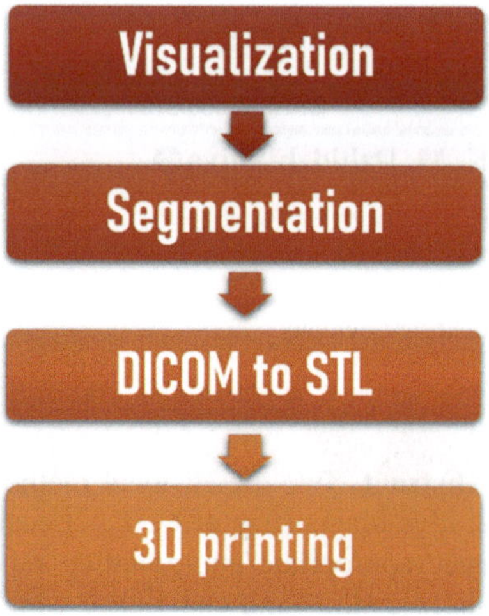

Fig. 1 Stages of 3D printing

Nowadays, 3D printing is an additional diagnostic tool which helps to visualize intracardiac structures from specific angles —the ones from which the revision of a heart is performed during the operation [18–20].

The results of the meta-analysis showed a high diagnostic accuracy of 3D heart models [21] and almost 100% correlation with CT data [17, 22]. In comparison with standard echo, 3D models have advantages in determining arterial trunks relationship, VSD location, projection and length of intraventricular tunneling, as well as the degree of the right ventricle reduction after the surgery [23].

In the field of congenital heart surgery, the 3D printing can be used for the following purposes:

- preoperative diagnostic and planning;
- surgical skills training;
- demonstrative models.

The process of 3D printing consists of four consecutive stages [24, 25] (Fig. 1):

1. visualization using one of the available standard 3D diagnostic tools (CT/MRI, 3D echo, rotational CT angiography);
2. computer segmentation using a special software;
3. conversion of DICOM format («digital imaging and communication in medicine») to one of the 3D printing formats: STL («stereolithography of standard tessellation language»), AMF (addictive manufacturing file format), OBJ (object), VRML (virtual reality modeling language);
4. 3D printing of a prepared computer model of a heart.

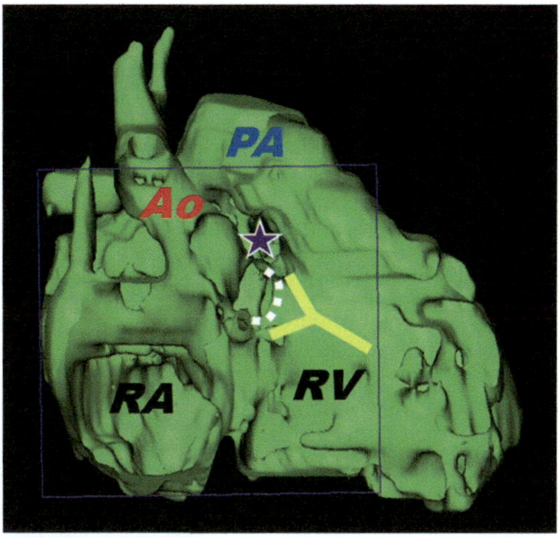

Fig. 2 3D computer model of DORV with subaortic VSD (white dotted line), view from the right ventricle. Dissecting plane through the right ventricle and right atrium. Spiral course of the arterial trunks (DP-aorta). The OS (violet asterisk) fuses with the aTS (yellow figure). *Ao—aorta; PA—pulmonary artery; RA—right atrium; RV—right ventricle*

Segmentation and printing of one heart specimen requires on average 75 ± 32 minutes and 35 hour respectively. Given the small size of a child's heart, printing of one specimen requires from 8 to 24 hour, and therefore, its preparation must be planned 2 days before the intended surgical intervention [17].

The use of 3D printing technology due to its relative high cost and labor intensity is justified only in cases of complex CHDs. Patients with DORV account for more than half of all cases of 3D printing in pediatric cardiac surgery [17, 24, 26]. On the one hand, types of DORV with subaortic and subpulmonary VSD does not represent a great challenge for the surgeon regarding preoperative assessment of anatomy and decision-making. In these types, standard diagnostic tools are sufficient. On the other hand, non-committed and subarterial (with the OS) VSD are very complex in anatomical terms and often precise heart anatomy may be obtained only during intraoperative revision.

During segmentation, it is possible to evaluate all major intracardiac structures of DORV by dissecting a heart in any individual planes, in particular: location and size of VSD; distance between superior rim of VSD and the arterial valves; VSD position relative to the septal leaflet of the tricuspid valve; the OS orientation; assessment of subarterial infundibulums; arterial trunks relationship; RVOT and LVOT obstruction; atrioventricular valve anomalies; characteristics of ventricles, and associated anomalies [27, 28] (Figs. 2, 3, 4, 5, and 6).

3D computer heart models can be printed both in accordance with the contour of blood filling heart chambers («blood model») and with the relief of endocardial surface («hollow model» or «wall model»).

The main factors which are recommended to be accessed on 3D computer or printed models for preoperative evaluation depending on the type of intervention are listed in the Table 1.

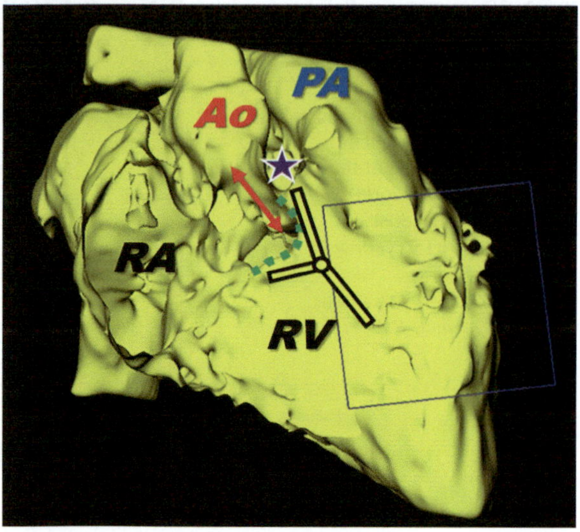

Fig. 3 3D computer model of DORV with not directly committed subaortic VSD (green dotted line), view from the right ventricle. Dissecting plane through the right ventricle and right atrium. Parallel course of the arterial trunks (D-aorta). The OS (violet asterisk) fuses with the aTS (yellow figure with black borders). Due to the elongated subaortic conus (double-headed red arrow) the aortic valve is remote from the superior rim of VSD. *Ao—aorta; PA—pulmonary artery; RA—right atrium; RV—right ventricle*

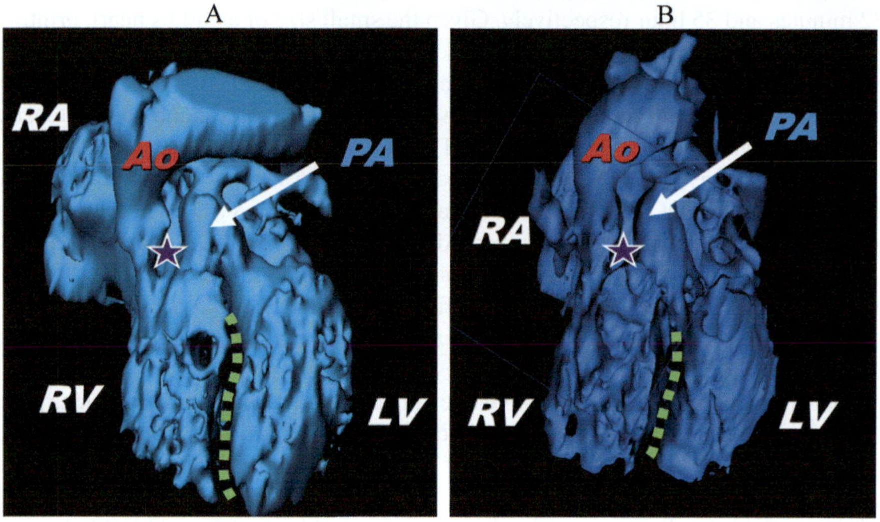

Fig. 4 3D computer model of DORV with subpulmonary VSD, parallel course of the arterial trunks (DA-aorta): **A**—left external view. Pulmonary artery overrides the IVS (green dotted line). The OS (violet asterisk) is deviated to the subaortic area causing subaortic obstruction; **B**—dissecting plane through the VSD and pulmonary artery. *Ao—aorta; PA—pulmonary artery; RA—right atrium; right ventricle; RV—right ventricle; LV—left ventricle*

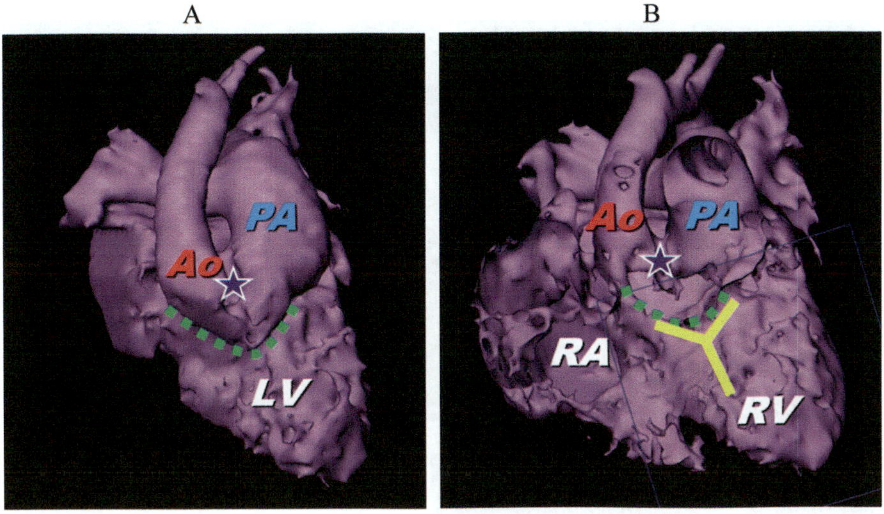

Fig. 5 3D computer model of DORV with subarterial VSD and the OS, parallel course of the arterial trunks (D-aorta): **A**—right heart chambers have been removed. The left ventricle communicates directly with the aorta and the pulmonary artery through the VSD (green dotted line); **B**—dissecting plane through the level of the arterial valves and VSD, view from the right ventricle. The OS (violet asterisk) does not fuse with any limbs of the TS (yellow figure) and is positioned superiorly and in the middle of VSD thus committing both subarterial infundibulums to the VSD. *Ao—aorta; PA—pulmonary artery; RA—right atrium; RV—right ventricle; LV—left ventricle*

Despite preoperative planning 3D printed heart models can be effective for improvement of manual skills both for residents and surgeons [29–32]. In this regard, the great advantage of 3D models is that they can be available during a routine diagnostic procedure compared to real heart specimens obtained from cadaver.

Also, the use of 3D models for communicative purposes as demonstrative material is very valuable. The employment of such models can help parents to understand the essence of CHD. So, specialist can demonstrate the anatomy of the disease and the principle of the upcoming surgery [33].

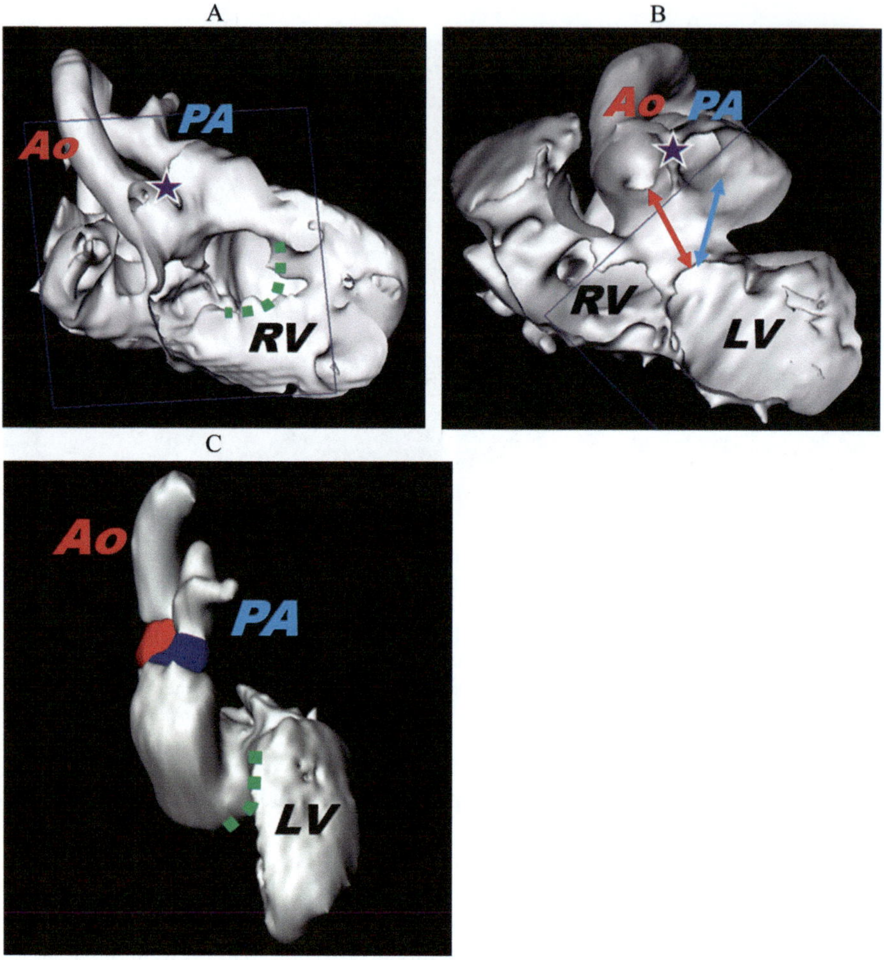

Fig. 6 3D computer model of DORV with non-committed VSD, parallel course of the arterial trunks (D-aorta): **A**—view from the right ventricle. VSD (green dotted line) locates in the inlet IVS and extends to the outlet part. The arterial valves «sit» high above the right ventricle; **B**—dissecting plane through the level of the arterial valves, rim of VSD and left ventricle. The distance between the superior rim of VSD and the arterial valves significantly exceeds the diameter of the aortic valve due to elongation of the subarterial infundibulums (red and blue arrows); **C**—the right ventricle and the right atrium have been removed. The arterial valves (color segments) are significantly remote from VSD. *Ao—aorta; PA—pulmonary artery; RV—right ventricle; LV—left ventricle*

Table 1 Preoperative 3D assessment protocol of intracardiac structures in DORV depending on the type of intervention

Type of repair	Structures to be assessed
DORV «tetralogy» and «VSD» types	–matching the size of VSD to the diameter of the aortic valve; –tricuspid-to-pulmonary valve distance; –abnormal attachment of the tricuspid valve chordae to the OS; –mitral-aortic continuity; –the OS; –pulmonary artery stenosis
DORV with non-committed VSD	–type and size of non-committed VSD; –proximity of VSD to the arterial valves; –pulmonary artery stenosis; –abnormal attachment of the tricuspid valve chordae; –subaortic obstruction; –tricuspid-to-pulmonary valve distance; –the OS
Pulmonary artery baffling and ASO	–coronary artery anatomy; –morphology of superior rim of VSD; –subaortic obstruction; –aortic arch obstructions
Rastelli/REV operation	–anatomy, size of the pulmonary valve and morphological substrate of pulmonary artery stenosis; –abnormal attachment of the atrioventricular valves; –size of VSD; –size of the OS; –a coronary artery branch crossing RVOT; –size of the right ventricle
Kawashima operation	–tricuspid-to-pulmonary valve distance; –relationship of the arterial trunks; –subaortic obstruction; –pulmonary artery stenosis; –morphology of superior rim of VSD; –attachment of the tricuspid valve chordae to the OS; –size of the right ventricle
Nikaidoh operation	–coronary artery anatomy—anomalous branching, proximal course to the aortic annulus (looping course); –size of the pulmonary annulus; –width of the OS; –abnormal chordal attachment of the atrioventricular valves to the OS
Half-turned truncal switch operation and double root translocation	–see Nikaidoh operation; –morphology of mitral-pulmonary continuity (fibrous/muscular continuity)

References

1. Vettukattil JJ, Nijres BM, Gosnell JM, Samuel BP, Haw MP. Three-dimensional printing for surgical planning in complex congenital heart disease. J Cardiac Surg. 2019;1–7. https://doi.org/10.1111/ocs.14180
2. J Xu Y Luo J Wang W Xu Z Shi J Fu Q Shu 2019 Patient-specific three-dimensional printed heart models benefit preoperative planning for complex congenital heart disease World J Pediatr. https://doi.org/10.1007/s12519-019-00228-4
3. S Mottl-Link M Hubler T Kuhne U Rietdorf JJ Krueger B Schnackenburg R Simone De F Berger A Juraszek H Meinzer M Karck R Hetzer I Wolf 2008 Physical models aiding in complex congenital heart surgery Ann Thorac Surg. 86 273 277
4. Z Sun I Lau YH Wong CH Yeong 2019 Personalized three-dimensional printed models in congenital heart disease J Clin Med. https://doi.org/10.3390/jcm8040522
5. L Kiraly 2018 Three-dimensional modelling and three-dimensional printing in pediatric and congenital cardiac surgery Transplant Pediatr. 7 129 138
6. Cantinotti M, Valverde I, Kutty S. Three-dimensional printed models in congenital heart disease. Int J Cardiovascul Imaging. https://doi.org/10.1007/s10554-016-0981-2
7. LM Meier M Meineri JQ Hiansen EM Horlick 2017 Structural and congenital heart disease interventions: the role of three-dimensional printing Neth Hear J. 25 65 75
8. Bramlet M, Olivieri L, Farooqi K, Ripley B, Coakley M. Impact of three-dimensional printing on the study and treatment of congenital heart disease. Circul Res. https://doi.org/10.1161/CIR CRESAHA.116.310546
9. JL Hersmen TM Burke SP Seslar DS Owens BA Ripley NA Mokadam ED Verrier 2017 Scan, plan, print, practice, perform: development and use of a patient-specific 3-dimensional printed model in adult cardiac surgery J Thorac Cardiovasc Surg. 153 132 140
10. BP Samuel C Pinto T Pietila JJ Vetukattil 2015 Ultrrasound three-dimensional printing in congenital heart disease J Digit Imaging 28 459 461
11. I Shiraishi M Yamagishi K Hamaoka M Fukuzawa T Yagihara 2010 Simulative operation on congenital heart disease using rubber-like urethane stereolithographic biomodels based on 3D datasets of multislice computed tomography Eur J Cardiothorac Surg. 37 302 306
12. LJ Olivieri A Krieger Y Loke DS Nath PCW Kim CA Sable 2015 Three-dimensional printing of intracardiac defects from three-dimensional echocardiographic images: feasibility and relative accuracy J Am Soc Echocardiogr. 28 392 397
13. S Yoo T Spray EH Austin T Yun GS Arsdell Van 2017 Hands-on surgical training of congenital heart surgery using 3-dimensional print models J Thorac Cardiovasc Surg. 153 1530 1540
14. R Javan D Herrin A Tangestanipoor 2016 Understanding spatially complex segmental and branch anatomy using 3D printing: liver, lung, prostate, coronary arteries, and circle of Willis Acad Radiol. 23 1183 1189
15. JP Costello LJ Olivieri L Su A Krieger F Alfares O Thabit MB Marshall SJ Yoo PC Kim RA Jonas DS Nath 2015 Incorporating three-dimensional printing into a simulation-based congenital heart disease and critical care training curriculum for resident physicians Congenit Heart Dis. 10 185 190
16. L Zhao S Zhou T Fan B Li W Liang H Dong 2018 Three-dimensional printing enhances preparation for repair of double outlet right ventricular surgery J Card Surg. https://doi.org/10.1111/jocs.13523
17. I Valverde G Gomez-Ciriza T Hussain C Suarez-Mejias MN Velasco-Forte N Byrne A Ordonez A Gonzalez-Calle D Anderson MG Hazekamp AAW Roest J Rivas-Gonzalez S Uribe I El-Rassi J Simpson O Miller E Ruiz I Zabala A Mendez B Manso P Gallego F Prada M Cantinotti L Ait-Ali C Merino C Merino A Parry N Poirier G Greil R Razavi T Gomez-Cia A Hosseinpour 2017 Three-dimensional printed models for surgical planning of complex congenital heart defects: an international multicenter study Eur J Cardiothorac Surg. 52 1139 1148
18. PB Dydynski C Kiper D Kozik BB Keller E Austin B Holland 2016 Three-dimensional reconstruction of intracardiac anatomy using CTA and surgical planning for double outlet right

ventricle: early experience at a tertiary care congenital center World J Pediatric Congen Heart Surg. 7 467 474
19. J Vodiskar M Kutting U Steinseifer JF Vazquez-Jimenez SJ Sonntag 2017 Using 3D physical modeling to plan surgical correction of complex congenital heart defects Thoracic Cardiovascul Surg. 65 31 35
20. P Bhatla JT Tretter S Chikkabyrappa S Chakravarti RS Mosca 2017 Surgical planning for a complex double-outlet right ventricle using 3D printing Echocardiography 34 802 804
21. IWW Lau Z Sun 2019 Dimensional accuracy and clinical value of 3D printed models in congenital heart disease: a systematic review and meta-analysis J Clin Med https://doi.org/10.3390/jcm8091483
22. Lau IWW, Liu D, Xu L, Fan Z, Sun Z Clinical value of Patient-specific three-dimensional printing of congenital heart disease: quantitative and qualitative assessments. PLOS ONE. 2018. https://doi.org/10.1371/journal.pone.0194333
23. S Garekar A Bharati M Chokhandre S Mali B Trivedi VP Changela N Solanski S Gaikwad V Agarwal 2016 Clinical application and multidisciplinary assessment of three-dimensional orienting in double outlet right ventricle with remote ventricular septal defect World J Pediatr Congen Heart Surg. 7 344 350
24. Yoo SJ, Thabit O, Kim EK, Die H, Yim D, Dragulescu A, Seed M, Grosse-Wortmann L, Van Arsdell G. 3D printing in medicine of congenital heart diseases. 3D Printing in Medicine. 2016;2:3. https://doi.org/10.1186/s41205-016-0004-x
25. RA Moore KW Riggs S Kourtidou K Shneider N Szugye W Troja G D'Souza M Rattan R Bryant III MD Taylor DLS Morales 2018 Three-dimensional printing and virtual surgery for congenital heart procedural planning Birth Defects Res. https://doi.org/10.1002/bdr2.1370
26. T Hoashi H Ichikawa T Nakata M Shimada H Ozawa A Higashida K Kurosaki S Kanzaki I Shiraishi 2018 Utility of a super-flexible three-dimensional printed heart model in congenital heart surgery Interact Cardiovasc Thorac Surg. 27 749 755
27. Yim D, Dragulescu A, Ide H, Seed M, Grosse-Wortmann L, Van Arsdell G, Yoo SJ. Essential modifiers of double outlet right ventricle. Revisit with endocardial surface images and 3-dimensional print models. Circul Cardiovascul Imaging. 2018;11ye006891. doi:https://doi.org/10.1161/CIRCIMAGING.117.006891.
28. SJ Yoo G Arsdell Van 2018 3D printing in surgical management of double outlet right ventricle Front Pediatr. https://doi.org/10.3389/fped.2017.00289
29. LJ Olivieri L Su CF Hunes A Krieger FA Alfares K Ramakrishnan D Zurakowski MB Marshall PCW Kim RA Jonas DS Nath 2016 «Just-in-time» simulation training used 3-D printed cardiac models after congenital cardiac surgery World J Pediatr Congen Heart Surg. 7 164 168
30. Hersmen JL, Yang R, Burke TM, Dardas T, Jacobs LM, Verrier ED, Mokadam NA. Development of a 3-D printing-based cardiac surgical simulation curriculum to teach septal myoectomy. J Thoracic Cardiovascul Surg. 2018. https://doi.org/10.1016/j.jtcvs.2017.09.136
31. SC White J Sedler TW Jones M Seckeler 2019 Utility of three-dimensional models in resident education on simple and complex intracardiac congenital heart defects Congenit Heart Dis https://doi.org/10.1111/chd.12673
32. Smerling J, Marboe CC, Lefkowitch JH, Pavlicova M, Bacha E, Einstein AJ, Naka Y, Glickstein J, Farooqi KM. Utility of 3D printed cardiac models for medical student education in congenital heart disease: across a spectrum of disease severity. Pediatric Cardiol. 2019. https://doi.org/10.1007/s00246-019-02146-8
33. Biglino G, Capelli C, Wray J, Schievano S, Leaver L, Khambadkone S, Giardini A, Derrick G, Jones A, Taylor AM. 3D-manufactures patient-specific models of congenital heart defects for communication in clinical practice: feasibility and acceptability. Br Med J Open. 2015.5.e007165. https://doi.org/10.1135/bmjopen-2014-007165

Treatment

Surgery

K. V. Shatalov and K. M. Dzhidzhikhiya

Abstract Despite more than 60-year world experience surgical repair of DORV remains a big challenge for the pediatric cardiac surgeons due to its anatomical variability, technical complexity and the absence of standard surgical approaches. In fact, main types of the malformation with subaortic, subpulmonary, subarterial and non-committed VSD are completely different in clinical, anatomical and surgical terms that allows to consider each of them as a CHDs. Thus, it is reasonable to describe methods of surgical repair of DORV in this chapter according to this division. Those extremely complex forms of DORV associated with atrioventricular valve anomalies are also discussed. The main goal of pre- and intraoperative assessment of patients with DORV is to obtain necessary anatomical details for correct decision-making. So, for the all surgical techniques described in this chapter «decision-making check-list» is also provided which will help in choosing optimal surgical strategy both at the stage of preoperative assessment and intraoperative revision.

Keywords Double-outlet right ventricle · Surgical treatment · Anatomical repair · Taussig-Bing anomaly · Univentricular palliation

DORV is itself an indication for surgical treatment. Surgical strategy is individual for each specific type of the disease and depends mainly on VSD location, the presence of pulmonary artery stenosis, as well as associated cardiac anomalies.

All types of DORV without pulmonary artery stenosis are characterized by pulmonary overcirculation due to left to right shunting, which over time leads to the development of pulmonary hypertension. In this regard, without surgery severe pulmonary hypertension develops mainly in patients with Taussig-Bing anomaly due to the direct entry of a large volume of blood under high left ventricular pressure into the pulmonary circulation. Surgical repair of all types of DORV can be safely

K. V. Shatalov · K. M. Dzhidzhikhiya (✉)
Departement of Emergency Surgery of Congenital Heart Diseases, A. N. Bakulev National Medical Investigation Center for Cardiovascular Surgery, Moscow, Russia
e-mail: d.m.konstantine@mail.ru

K. V. Shatalov and K. M. Dzhidzhikhiya (eds.), *Double-Outlet Right Ventricle*,
https://doi.org/10.1007/978-3-031-49707-0_10

performed with satisfactory clinical results with average pressure in the pulmonary artery up to 40 mmHg [1].

Depending on the possibility to restore segmental anatomy of a heart all existing methods of surgical correction of DORV can be divided into the methods of biventricular and univentricular repair.

1 Biventricular Repair

The mail goal of biventricular (anatomical) repair of DORV is to restore ventricular-arterial concordance by shifting the aorta to the left ventricle. In some cases, this is achieved only by intraventricular tunneling, in others—in combination with extracardiac procedures such as ASO, aortic or/and pulmonary root translocation and half-turned truncal switch operation.

In patients with DORV and concomitant pulmonary artery stenosis after aortic tunneling and elimination of the stenosis pulmonary blood flow increases as well as blood return to the left heart. Accordingly, the general indications for biventricular correction for all types of DORV with pulmonary artery stenosis is adequate pulmonary arterial index (Nakata index—330 ± 30 mm^2/m^2) along with normal size of the left ventricle.

Anatomical correction of DORV implies either one-stage repair in the first six month of life or two-stage approach. Early one-stage repair contributes to an earlier restoration of normal intracardiac hemodynamics and is characterized by the prevention of significant remodeling of the heart and the negative effect of chronic hypoxemia on other organs and tissues. But at the same time, there is a risk of reinterventions due to tunnel obstruction in a growing organism [2]. In this regard, some surgeons prefer two-stage approach when the risk of tunnel obstruction is lower because anatomical repair is performed at an older age. As a first palliative stage either systemic-to-pulmonary shunt or pulmonary artery banding is performed depending on the pulmonary circulation. With two-stage approach, it is necessary to take into account inter-stage mortality as well as complications associated with a palliative procedure itself.

One-stage correction is advisable for patients with DORV and committed VSDs, whereas in other cases two-stage approach is preferable [2], although some centers adhere to one-stage approach in all cases of DORV regardless of VSD type with satisfactory outcomes [3]. In Taussig-Bing anomaly due to the high risk of pulmonary hypertension, surgical intervention should be performed in the first weeks of life.

Before anatomical correction of DORV, it is recommended to evaluate the following anatomical structures [4]: the OS and type of its connection to the limbs of the TS, the VIF, VSD and its proximity to the arterial trunks, arterial trunks relationship, tricuspid-to-pulmonary valve distance.

According to the classification proposed in 2000 by «The Congenital Heart Surgery Nomenclature and Database Project Committee» all types of DORV are divides on the bases of clinical, anatomical and hemodynamic features [5]. So, the following description of the methods of surgical treatment of DORV will be given in accordance with this classification.

2 DORV «Tetralogy» and «VSD» Types

Generally surgical intervention in DORV «tetralogy» and «VSD» types is analogous to the corresponding isolated malformations. The main difference is that in case of DORV it is necessary to shift the aorta to the left ventricle by constructing intraventricular tunnel, and not just a simple VSD closure as it is routinely performed in tetralogy of Fallot and isolated VSD. For this purpose, a larger patch is required.

When performing intraventricular tunnelling the surgeon needs to understand that the bigger VIF between the mitral and aortic valves the more dextraposition of aorta and the larger patch is needed [6] (Fig. 1).

Accordingly, the size of intraventricular patch being located in the right ventricle, determines the reduction of the right ventricular volume. This is especially important to take into account in «VSD» type of DORV when deciding whether to augment RVOT with a patch or not, since in «tetralogy» type such an augmentation is performed routinely in order to eliminate pulmonary artery stenosis.

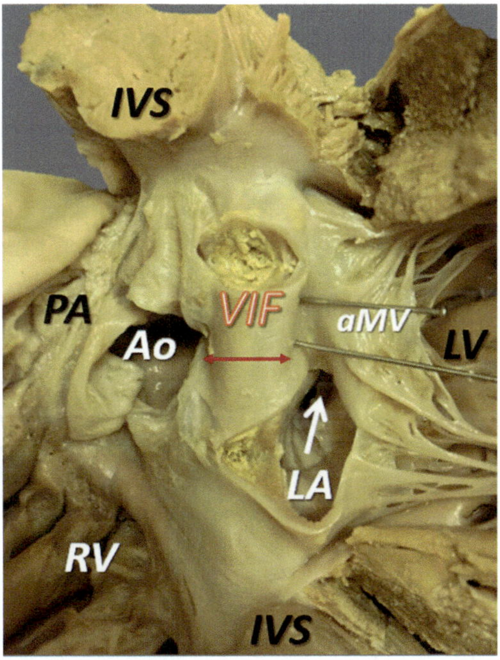

Fig. 1 DORV with subaortic VSD (autopsy specimen). IVS is dissected to the apex; the anterior leaflet of the mitral valve is partially detached from the annulus. The presence of prominent VIF between the mitral and aortic valves causes mitral-aortic muscular continuity. *Ao—aorta; PA—pulmonary artery; RV—right ventricle; LV—left ventricle; LA—left atrium; VIF—ventriculo-infundibular fold; IVS—interventricular septum; aMV—anterior leaflet of the mitral valve*

Timing

The optimal time for repair is 3–6 months of age.

Approach

The correct determination of the anatomical structures of the right ventricle is a key part of the operation and is a main goal of intraoperative revision. In «VSD» type of DORV transatrial approach is often sufficient for revision, which, if necessary, can be supplemented with approach through the pulmonary artery trunk [7] (especially in case of subarterial VSD) or aorta [8], avoiding ventriculotomy, in young children in particular. In «tetralogy» type transatrial and transventricular approaches provide excellent exposition of all right ventricle structures (Fig. 2). In some cases of subaortic VSD without pulmonary artery stenosis for better visualization the anterior tricuspid leaflet may be detached from the annulus [9]. In other cases transventricular approach is advisable. When performing ventriculotomy, it is necessary to consider any coronary arteries crossing RVOT.

Revision

Structures to be assessed [10]:

- size of VSD;
- tricuspid-to-pulmonary valve distance;
- anomalous attachment of tricuspid valve chordae to OS;
- mitral-aortic muscular continuity;
- OS;
- parietal and septal insertions of OS;
- morphology of postero-inferior rim of VSD;
- pulmonary artery stenosis.

Size of VSD. Restrictive nature of VSD does not preclude biventricular repair as it may always be enlarged anterosuperiorly up to the required size (Fig. 3). VSD enlargement does not necessarily imply massive tissue resection since it may be achieved by a simple incision of IVS. The possible damage to the anterior leaflet of

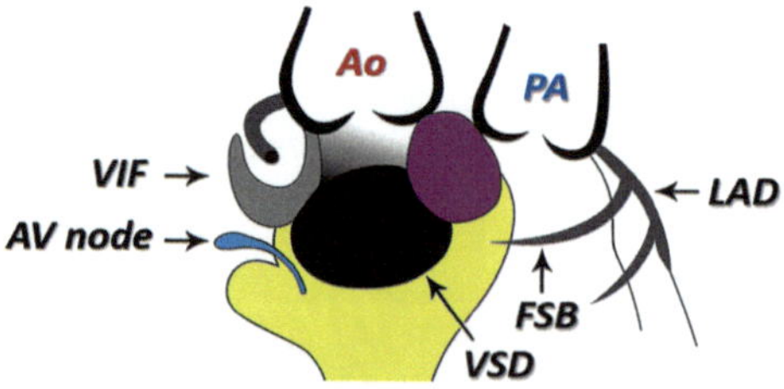

Fig. 2 Relationship of subaortic VSD with important intracardiac structures (view through the right ventriculotomy). *Ao—aorta; PA—pulmonary artery; VIF—ventriculo-infundibular fold; AV node—atrioventricular node; LAD—left anterior descending artery; FSB—first septal branch; VSD—ventricular septal defect*

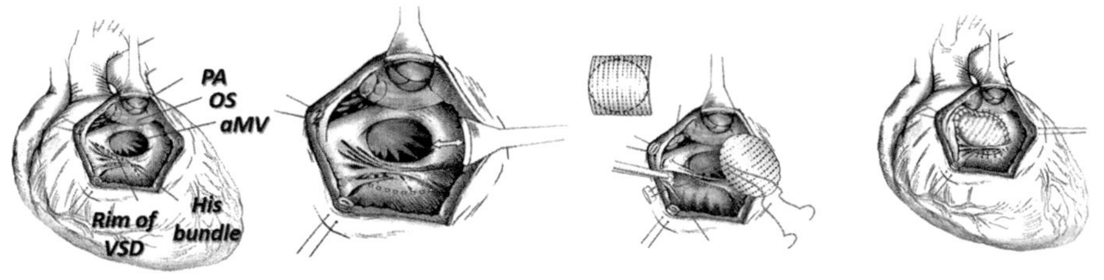

Fig. 3 Intraventricular tunneling in DORV «tetralogy» and «VSD» types with VSD enlargement. In Figure B, the arrow indicates anterosuperior direction of incision. *PA—pulmonary artery; OS—outlet septum; aMV—anterior leaflet of the mitral valve*

the mitral valve, right ventricular anterior wall and coronary artery should be avoided. During cardiac arrest VSD size should exceed aortic valve annulus diameter at least by 2 mm. In all cases of restrictive VSD the enlargement should always be done without a risk of damage of important intracardiac structures.

When comparing the results of surgical treatment of DORV with and without VSD enlargement, it was shown that VSD enlargement does not increase the risk of left ventricular failure, heart block as well as early and late survival [11].

Tricuspid-to-Pulmonary Valve Distance. For save biventricular repair, tricuspid-to-pulmonary valve distance plays a significant role. This distance must be at least equal to the aortic valve diameter to create a tunnel of sufficient width and without left ventricle outflow obstruction (i.e. subaortic obstruction). For the first time, the significance of tricuspid-to-pulmonary valve distance in DORV was pointed out by Sakata et al. in 1988 [12].

As mentioned above, the length of subaortic conus depends on the size of VIF between the mitral and aortic valves—the greater mitral-aortic muscular continuity, the longer the subaortic conus. The latter determines the relationship of the arterial trunks—with an increased length of subaortic infundibulum, the aorta shifts to the right and then anteriorly to the pulmonary artery. Until aorta locates posterior or to the right to the pulmonary artery, tricuspid-to-pulmonary valve distance does not affect the construction of a wide intraventricular tunnel. Further shifting of the aorta anteriorly to the pulmonary artery-A position-leads to pulmonary valve being interposed between the aortic valve and VSD, thereby complicating tunnel construction [10] (Fig. 4).

Usually, in DORV with subaortic VSD and normal arterial trunks relationship tricuspid-to-pulmonary valve distance is always greater than the diameter of the aortic valve [13]. If the pulmonary valve is interposed between the aortic valve and VSD, then the following surgical techniques are available to create a nonobstructive tunnel from the left ventricle [10]:

- without pulmonary artery stenosis—conversion of the disease into «TGA» form by tunneling of the pulmonary artery to the left ventricle followed by ASO (Jatene operation);

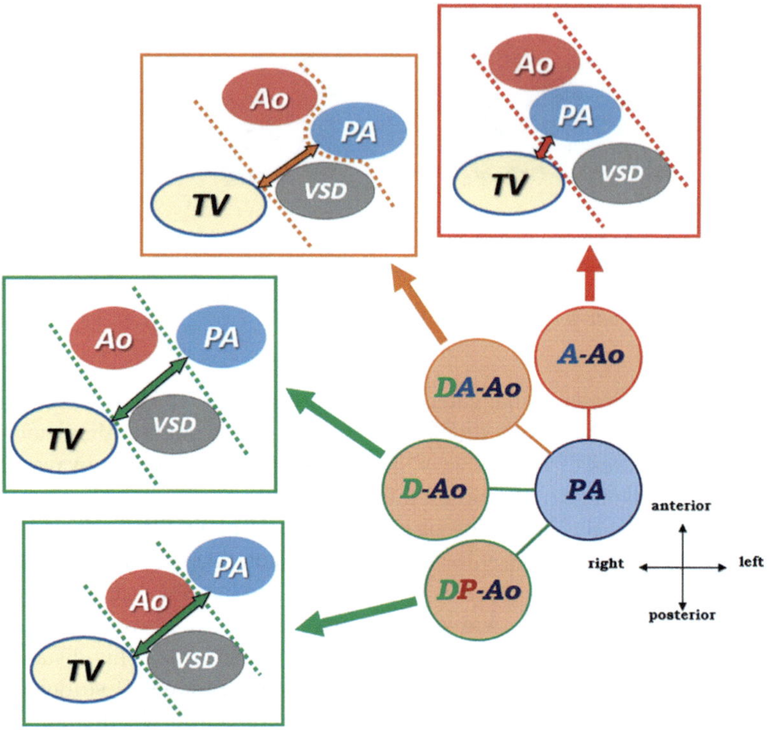

Fig. 4 Influence of the tricuspid-to-pulmonary valve distance (double-headed arrows) on the construction of intraventricular tunnel with the aorta (dotted lines) in different types of arterial valves relationships (bottom view). Until the aorta locates to the right and posterior to the pulmonary artery, the tricuspid-to-pulmonary valve distance is sufficient to construct nonobstructive intraventricular tunnel with the aorta (green arrows). As soon as the aorta is slightly anterior to the pulmonary artery, the pulmonary valve becomes partially interposed between the aortic valve and VSD (orange arrow). With further displacement of the aorta anteriorly, the pulmonary valve fully interposes between the aortic valve and VSD thus precluding aortic tunneling (red arrow). *Ao—aorta; PA—pulmonary artery; TV—tricuspid valve; VSD—ventricular septal defect*

- with pulmonary artery stenosis—Rastelli/REV operation with complete or partial exclusion of the pulmonary valve from hemodynamics.

Anomalous Attachment of Tricuspid Valve Chordae to OS. If malinserted tricuspid valve chordae to the OS crosses intraventricular tunnel projection, then in order to translocate the aorta to the left ventricle, the base of the abnormally attached papillary muscle should be cut off with a myocardial flap and subsequently reimplanted onto the intraventricular patch [14] (Fig. 5).

Mitral-Aortic Muscular Continuity. The longer mitral-aortic muscular continuity (i.e. VIF) the greater aortic dextraposition and the larger the patch size is required.

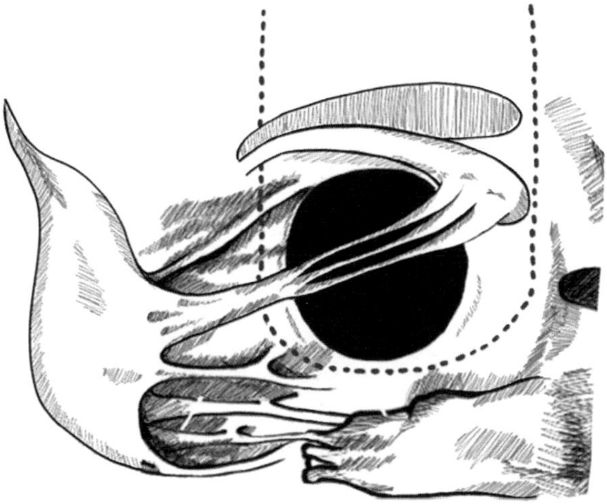

Fig. 5 Abnormal attachment of the tricuspid valve chordae to the OS. Dotted line indicates the excision areas for a myocardial flap bearing abnormal chordal attachment with its subsequent reimplantation on the intraventricular patch

OS. In «tetralogy» and «VSD» types of DORV the initial subaortic obstruction, which is responsible for pressure gradient between the right ventricle and the aorta, is rarely seen. Anatomical substrate of the obstruction may be presented by the hypertrophied OS, VIF, TS or their combination [15–18].

Before tunneling, an optimal resection of OS and VIF (if needed) must be performed to create nonobstructed tunnel. Usually, subaortic obstruction due to hypertrophied VIF is rare, but the surgeon needs to know that with its excessive resection there is a risk of getting out of the heart as well as damage to the coronary artery in the right atrioventricular groove [7]. Most often, the subaortic obstruction develops secondarily after pulmonary artery banding (mainly in «VSD» type) in response to increased postload on the right ventricle and subsequent concentric hypertrophy [19].

Parietal and septal insertions of the OS, morphology of posteroinferior rim of VSD and pulmonary stenosis. See text below.

Technique

Since the real exit from the left ventricle in DORV is an opening restricted by the crest of IVS and VIF located between the mitral and aortic valves, intraventricular tunnel does not augment this exit, but only shifts the aorta to the left ventricle.

OS with pulmonary valve and the anterior limb of TS are the most remote structures when approached through the right atrium. In practice, tricuspid-to-pulmonary valve distance with these types of DORV is always sufficient to create nonobstructive intraventricular tunnel when the aorta locates posterior to the pulmonary artery. If necessary, the tunneling zone can be augmented by additional resection through the anterior limb of TS and/or by shifting the suture line towards the pulmonary valve taking care not to cause subpulmonary obstruction. A segment 1/2–3/5 of a vascular graft diameter can be used as a patch, slightly exceeding the diameter of the aortic

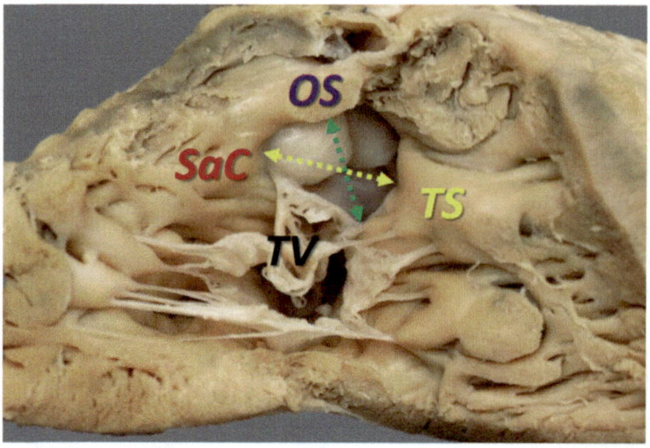

Fig. 6 DORV «tetralogy» type, view from the right ventricle (autopsy specimen). Calculation of a patch size. Length of a patch (yellow dotted arrow) exceeds the distance between the anterior rim of VSD and the most lateral aspect the subaortic conus. Width of a patch (green dotted arrow) slightly exceeds the distance between the basement of the tricuspid septal leaflet and the OS. *OS—outlet septum; SaC—subaortic conus; TS—trabecula septomarginalis; TV—tricuspid valve*

valve [20], or a diamond-shaped PTFE patch or autopericardium/xenopericardium [21].

The length of a patch is determined by the distance from the anterior rim of VSD to the most lateral aspect of the aortic conus [20]; in other words—the distance between the crest of IVS and distal conus [22]. The width of a patch should slightly exceed the distance from the basement of the tricuspid septal leaflet to the OS [7] (Fig. 6). Given the dextraposition of the aorta, a patch after the tunnel construction should bulge somewhat into the right ventricle. For this, a patch should slightly exceed calculated dimensions, because a too small patch may cause subaortic obstruction.

In case of subaortic VSD suture line follows inferior rim of defect, represented by TS and its limbs, with a continuation upward to the anterior aspect of the subaortic conus. From the body of TS, suture line continues up on the posterior limb of TS and VIF posteriorly and on the anterior limb of TS and the OS anteriorly (Fig. 7). If the pTS fuses with the VIF, then the His bundle is protected by this muscle band, therefore sutures in this area can be placed relatively deeply and safely.

In case of fibrous postero-inferior rim His bundle becomes vulnerable, so suture line should be performed 2–3 mm away from the rim of VSD. Near the tricuspid annulus sutures are placed through the base of the septal leaflet in a mattress manner (Figs. 3, 8).

In subarterial VSD intraventricular tunneling is more complex due to the absence of OS as a muscular structure along which suture line follows. In this regard, the key difference in tunneling of such type of VSD is the necessity to create «neo-outlet septum» [15]. As in subaortic VSD, the most distant point through the transatrial approach is the anterior rim of VSD represented by the continuation of the anterior limb of TS and fibrous remnants of OS. Initially suture line follows TS and its limbs and then continues in the back direction through the VIF upward to the free wall of

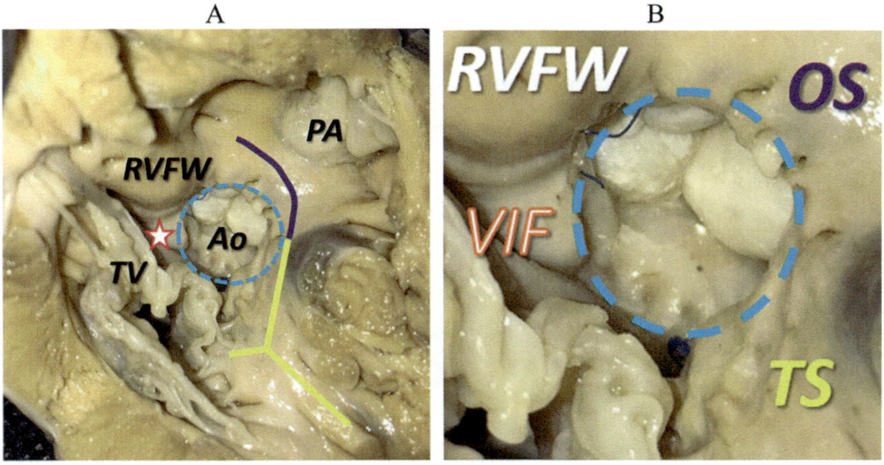

Fig. 7 DORV with subaortic VSD, view from the right ventricle (autopsy specimen after anatomical correction; intraventricular patch has been removed): **A**—tricuspid-to-pulmonary valve distance allows save intraventricular tunneling; **B**—suture line (blue figure) follows TS, OS, VIF and right ventricle free wall. *Ao—aorta; PA—pulmonary artery; VIF—ventriculo-infundibular fold; OS—outlet septum; TS—trabecula septomarginalis; RVFW—right ventricle free wall; TV—tricuspid valve*

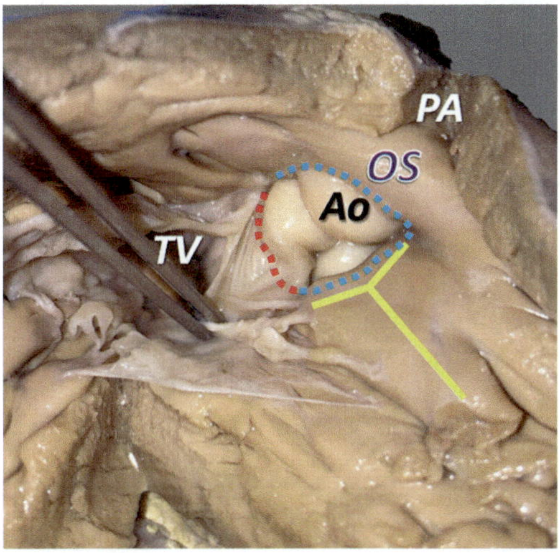

Fig. 8 DORV «tetralogy» type, view from the right ventricle (autopsy specimen). Tricuspid-aortic fibrous contact (red dotted line) between the tricuspid septal leaflet and the noncoronary cusp of the aortic valve is responsible for fibrous nature of postero-inferior rim of subaortic VSD. In this area sutures are placed through the base of the tricuspid septal leaflet (red dotted line). Anterior deviation of OS causes pulmonary artery stenosis. *Ao—aorta; PA—pulmonary artery; OS—outlet septum*

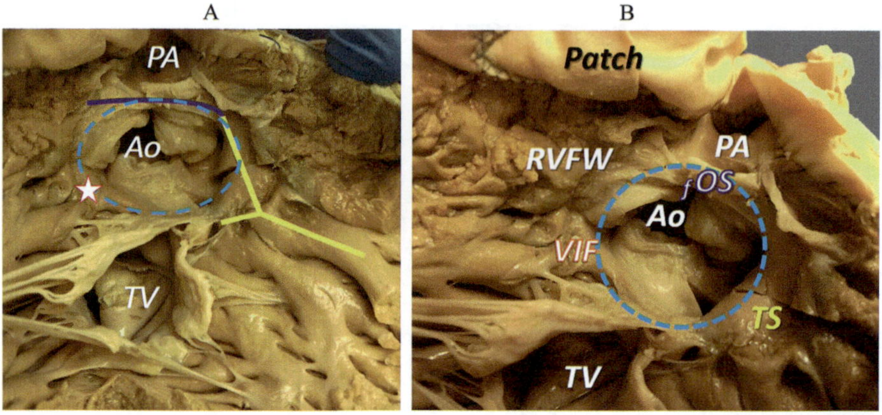

Fig. 9 DORV with subarterial VSD without OS as a muscular structure, view from the right ventricle (autopsy specimen after anatomical correction; intraventricular patch has been removed; monocusp patch on RVOT): **A**—projection of suture line (blue oval); **B**—suture line follows TS, fibrous remnants of OS, right ventricle free wall and VIF (also asterisk in the panel A). *Ao—aorta; PA—pulmonary artery; VIF—ventriculo-infundibular fold; fOS—fibrose outlet septum; TS—trabecula septomarginalis; RVFW—right ventricle free wall; TV—tricuspid valve*

the right ventricle (Fig. 9). In antero-superior area a patch is oriented in such a way as to completely separate the aortic and pulmonary valves. For this purpose, sutures are placed through the pulmonary valve fibrous annulus near the base of its cusps [22]. At this stage, there is a high risk of subpulmonary obstruction by patch bulging and therefore RVOT augmentation should be considered. In postero-inferior area, the suture line follows the same structures as in subaortic VSD.

In case the right ventricle is heavily trabeculated sutures in subaortic area should be placed directly on VIF and right ventricle free wall as closer to the aortic annulus as possible (Fig. 10A). If suture line is carried out through the muscular trabeculae, then there is a risk of residual shunting through the space under the trabeculae with the formation of the so-called intramural defect [24] (Fig. 10B). If possible, such trabeculae should be resected, but the surgeon should bear in mind that such resected areas are potentially weak and the risk of suture instability and subsequent left to right shunting is high in comparison with the intact myocardium. In this regard, areas of muscle resections are preferably reinforced with pledged sutures [21]. Intramural defects complicate early postoperative period due to their large size (>2 mm) compared to common residual VSDs formed along the suture line [25]. The routine use of intraoperative transesophageal echo reduces the risk of this complication [26].

When enlargement of restrictive VSD is intended it is important to perform an optimal incision on IVS not exceeding the required left ventricle outflow egress. There is a direct correlation of the distance between the crest of IVS and the aortic valve with the results of tunneling. If «aortic-IVS» distance account for more than 80% of left ventricle end-diastolic diameter the risk of mortality, subaortic obstruction and arrhythmias increases. It was also shown that in patients with right ventricle

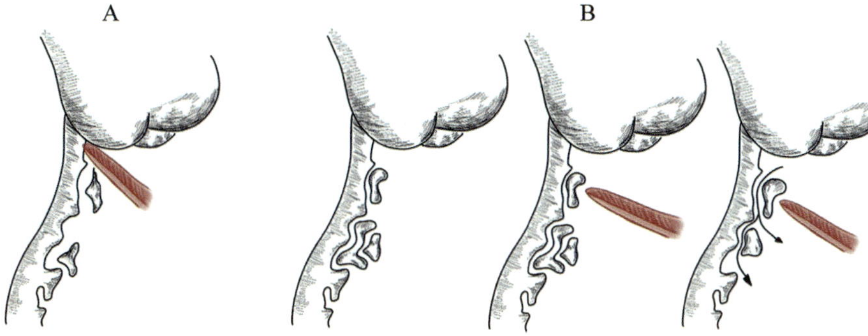

Fig. 10 Mechanism of intramural residual defect with left-to-right shunting: **A**—correct placement of a patch to the subaortic conus; **B**—incorrect placement of a patch to right ventricle trabeculae

end-diastolic volume ≥ 120% survival was higher compared to the control group [27].

Thus, the length of intraventricular tunnel and the right ventricle volume are important parameters on which the results of surgical treatment of DORV depend.

Reconstruction of Pulmonary Arteries

As a rule, pulmonary artery stenosis in DORV is multilevel and more often affects valvular and subvalvular levels (Fig. 11A). Valvular stenosis is usually represented by the fusion of the commissures. If pulmonary valve leaflets are dysplastic and deformed, then they should be excised and transannular repair should be implemented. In rare cases, imperforated pulmonary valve may be encountered (Fig. 11B).

Infundibular stenosis in «tetralogy» type is mainly caused by the parietal and septal insertions of the OS. Sometimes stenosis may be due to hypertrophy of TS, the moderator band (or its high origin), as well as hypertrophied or abnormal RVOT muscles, which narrow the exit from the right ventricle. Optimal resection of these muscle structures is a main goal for elimination of stenosis (Fig. 11A). When resecting OS insertions through the right ventriculotomy, it is necessary to control aortic valve leaflets (which locate just behind OS) in order to avoid their accidental damage. Also, it is necessary to resect all the trabecular elements of the right ventricle, which can potentially cause residual stenosis. When resecting the moderator band, it should be remembered that this structure contributes to the maintenance of the right ventricle systolic function, and therefore, if necessary, its resection should be optimal.

RVOT reconstruction can be performed using transannular or valve-sparing technique (within the RVOT itself).

Transannular Technique. Transannular approach is indicated if Z-score of pulmonary annulus is <−2 [28] (according to the scale of Petterson et al. [29]) or if residual right ventricle pressure is more than 2/3 of the systemic one after RVOT reconstruction [30]. If the pulmonary valve/aortic valve ratio is more than 0.3 there is

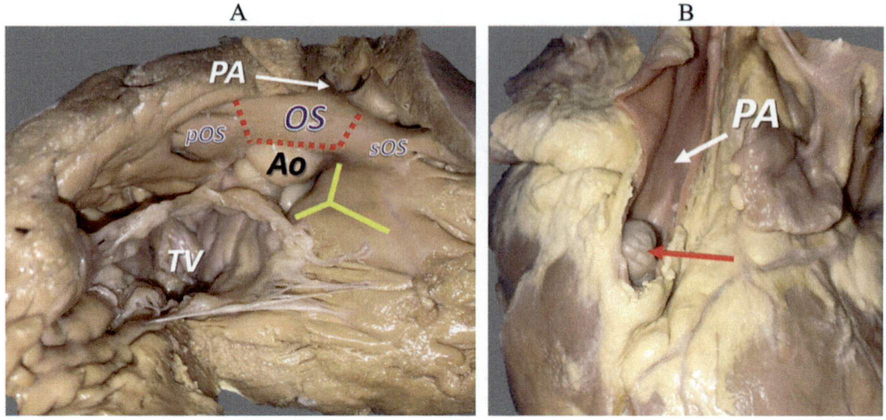

Fig. 11 DORV «tetralogy» type (autopsy specimen): **A**—view from the right ventricle. Severe infundibular (subvalvular) stenosis due to anterolateral deviation of the OS compromising pulmonary circulation (white arrow). The red dotted line indicates block of OS resection for elimination of infundibular stenosis; **B**—external view of the heart (another specimen). The pulmonary valve is imperforated (red arrow)—DORV with pulmonary valve atresia. *Ao—aorta; OS—outlet septum with its parietal (pOS) and septal (sOS) insertions; PA—pulmonary artery; TV—tricuspid valve; yellow figure—trabecula septomarginalis*

a chance to perform RVOT reconstruction without a transannular incision provided by normal morphology of pulmonary leaflets [31].

The transannular incision extends from RVOT to the pulmonary trunk through the anterior leaflet or anterior commissure of the pulmonary valve. It is advisable to leave the posterior leaflet intact. The length of the incision varies in each individual case, but should be optimal for proper RVOT augmentation. To preserve the systolic function of the right ventricle, it is important that the ventriculotomy does not extend below the inferior point of OS.

In some cases, when the transannular incision is limited by the coronary artery crossing RVOT, an extracardiac conduit implantation is indicated (Rastelli/REV operation). In this case, there are alternative surgical methods by translocation of the pulmonary artery anteriorly to the abnormal coronary artery (in fact REV procedure), transannular patch implantation under the coronary artery, as well as performing vertical ventriculomy in the area free of coronary arteries, which allows to avoid conduit implantation [32] (Fig. 12).

Transannular repair can be performed using both simple or monocusp patch made of biological or synthetic materials as well as homograft patch. Using a simple patch compared with a monocusp one contributes to the development of pulmonary valve insufficiency, which leads to right ventricle overload in the early postoperative period and increases total stay in ICU [33].

Valve-sparing Technique. Chronic pulmonary regurgitation and volume overload in the long-term after surgery, which occurs with transannular repair, can lead to

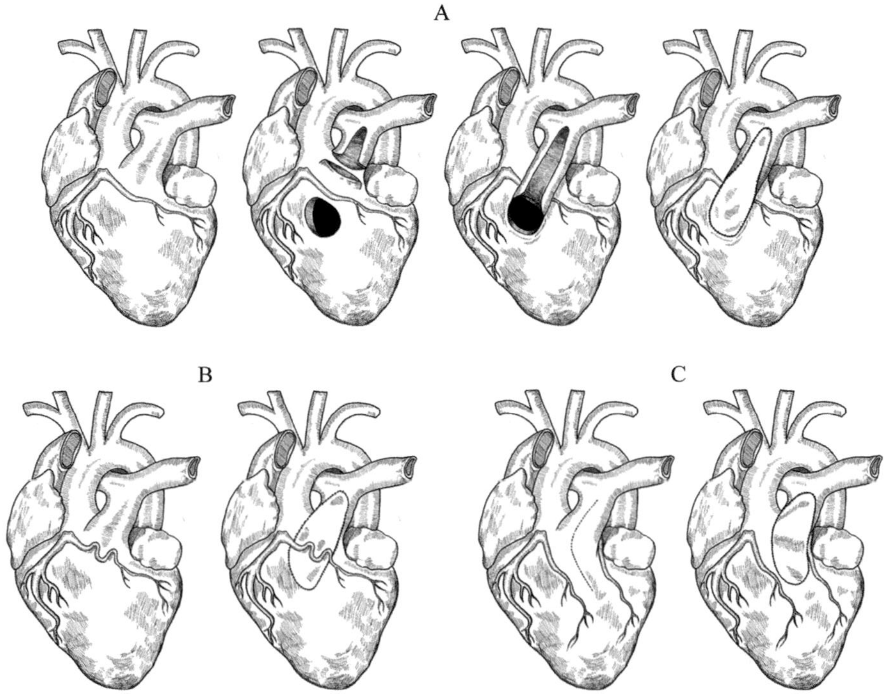

Fig. 12 Surgical techniques available in case of coronary artery crossing RVOT in order to avoid implantation of an extracardiac conduit according to Tchervenkov C.I. et al.: **A**—translocation technique; **B**—coronary artery mobilization technique; **C**—shifting of the incision line

right ventricle dilation, tricuspid valve insufficiency and the development of arrhythmias [34]. Pulmonary regurgitation also contributes to the development of diastolic dysfunction of the right ventricle, which is associated with a poor long-term prognosis [35]. In addition, the elimination of infundibular stenosis through a transannular approach supplemented with ventriculotomy leads to a decreased ejection fraction of both ventricles in the long-term after surgery compared to the transpulmonary approach without ventriculotomy due to the development of fibrosis and zone of akinesia represented by the patch itself [36]

Nowadays to solve these problems the valve-sparing techniques for RVOT reconstruction in tetralogy of Fallot and DORV «tetralogy» type are increasingly used when it is possible. These techniques imply the preservation of, albeit degenerated, but native leaflets to prevent pulmonary valve insufficiency without a transannular incision.

The indication for the valve-sparing technique is Z-score of the pulmonary annulus > -2 as long as absence of unicuspid valve and significant dysplasia of the leaflets. With the valve-sparing technique relief from infundibular stenosis is performed through a transatrial or transpulmonary approaches [37].

Pulmonary leaflet repair implies mainly commissurotomy, and in rare cases suspension of the commissures. Intraoperative balloon valvuloplasty can be performed under direct visual control to dilate the annulus [38–40].

Despite the presence of a higher residual pressure gradient on RVOT compared to the transannular technique, the main advantage of the valve-sparing technique is the absence of pulmonary regurgitation and its adverse consequences on the right ventricle performance after surgery.

3 DORV «TGA» Type

DORV with subpulmonary VSD is a type of malformation, which in anatomical and hemodynamic terms approaches TGA.

Timing

The optimal time for correction mainly depends on the presence of pulmonary artery stenosis, aortic arch obstruction and associated lesions.

Surgical Tactics

The following determining factors in choosing the type of surgical intervention in DORV «TGA» type are distinguished [23]:

- presence of pulmonary artery stenosis;
- presence of subaortic obstruction;
- tricuspid-to-pulmonary valve distance;
- arterial valves relationship;
- anatomy of coronary arteries.

When planning ASO as the most anatomical method of repair of DORV «TGA» type, the presence of uncorrectable pulmonary artery stenosis is a main contraindication. In this regard if tricuspid-to-pulmonary valve distance is enough, the Kawashima (when «side-by-side» relationship of the arterial trunks) or Rastelli/REV (when no «side-by-side» relationship) operations are indicated. If tricuspid-to-pulmonary valve distance is less than the diameter of the aortic valve, then the Rastelli/REV operation is indicated which implies pulmonary valve oversewing and switching it off from circulation (Fig. 13). In some cases, tricuspid-to-pulmonary valve distance can be increased by OS resection, which will be enough for Kawashima operation.

After Kawashima/Rastelli/REV operations the intraventricular tunnel, and hence the exit from the left ventricle, is Z-shaped due to aortic dextraposition, despite the fact that the OS is almost completely resected. In this regard, the risk of subaortic obstruction during these operations remains high. Kawashima/Rastelli/REV operations can also be performed as alternative techniques to ASO in case of complex coronary artery anatomy.

To prevent the formation of a curved intraventricular tunnel in DORV «TGA» type associated with pulmonary artery stenosis, there have been developed another

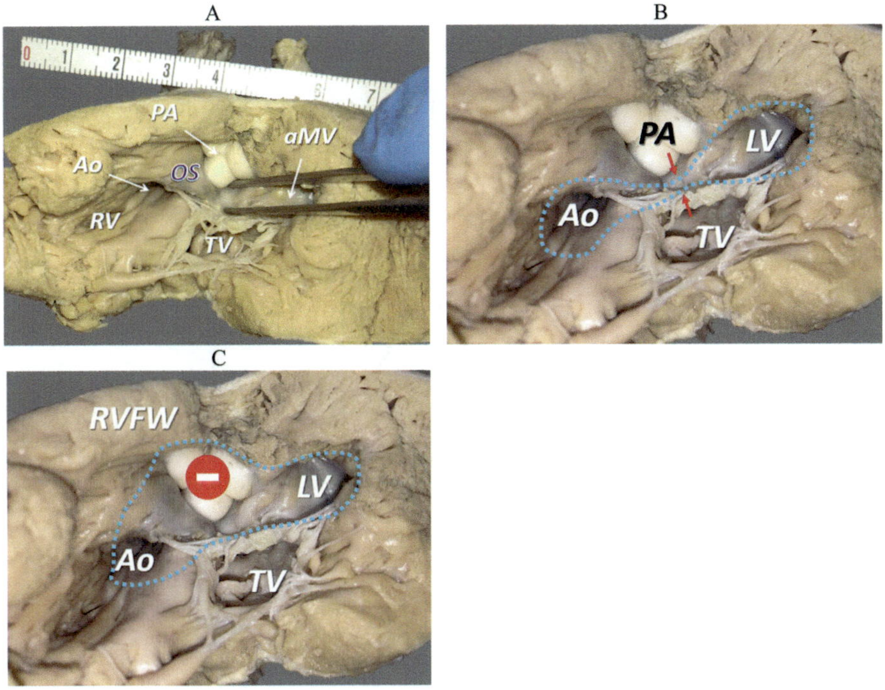

Fig. 13 DORV «TGA» type with anterior and right aorta (autopsy specimen; view from the right ventricle): **A**—there is a short tricuspid-to-pulmonary valve distance (between the tips of the forceps); **B**—Kawashima operation (blue dotted line) in this case will inevitably lead to tunnel obstruction due to its hourglass shape; **C**—if ASO is contraindicated, then the Rastelli/REV operation may be implemented (blue dotted line) or alternative surgical techniques. *Ao—aorta; PA—pulmonary artery; LV—left ventricle; RV—right ventricle; OS—outlet septum; aMV—anterior leaflet of the mitral valve; RVFW—right ventricle free wall; TV—tricuspid valve*

surgical approaches, which result in construction of a direct and thus more anatomical exit from the left ventricle to the aorta. Such methods may be performed both with pulmonary valve preservation (half-turned truncal switch operation and double root translocation) and without (Nikaidoh operation). The routine use of these techniques is limited by their surgical complexity and the need for reimplantation of coronary arteries (Fig. 14).

Approach

A transatrial approach does not allow full assessment of anatomy and relationship of all the intracardiac structures. It is more preferable to approach through the pulmonary trunk, which is almost always enlarged [41, 42]. If it is planned to construct an intraventricular tunnel with the aorta, then ventriculotomy provides access to the posterior-inferior rim of VSD. In a number of cases of ASO intraventricular tunneling can also be performed through the ascending aorta.

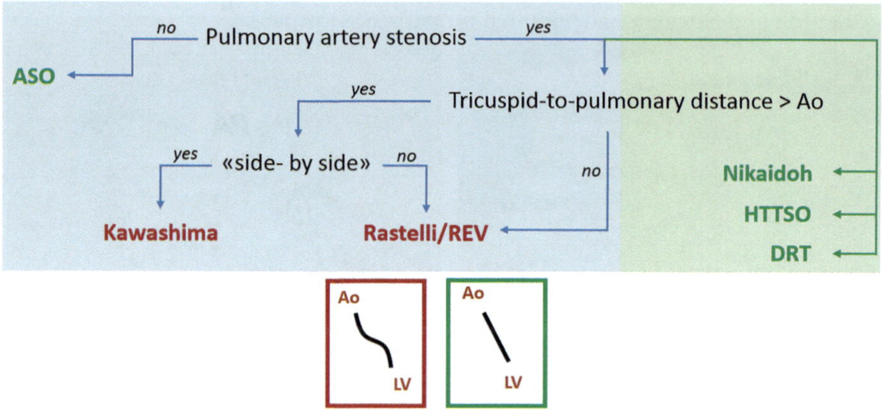

Fig. 14 Surgical strategy for DORV with subpulmonary VSD. The red and green squares indicate the geometric shape of the exit from the left ventricle after the techniques of anatomical correction indicated by the corresponding color spheres. *Ao—aorta; LV—left ventricle; ASO—arterial switch operation; HTTSO—half-turned truncal switch operation; DRT—double root translocation*

Revision

Structures to be assessed:

- presence of pulmonary artery stenosis;
- anatomy of coronary arteries;
- OS and its deviation to the subaortic or subpulmonary area;
- arterial valves relationship;
- tricuspid-to-pulmonary valve distance;
- anomalous attachment of atrioventricular valves.

Because ASO is a method of choice in DORV «TGA» type without pulmonary artery stenosis, the evaluation of the pulmonary valve, coronary arteries and the OS is of paramount importance.

3.1 Standard Surgical Techniques

Jatene Operation

Jatene operation is ASO with coronary arteries reimplantation into the neoaorta. In Taussig-Bing anomaly this is supplemented by tunneling of the pulmonary artery to the left ventricle [43–45]. An important condition for performing the operation is a normal-sized pulmonary valve and its normal morphology.

Indications: Taussig-Bing anomaly; TGA; TGA with VSD without or with correctable pulmonary artery stenosis.

Timing and Surgery. The optimal time for ASO is the first month of life due to the further risk of pulmonary hypertension, the negative impact of chronic arterial hypoxemia, as well as an increase in the discrepancy between the sizes of arterial trunks [46]. However, when comparing the results of primary ASO in Taussig-Bing anomaly and TGA in patients younger and older than 6 months and with an average pressure in the pulmonary artery before surgery of 46.5 ± 16.3 mmHg there were no differences in the mortality rate, hospital and ICU stay [47].

Surgical tactics in patients with Taussig-Bing anomaly who are candidates for ASO depends on the presence or absence of concomitant obstructive lesions of the aortic arch. With their combination, surgical treatment may involve early one-stage or staged correction. As a first stage aortic arch reconstruction with pulmonary artery banding and ligation of patent ductus arteriosus are carried out. Later ASO should be provided as a second stage of surgery. One stage repair should be performed in the first 2 months of life [48–50]. The main advantages of this approach compared to staged approach are a lower risk of surgery, no risk of pulmonary hypertension, better exposure of the aortic arch through the median sternotomy compared to lateral thoracotomy, as well as a lower frequency of postoperative complications and reinterventions [51].

In some cases, for preoperative stabilization of a patient's clinical condition balloon atrioseptostomy may be utilized to improve the mixing of arterial and venous blood at the atrial level and, thereby, increase systemic oxygenation due to the partial redirection of arterial blood from the left atrium to the right ventricle (Fig. 15). With severe aortic arch obstruction, infusion of prostaglandin provides perfusion of lower part of body.

In symptomatic patients with pulmonary overcirculation pulmonary artery banding may be implemented, but it should be noted that with subsequent ASO there is a risk of neoaortic valve insufficiency in the long-term after surgery due to hemodynamic load on the pulmonary valve annulus after banding [52].

Approach. The main stages of ASO in Taussig-Bing anomaly can be performed without ventriculotomy. Tunneling of the pulmonary artery is performed through the pulmonary trunk [51, 53] or right atrium [50], while elimination of subaortic obstruction through the aortic valve [50, 53]. In rare cases of inadequate visualization of VSD, right ventriculotomy may be necessary [49, 54].

Revision. Structures to be assessed:

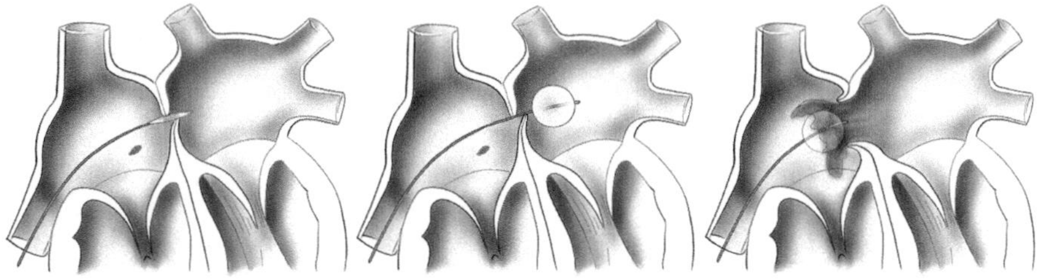

Fig. 15 Atrioseptostomy (Rashkind procedure)

- anatomy of coronary arteries;
- morphology of the upper rim of VSD;
- subaortic obstruction;
- aortic arch obstruction.

Anatomy of Coronary Arteries. Evaluation of coronary arteries should include detection of their anomalous course, single and intramural coronary artery. The presence of a single or intramural coronary artery is associated with high risk of adverse coronary events after surgery, and therefore, in some cases, an alternative surgical option may be required (Fig. 14).

Morphology of the Upper Rim of VSD. Determining the morphology of the upper rim of VSD is important in relation to eliminating the risk of pressure gradient in LVOT immediately after the correction, or in the long-term period. If the upper rim of VSD is muscular and is represented by the subpulmonary conus (the left part of VIF between the mitral and pulmonary valves—mitral-pulmonary muscular continuity), then the muscular elements of the conus can be optimally resected to create a nonobstructive tunnel [55]. During this, care should be taken not to exit out of the heart and damage left coronary artery.

Subaortic Obstruction. Subaortic obstruction in Taussig-Bing anomaly usually develops due to deviation of the OS to the right when aorta becomes "squeezed" between the OS and VIF (Fig. 16). Since after the Lecompte maneuver (if performed) the pulmonary artery will be translocated to the aortic position, this area is not critical for subaortic stenosis after correction. Optimal resection of the OS and/or the right half of VIF reliefs the obstruction.

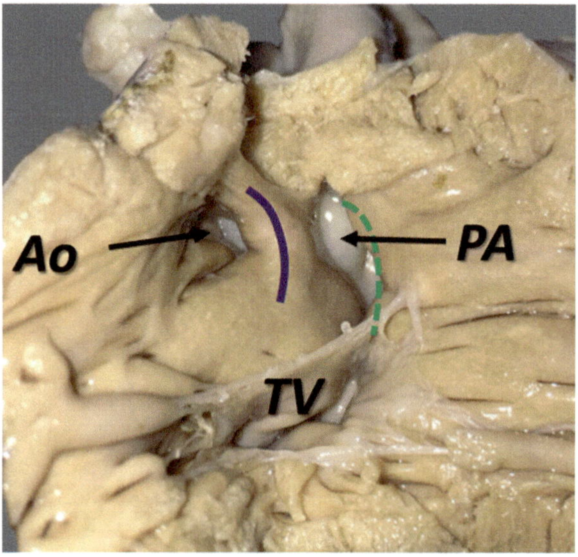

Fig. 16 DORV «TGA» type, view from the right ventricle (autopsy specimen). The OS deviates to the right causing subaortic obstruction. *Ao—aorta; PA—pulmonary artery; TV—tricuspid valve; purple figure—outlet septum; green figure—VSD crest*

Aortic Arch Obstruction. Surgical treatment depends on type of aortic arch obstruction. Arch reconstruction is similar to the standard techniques used in the isolated lesions.

Technique. After the median sternotomy, autopericardium is harvested. Before the ascending aorta is cross-clamped both pulmonary arteries are widely mobilized and ductus arteriosus is ligated and transected. Coronary anatomy is assessed. If there are no contraindications to ASO then the operation can be proceeded. The pulmonary trunk is transected just below the bifurcation site and the ascending aorta 3–5 mm above the sinotubular junction. Coronary arteries are mobilized and detached from the aortic wall. If detected, subaortic obstruction is eliminated by optimal resection of the OS and/or VIF [56].

After intracardiac revision the operation proceeds with intraventricular tunnel construction. The length of tunnel corresponds to the distance from TS to the OS located to the right to the pulmonary artery, and the width corresponds to the distance between the limbs of TS. Accordingly, the more the pulmonary artery is displaced to the right ventricle, the longer the patch length required. Also, the diameter of the pulmonary artery during systole can serve as a reliable indicator of the patch size [57].

To increase the exit from the left ventricle, a suture line can be lead along the right edge of IVS. The suture line follows anteriorly along TS and its anterior limb and continues up to the free wall of the right ventricle until the anterior edge of VIF. Posteriorly the suture line follows posterior limb of TS until the posterior edge of VIF. After that, a patch can be trimmed, adapting it to the size of VSD. The upper part of a patch is sewn along the OS and the free wall of the right ventricle just below the pulmonary valve leaflets attachment (Fig. 17).

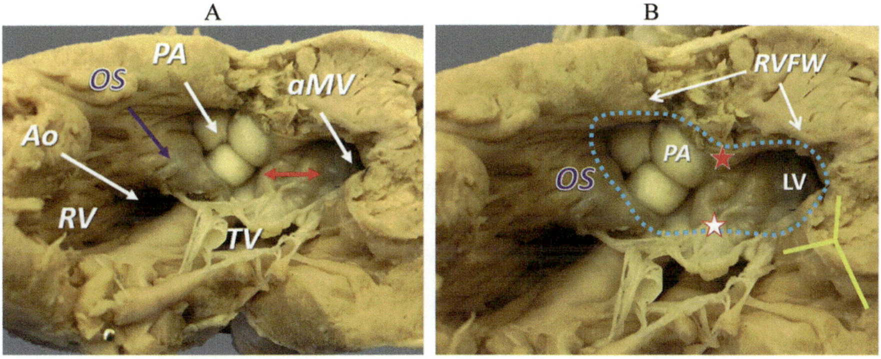

Fig. 17 Taussig-Bing anomaly (autopsy specimen): **A**—view from the right ventricle. Between the anterior leaflet of the mitral valve and the pulmonary valve there is a prominent VIF (double-headed red arrow); **B**—the line of intraventricular tunneling of the pulmonary artery (see text). *Ao—aorta; OS—outlet septum; PA—pulmonary artery; LV—left ventricle; RV—right ventricle; RVFW—right ventricle free wall; TV—tricuspid valve; yellow figure—trabecula septomarginalis; blue dotted line—intraventricular tunneling line; red asterisk—anterior edge of VIF; white asterisk—posterior edge of VIF*

ASO in Taussig-Bing anomaly can be performed both with and without the Lecompte maneuver [56]. Coronary arteries are reimplanted to the corresponding sinuses of the neoaorta, and the ascending aorta is reconstructed. With a great discrepancy between the diameter of the neoaortic valve and the ascending aorta, resection of the triangular segment of the noncoronary sinus helps to reduce the diameter of the neoaorta and its adaptation to the diameter of ascending aorta [46, 48]. Defects in the wall of the neopulmonary trunk are replaced by autopericadial or xenopericadial patches.

The operation completes with neopulmonary trunk restoration. If left anterior descending or circumflex artery pass behind the pulmonary annulus, then after the Lecompte maneuver there is a risk of their compression by the neopulmonary trunk. In this regard, the incision from the pulmonary artery bifurcation can be extended to the right and thus perform anastomosis with the right pulmonary artery [46, 49, 51, 54, 58, 59], which allows to shift the neopulmonary trunk to the right to the coronary artery.

Jatene operation may be performed with good clinical results in almost all cases of Taussig-Bing anomaly regardless of the anatomy of coronary arteries and arterial trunks relationship [47, 49, 54, 60].

Advantages: straight exit from the left ventricle to the neoaorta; no need for ventriculotomy; better hemodynamic profile compared to aortic tunneling.

Disadvantages: the need for reimplantation of coronary arteries; neoaortic valve insufficiency after previous pulmonary artery banding (if performed).

3.1.1 Kawashima Operation

Kawashima operation—tunneling of D-aorta to the left ventricle with an intraventricular patch behind the pulmonary valve [61].

Indications: Taussig-Bing anomaly; DORV with subpulmonary VSD and pulmonary artery stenosis with «side by side» arterial trunks and tricuspid-to-pulmonary artery distance greater than the diameter of the aortic valve.

Timing. If without pulmonary artery stenosis—see Jatene operation. In the presence of severe pulmonary artery stenosis and arterial hypoxemia, the modified systemic-to-pulmonary shunt may be indicated with subsequent Kawashima operation in 6–12 months of life.

Approach. Through the right atrium in combination with ventriculotomy under the pulmonary artery.

Revision. Structures to be assessed:

- tricuspid-to-pulmonary valve distance;
- arterial valves relationship;
- subaortic obstruction;
- pulmonary artery stenosis;
- anomalous attachment of tricuspid valve chordae to OS.

Tricuspid-to-Pulmonary Valve Distance. Since aortic tunneling is performed behind the pulmonary valve, the main determining factor in performing the operation is a sufficient tricuspid-to-pulmonary valve distance, which should be greater than or at least equal to the diameter of the aortic valve. Otherwise, there is a high risk of narrowing of intraventricular tunnel. On the one hand, insufficient tricuspid-to-pulmonary valve distance is not always an obstacle for construction of a nonobstructive intraventricular tunnel. On the other hand, performing a standard resection of the OS and the length of tricuspid-to-pulmonary valve distance of 3–4 mm is not enough to prevent tunnel obstruction [62]. If tricuspid-to-pulmonary valve distance is short, additional tunnel width can be achieved by resection of the adjacent pulmonary valve with the formation of part of the suture line along the inner wall of the pulmonary artery [61, 62].

Arterial Valves Relationship. Kawashima operation can be performed not only when the arterial trunks are «side by side», but also when the aorta is slightly anterior to the pulmonary artery. It should be mentioned that the more aorta is displaced anterior, the more difficult to construct intraventricular tunnel behind the pulmonary valve and the higher risk of subaortic obstruction subsequently.

Subaortic Obstruction. See Jatene operation.

Pulmonary Artery Stenosis. The presence of pulmonary artery stenosis requires RVOT reconstruction by one of the known methods (see DORV «tetralogy» and «VSD» types).

Anomalous Attachment of Tricuspid Valve Chordae to the OS. If anomalous chordae of the tricuspid valve is attached to the OS (Fig. 18A), it can be detached and subsequently reimplanted onto the intraventricular patch.

Technique. After evaluation of the intracardiac structures, the aorta is tunneled to the left ventricle. Because intraventricular tunnel is constructed behind the pulmonary artery (Fig. 19A), it is necessary to resect OS through ventriculotomy [21] (Fig. 19B). It is important to clearly visualize the aortic valve in order to avoid its unintentional

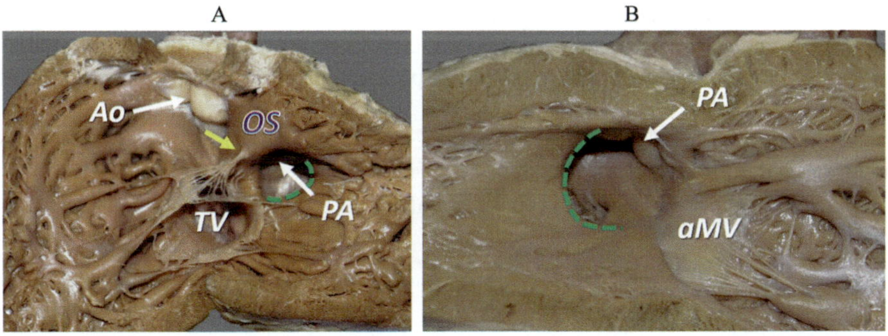

Fig. 18 Taussig-Bing anomaly (autopsy specimen): **A**—view from the right ventricle. The chordae of the tricuspid septal leaflet are attached to the OS (yellow arrow); **B**—view from the left ventricle. *Ao—aorta; OS—outlet septum; PA—pulmonary artery; aMV—anterior leaflet of the mitral valve; TV—tricuspid valve; green dotted line—rim of VSD*

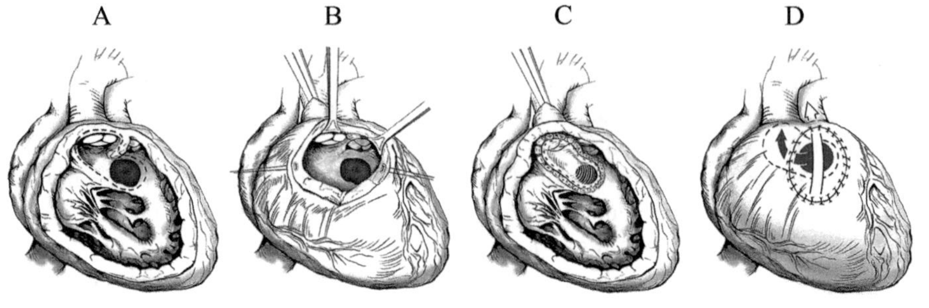

Fig. 19 Kawashima operation. See text

damage. Insufficient resection of the OS contributes to the curved configuration of tunnel. A patch is usually trimmed oval or diamond-shaped. The use of a complex-shaped patch is accompanied by the risk of subaortic obstruction, which results in the inevitable turbulence of the blood with subsequent fibrous intimal proliferation [62].

The right half of VIF and the myocardium of the free wall of the right ventricle, constituting the subaortic conus, also take part in the formation of subaortic obstruction, and must be optimally resected [63].

The suture line follows TS and its anterior limb, continues upward to the free wall of the left ventricle and the left half of VIF (behind the pulmonary valve and in front of the mitral valve). After that, the suture is carried out backward to the anterior aspect of the resected OS and then follows in front of the aortic valve (from the left) until the free wall of the right ventricle (Fig. 19A). On the opposite side, the suture line is conducted along the posterior limb of TS, to the right aspect of VIF and then it follows in front of the aortic valve (from the right) (Fig. 19B).

When suturing, it is necessary to take into account the relief of the muscular trabeculae of the right ventricle free wall to prevent residual left to right shunting due to intramural VSD [21]. Superficial stitches within the myocardium without involving fibrous elements of the aortic valve more prone to residual shunting [13].

RVOT reconstruction in the presence of pulmonary artery stenosis is performed (Fig. 19D).

Advantages: aortic valve remains a systemic one in comparison with ASO; no need for coronary arteries reimplantation.

Disadvantages: long and curved intraventricular tunnel.

3.1.2 Patrick–McGoon Operation

Patrick–McGoon operation—tunneling of A-aorta to the left ventricle with an intraventricular patch positioned anterior and left to the pulmonary valve [64].

Indications: Taussig-Bing anomaly; DORV with subpulmonary VSD and pulmonary artery stenosis with A-aorta.

The operation was developed for the treatment of DORV with subpulmonary VSD and anterior aorta, but due to the high risk of tunnel obstruction, this method has lost its value. Nowadays with such an anatomy the operation of choice is ASO.

3.1.3 Rastelli Operation

Rastelli operation—tunneling of aorta to the left ventricle through the VSD with an intraventricular patch involving the orifice of the pulmonary valve [65, 66] (Fig. 20).

Indications: DORV with subpulmonary VSD, pulmonary artery stenosis if Kawashima operation is not feasible.

Timing. The most optimal age for the operation is 6–12 months.

Approach. Combination of atrial approach and ventriculotomy.

Revision. Structures to be assessed:

- anatomy, size and morphological substrate of pulmonary valve stenosis;
- anomalous attachment of atrioventricular valves;
- VSD size;
- OS;
- coronary artery crossing RVOT;
- size of the right ventricle.

Anatomy, Size and Morphological Substrate of Pulmonary Valve Stenosis. Evaluation of the pulmonary valve morphology and the substrate of its stenosis is important in terms of whether it is possible to proceed with ASO or not. If pulmonary stenosis may be eliminated or Z-score of the pulmonary valve is > −1.8, ASO is not contraindicated [67].

The intraventricular tunnel constructed during the Rastelli procedure is characterized by a curved shape, which depends on and directly correlates with the diameter of the pulmonary valve. In this regard, the ideal candidate for Rastelli operation is

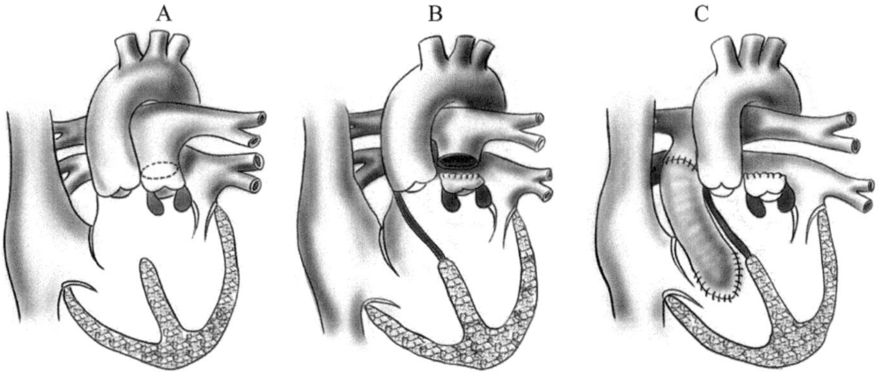

Fig. 20 Rastelli operation. An extracardiac conduit is placed to the right to the aorta. See text

a patient with severe hypoplasia of the pulmonary valve annulus. With moderate hypoplasia, it is recommended to consider Nikaidoh operation or other alternative surgical approaches, since they provide a straight exit from the left ventricle to the ascending aorta.

Anomalous Attachment of Atrioventricular Valves. In case of abnormal attachment of the tricuspid valve, it can be detached at the base and subsequently reimplanted onto the intraventricular patch [68].

VSD size. As a rule, VSD in DORV «TGA» type is quite large and there is rarely a need to its extension.

OS. Regardless of the size of the OS, it must be resected to provide straight exit from the left ventricle.

Coronary Artery Crossing RVOT. Before ventriculotomy it is necessary to make sure that there are no large infundibular coronary branches crossing RVOT.

Size of the Right Ventricle. Because intraventricular tunnel occupies a relatively large space of the right ventricle, Rastelli operation is contraindicated in patients with borderline right ventricle.

Technique. The pulmonary artery is transected above the level of commissures. The pulmonary valve and the morphological substrate of stenosis are evaluated. If severe annulus hypoplasia and/or dysplastic leaflets are observed, pulmonary artery is oversewn involving valve leaflets to prevent further thrombosis, thus switching off the pulmonary valve from circulation (Fig. 20B). OS is resected as much as possible to create a straight exit from the left ventricle to the aorta.

Intraventricular tunnel construction is conducted through the ventriculotomy. The suture line follows the same anatomical structures as in Kawashima operation, with the difference that the upper part of a patch is sewn anterior to pulmonary valve along the free wall of the right ventricle, constituting the subpulmonary conus (Fig. 13C). As a result, both orifices of the arterial valves are tunneled to the left ventricle. The connection between the right ventricle and the pulmonary artery is restored using an extracardiac conduit which, if possible, should be positioned to the left to the ascending aorta in order to prevent its compression by the sternum after closing the chest (Fig. 20C).

Advantages: the only possible technique in case of pulmonary artery stenosis and tricuspid-to-pulmonary valve distance less than diameter of the aorta (except for alternative surgical methods—see below).

Disadvantages: long and curved intraventricular tunnel; reduction of the right ventricular cavity; implantation of an extracardia conduit.

3.1.4 REV Operation

REV operation (*repair à l'etage ventriculaire*) is a modification of Rastelli procedure with RVOT reconstruction by native pulmonary trunk [4, 69].

REV was developed as an alternative to Rastelli operation in order to avoid late complications related to conduit implantation and thereby to eliminate the risk of reinterventions.

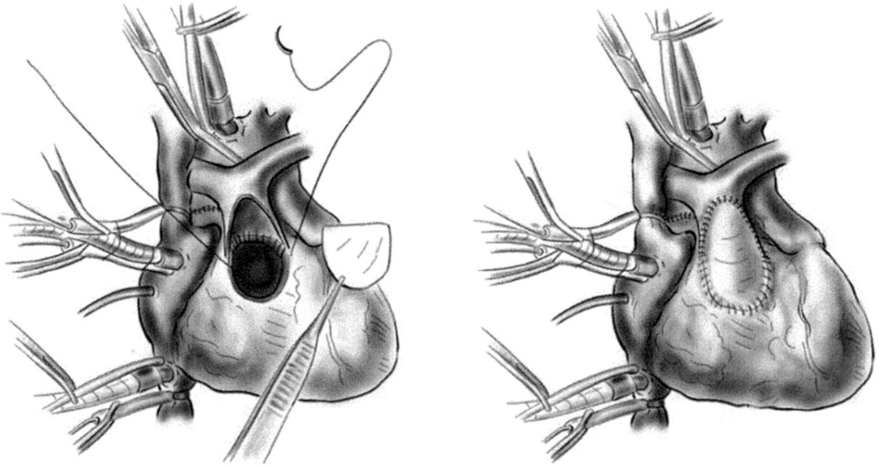

Fig. 21 REV (repair à l'etage ventriculaire) operation. See text

Technique. The pulmonary artery is transected above the level of commissures and its proximal part is ovrsewn involving leaflets to prevent thrombus formation. The intracardiac part of the operation is similar to Rastelli procedure. The aorta is transected above the commissures, and the Lecompte maneuver is performed (Fig. 21A). RVOT reconstruction is performed with native pulmonary trunk and a monocusp patch (Fig. 21B).

The key points of REV operation are extensive resection of OS to create a straighter exit from the left ventricle to the aorta, as well as wide mobilization of the pulmonary artery branches to prevent their tension after the Lecompte maneuver [70]. The modified REV operation is performed without the Lecompte maneuver [71].

Advantages: see Rastelli operation.

Disadvantages: long intraventricular tunnel; reduction of the right ventricle cavity; tension of the pulmonary artery branches.

3.1.5 Atrial Switch with Pulmonary Artery Tunneling

Atrial switch operation is a method of physiological correction of DORV «TGA» type with pulmonary artery tunneling to the left ventricle additioned by Musturd or Senning procedures [72–77]. As a result of the operation, the left ventricle provides pulmonary, while the right ventricle provided systemic circulation. Earlier the operation also used in DORV with noncommitted VSD [74].

The operation had a value at the early stages of pediatric cardiac surgery, when ASO had not yet been introduced into clinical use. At later stages, the indication for atrial switch was the complex anatomy of the coronary arteries, which did not allow ventriculotomy or ASO. To date, the operation has lost its practical value.

3.1.6 Damus–Kaye–Stansel Operation

Damus–Kaye–Stansel operation is a method of translocation of the pulmonary artery to the left ventricle, connection of the pulmonary artery to the ascending aorta, and RVOT reconstruction using an extracardiac conduit [78–81].

Indications: DORV with subpulmonary VSD and aortic valve hypoplasia or severe subaortic obstruction; with deformation of the proximal part of the pulmonary trunk [81].

3.1.7 Abe and Dotty Operations

Abe and Doty operations are method of aortic tunneling to the left ventricle by various techniques of intraventricular conduit. To date, these operations are no longer used [82, 83].

3.2 Alternative Surgical Techniques

The general requirements for each of the surgical techniques described below is the wide mobilization of the pulmonary artery branches for the Lecompte maneuver as well as the coronary arteries due to the need for their reimplantation.

The factors that prevent intraventricular tunneling during Rastelli procedure, such as anomalous attachment of the tricuspid valve chordae, insufficient tricuspid-to-pulmonary valve distance etc., do not affect these operations. On the one hand, these techniques result in straight exit from the left ventricle to the aorta, which is beneficial in anatomical and hemodynamic terms. On the other hand, they all are technically difficult to perform, requiring specific high surgical skills.

3.2.1 Nikaidoh Operation

Nikaidoh operation is a posterior translocation of the aorta without pulmonary valve preservation.

Indications: DORV with subpulmonary VSD and pulmonary artery stenosis. Initially, Nikaidoh procedure was proposed for surgical correction of TGA with VSD and pulmonary artery stenosis [84], but later it found its application in DORV «TGA» type [85].

Timing. The optimal age for the operation is 6–12 months of life.

Approach. Due to excellent exposure of all intracardiac structures after aortic root detachment from the myocardium of the right ventricle, only standard transatrial approach is performed.

Revision. Structures to be assessed:

- anatomy of coronary arteries;
- distance of aortic translocation;
- anomalous attachment of atrioventricular valve chordae to the OS.

Anatomy of Coronary Arteries. Evaluation of coronary anatomy is necessary to choose the technique for their reimplantation. When single coronary anatomy the risk of adverse coronary events is increased several times.

The proximal course of the main coronary arteries to the aortic annulus complicates harvesting of the aortic root from the right ventricle, and in some cases makes it impossible. Such a scenario is observed in looping coronary arteries—E and F types of coronary anatomy according to the Yacoub classification [86] (Fig. 22). The operation is also precluded in type B, when the right coronary artery passes between the arterial trunks.

Distance of Aortic Translocation. It is important to understand that the distance of the aortic translocation depends on the sum of OS width and the diameter of the pulmonary valve, which is critical in terms of the risk of tension of the coronary arteries after their reimplantation (Fig. 23). When the diameter of the pulmonary valve is < 5 mm Nikaidoh operation will not provide sufficient LVOT augmentation, therefore Rastelli/REV operation is good alternative (Fig. 23B). If pulmonary annulus is big (80% of the diameter of the aorta) and the risk of coronary artery reimplantation

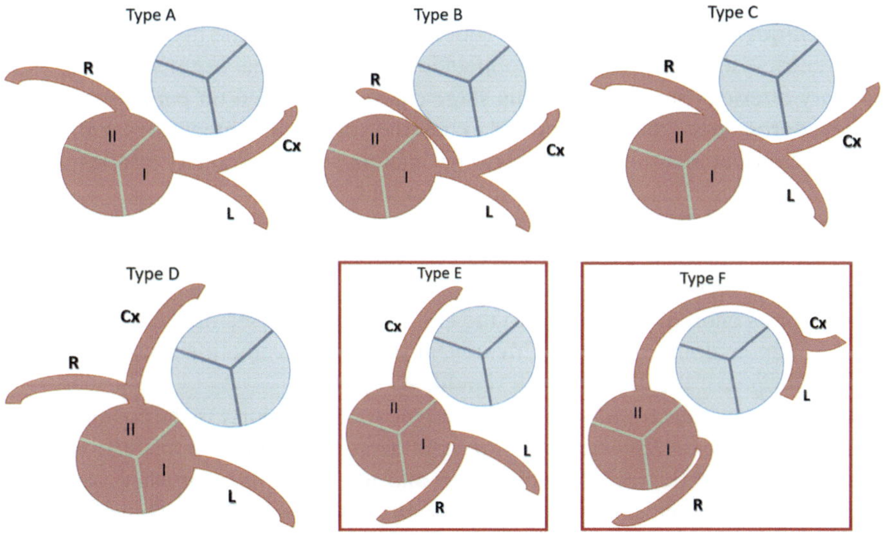

Fig. 22 Coronary artery anatomy according to the Yacoub classification. E and F types are characterized by looping right coronary artery passing in front of the aortic valve thus complicating its harvesting from the myocardium of the right ventricle during Nikaidoh procedure. In type B aortic translocation cannot be done because of the right coronary artery passing between the arterial trunks. *R—right coronary artery; L—left coronary artery; Cx—circumflex artery*

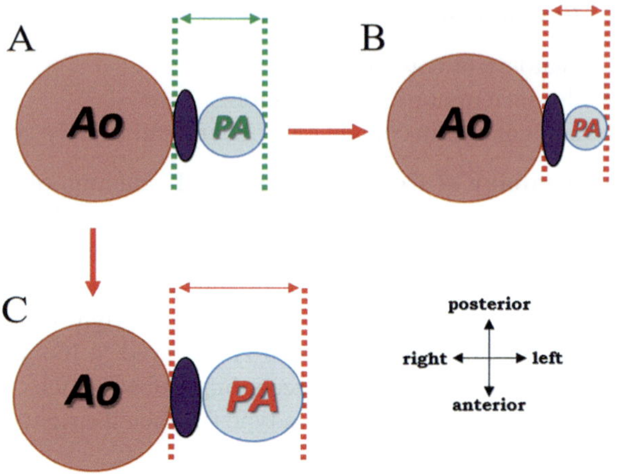

Fig. 23 Distance of translocation and its dependence on the diameter of the pulmonary artery (OS is designated as a violet figure): **A**—the optimal distance without the risk of coronary artery tension (approximately 6–12 mm); **B**—too small distance which will not allow to construct a straight exit from the left ventricle; **C**—too long distance with the risk of tension of the coronary arteries. *Ao—aorta; PA—pulmonary artery*

seems to be high due to long distance of translocation, then ASO may be considered if pulmonary valve stenosis is correctable (Fig. 23C).

Anomalous Attachment of Atrioventricular Valve Chordae to OS. Anomalous attachment of atrioventricular valves is not a contraindication to the operation. On the contrary, Nikaidoh procedure is the only possible technique (along with the ones described below) that allows performing biventricular repair with anomalous chordal attachment of atrioventricular valves, especially mitral one.

Technique. First of all, the aortic root is harvested from the myocardium of the right ventricle along with a wide mobilization of the proximal segments of the main coronary arteries (Fig. 24A,B). This stage can be performed on parallel perfusion without aortic cross-clamping, provided that the aortic valve function is competent. The key factor at this stage is the favorable anatomy of the coronary arteries, which allows a surgeon to safely mobilize the aortic root.

The right and left pulmonary arteries are extensively mobilized, pulmonary trunk is transected above the level of the commissures, and the valve leaflets are excised. After that, the OS is dissected towards subpulmonary VSD (Fig. 24C). In the presence of anomalous chordal attachment to the OS, the latter may be dissected anterior to the site of anomalous attachment. To prevent subaortic obstruction after surgery, the muscular edges of the dissected OS should be resected.

The next step is the translocation of the aortic root posteriorly to the position of the pulmonary artery, thereby creating a straight exit to the aorta from the left ventricle. Depending on the degree of mobilization and tension of the coronary arteries in couple with the distance of translocation it may be necessary to detach the coronary arteries from the aortic wall. The aortic root should be oriented in the plane of the truncal block, avoiding its deviation above or below this level (Fig. 25). To reduce the tension of the coronary arteries, the aortic root can be rotated 180°, after which the ostia of the coronary arteries are better match the contralateral defects of the aortic wall. After that, VSD closure is performed sewing a patch in its upper part to the right-anterior aspect of the aortic root (Fig. 24D).

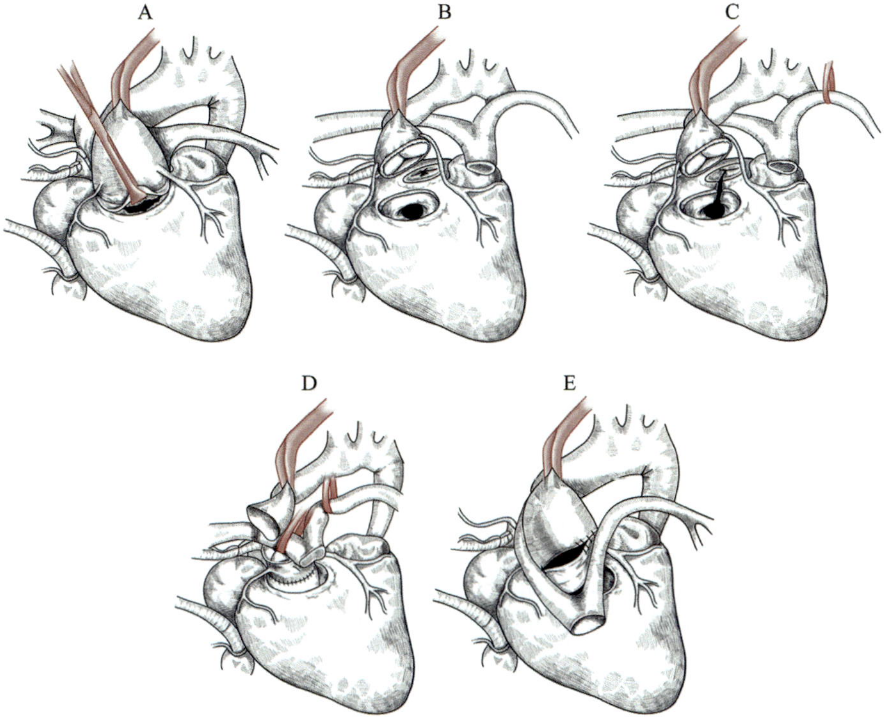

Fig. 24 Nikaidoh operation. See text

Fig. 25 Correct orientation of the aortic root in LVOT. See text

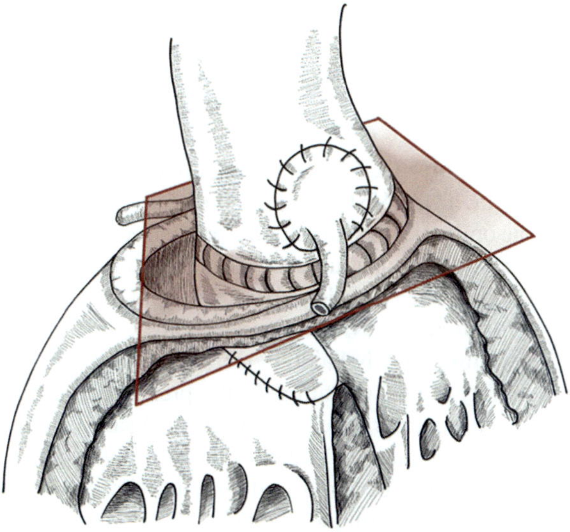

A patch for VSD closure must be correctly matched both in height and width. A too short in height patch can lead to tension between the aortic annulus and VSD, while a too long patch will bulge into the right ventricle during the systole. If a patch is short in width, there is a risk of LVOT narrowing, while an excessively wide patch can contribute to aortic valve insufficiency in the long-term after surgery.

After translocation the ascending aorta may bend in the anterior direction and lead to compression of the pulmonary arteries after the Lecompte maneuver. In this case, a cylindric segment of the ascending aorta can be resected in order to reduce its length.

The pulmonary artery can be translocated anteriorly by the Lecompte maneuver (Fig. 24E). In this case, the ascending aorta is transected, and the pulmonary artery bifurcation is translocated anteriorly to the aorta [87, 88].

RVOT reconstruction is performed with a patch [85, 89] or an extracardiac conduit [89, 90].

A contraindication to the Nikaidoh operation is a looping course of the coronary arteries precluding the harvesting of the aortic root [91]. The presence of a single coronary artery is a relative contraindication. In these cases Kawashima or Rastelli/REV operation may be an alternative choice [85, 96].

Advantages: anatomically straight exit from the left ventricle to the aorta; no need for ventriculotomy; orthotopic implantation of an extracardiac conduit; no reduction of the right ventricular cavity [92].

Disadvantages: need for coronary artery reimplantation; no pulmonary leaflets preservation; risk of aortic valve insufficiency after correction.

3.2.2 Half-Turned Truncal Switch Operation

Half-turned truncal switch operation—harvesting of the aorta and pulmonary artery within a truncal block from the base of the heart followed by its 180° rotation and reimplantation.

Indications: DORV with subpulmonary VSD and pulmonary artery stenosis with DA-aorta; TGA, VSD and pulmonary artery stenosis with A-aorta.

The optimal indication for the procedure is pulmonary artery/aortic valve diameter ratio 0.3–0.8 for adequate LVOT augmentation.

Timing. See Nikaidoh operation.

Approach. See Nikaidoh operation.

Revision. See Nikaidoh operation. Also, it is necessary to assess mitral-to-pulmonary valve continuity. In the presence of muscular continuity, the harvesting of the pulmonary root can be performed safely, while fibrous continuity may cause damage to the anterior leaflet of the mitral valve.

Technique. The aorta is transected above the sinotubular junction (Fig. 26A). In the original technique, the pulmonary artery is transected by an oblique incision from its bifurcation (anteriorly) to the level just above the commissures (posteriorly), thereby preserving its anterior wall [94]. In the later modification, the pulmonary artery is transected below the bifurcation [93]. The aorta and pulmonary artery are harvested from the base of the heart as a common block using the incision running along their fibrous annuli leaving the muscular cuff under the aortic component (Fig. 26B).

The one of the most important parts of the operation is harvesting of the pulmonary component of the truncal block at the site of mitral-pulmonary continuity (Fig. 26C). In case of fibrous continuity there is a risk of damage to the anterior leaflet of the mitral valve. Moreover, it is necessary to leave some tissue in this area to allow implantation of the aortic component of the truncal block after its rotation. In this regard, it is recommended to carry out dissection of mitral-pulmonary continuity at 45° angle [95] (Fig. 27).

After detachment from the OS, the truncal block is completely removed from the base of the heart. The OS is dissected vertically towards VSD (Fig. 26D). If dissection is complicated by anomalous attachment of atrioventricular valves to the OS, then the vertical incision should be done anteriorly (Fig. 28) [96–98].

The truncal block rotates 180° thus positioning the aortic and pulmonary components above the appropriate ventricles. Next, the aortic component is sewn to LVOT with simultaneous VSD closure in the manner as described for Nikaidoh procedure (Fig. 26E,F).

Once implantation of the aortic component and VSD closure are completed, the coronary arteries are reimplanted to the contralateral (after block rotation) sinuses—the left coronary artery to the right coronary sinus, and right coronary artery to the left coronary sinus. After that, the Lecompte maneuver is performed, and the ascending aorta is reconstructed (Fig. 26G). If needed, the ascending aorta may be shortened by

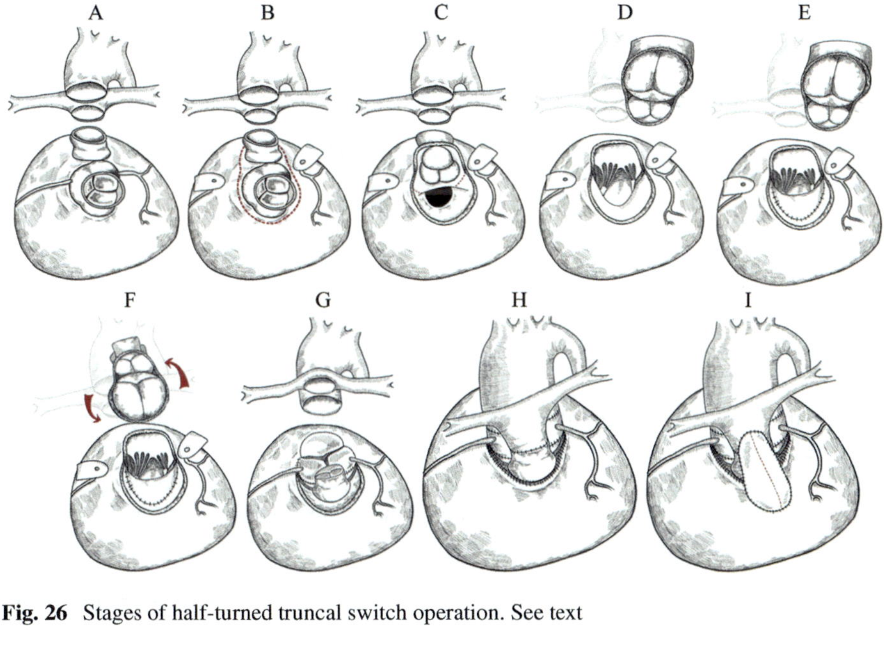

Fig. 26 Stages of half-turned truncal switch operation. See text

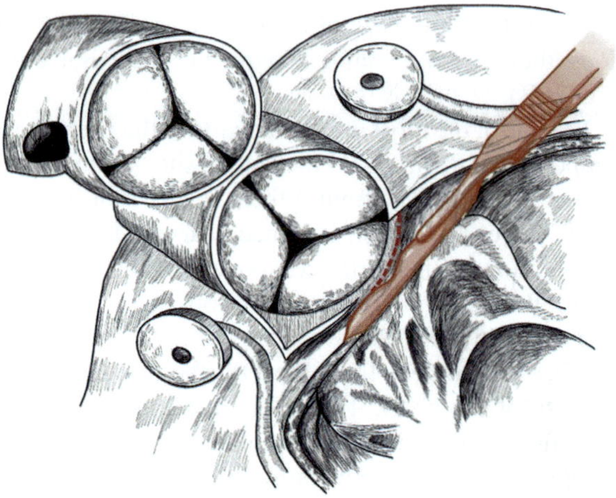

Fig. 27 Technique of detachment of the pulmonary root from the anterior leaflet of the mitral valve

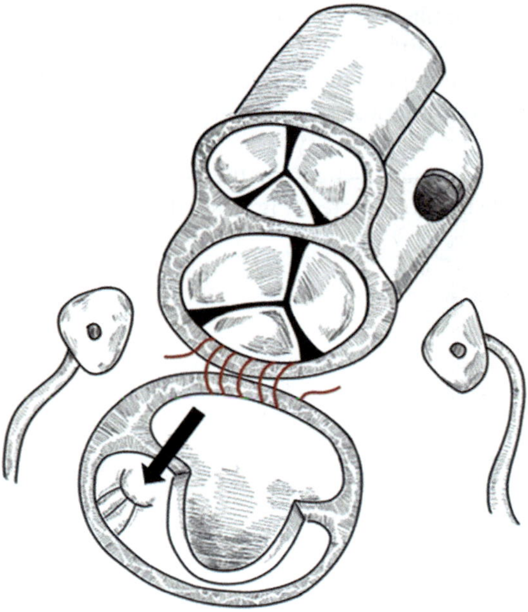

Fig. 28 Dissection of the OS anteriorly to the abnormally attached tricuspid valve chordae (arrow)

excising its cylindric or triangular segment to prevent bending and thus compression of the pulmonary artery.

If the pulmonary artery was initially transected as in the original description, the preserved anterior wall after rotation becomes the posterior one to which bifurcation is anastomosed. An anterior wall of the pulmonary artery is reconstructed with a monocusp patch. If pulmonary artery was transected transversely, then RVOT reconstruction may be performed with or without a patch depending on the degree of pulmonary stenosis (Fig. 26H,I).

Like in Nikaidoh procedure, the proximal course of the coronary arteries to the aortic annulus makes the operation very difficult or even impossible. Contraindications to the operation are E and F type of coronary arteries anatomy according to the Yacoub classification (Fig. 26). As an alternative Rastelli/REV operation may be considered [96].

Advantages: preservation of the native pulmonary valve and its potential to grow; no need for an extracardiac conduit; less tension of the pulmonary arteries after the Lecompte maneuver; less tension of the coronary arteries due to their reimplantation over a short distance [93].

Disadvantages: need for coronary artery reimplantation; risk of damage to the mitral valve.

3.2.3 Double Root Translocation

Double root translocation—separate harvesting of the aortic and pulmonary roots from the base of the heart with their subsequent translocation. The operation does not require the construction of a long intraventricular tunnel and the native pulmonary valve is preserved [99–101]. This technique is also a modification of Nikaidoh operation.

Indications: DORV with subpulmonary VSD and pulmonary artery stenosis; DORV with non-committed VSD and pulmonary artery stenosis [100]. Initially, the operation was proposed for TGA with VSD and pulmonary artery stenosis [99]. An important condition for its implementation is the presence of a fully muscular conus of the aortic and pulmonary valves.

Timing. See Nikaidoh operation.

Approach. See Nikaidoh operation.

Revision. See half-turned truncal switch operation.

Technique. The operation starts with harvesting of the aortic and pulmonary roots separately (Fig. 29A). The ascending aorta is transected 3–5 mm above the sinotubular junction and is detached from the myocardium of the right ventricle leaving 5–6 mm muscular cuff below the aortic valve. Detachment of the coronary arteries is required when «side-by-side» arterial trunks, while with antero-posterior relationship the coronary arteries can be translocated together with the aortic root without their detachment.

To dissect free the pulmonary artery, an incision is made 5 mm below the pulmonary valve. The longer the subpulmonary infundibulum, the safer the harvesting of the pulmonary artery (Fig. 30). In the presence of mitral-pulmonary fibrous continuity the procedure is complicated by the risk of damage to the anterior leaflet of the mitral valve.

Having harvested both arterial trunks, the Lecompte maneuver is performed—in fact, posterior translocation of the aorta and anterior translocation of the pulmonary

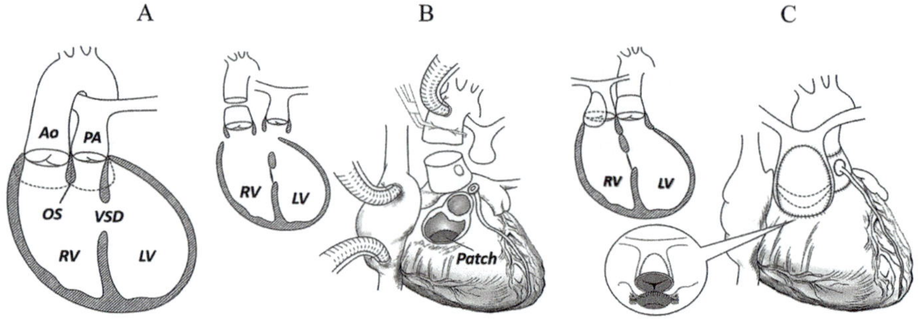

Fig. 29 Double root translocation. See text. *Ao—aorta; PA—pulmonary artery; RV—right ventricle; LV—left ventricle; OS—outlet septum; VSD—ventricular septal defect*

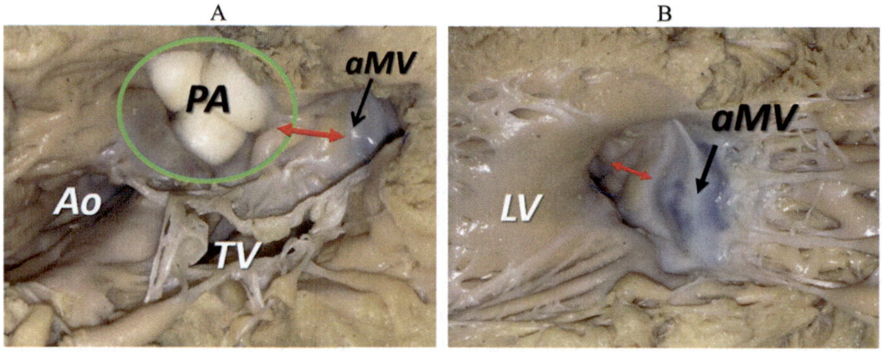

Fig. 30 DORV «TGA» type (the same specimen as in Fig. 17) Due to the presence of VIF between the mitral and pulmonary valves (red arrows), complete muscular subpulmonary conus (green circle) is formed, which makes it possible to harvest the pulmonary root more safely without the risk of damage to the anterior leaflet of the mitral valve: **A**—view from the right ventricle; **B**—view from the left ventricle. *Ao—aorta; PA—pulmonary artery; aMV—anterior leaflet of the mitral valve; TV—tricuspid valve*

artery. After VSD closure, the aortic root is sewn to LVOT, and the coronary arteries are reimplanted into the corresponding sinuses (if they were detached) (Fig. 29B). As in Nikaidoh procedure, the ascending aorta can be shortened in cylindrical or triangular fashion to prevent its anterior bending and compression of the pulmonary arteries. Anterior wall of the pulmonary artery is longitudinally incised after which it is sewn to RVOT and a monocusp patch is used to complete pulmonary artery reconstruction [100] (Fig. 29C).

Advantages: straight exit from the left ventricle to the aorta with a simple VSD closure instead of tunnel construction; preservation of the growth potential of both arterial trunks.

Disadvantages: need for coronary artery reimplantation.

4 DORV with Non-committed VSD

In case of not directly committed VSD surgical correction does not differ significantly from that of DORV with subaortic VSD, since these VSDs are conoventricular. The only difference is a need to construct a longer intraventricular tunnel due to larger subaortic conus in not directly committed VSD. In this case, the tunnel occupies a larger space of the right ventricle in compared to tunneling committed VSDs.

Among all the morphological variants DORV with non-committed (inlet) VSD is the most extreme form of the malformation in surgical terms and is associated with higher early and late mortality, as well as more frequent tunnel obstruction compared with committed VSDs [2, 102, 103].

The polymorphism of VSDs coupled with different types of arterial trunks relationship do not allow to develop a standard surgical approach for the malformation.

Because non-committed VSDs are located in the inlet part of IVS and significantly remote from the arterial valves, biventricular repair requires the formation of a long intraventricular tunnel, which is associated with the risk of its obstruction, especially in a growing child. The construction of such a tunnel can lead to a significant reduction of the right ventricle cavity and compromise the function of the tricuspid and pulmonary valves. In addition, a long tunnel increases the hemodynamic load on the left ventricle due to a large zone of akinesia represented by a non-contracting intraventricular patch. Also, in abnormal attachment of tricuspid valve chordae in the tunneling projection is common in DORV with non-committed VSD [103, 104].

The main goal of biventricular repair of DORV with non-committed VSD is to construct as straight and short tunnel as possible to one of the arterial trunks. For this, the following principles should be taken into account. First, the reasonable length of the tunnel. Thus, apical trabecular VSD is unlikely to allow performing biventricular repair without high surgical risk. Second, the elimination of subaortic obstruction by resecting muscles constituting subaortic conus. This manipulation is usually done from ventriculotomy, providing access to the tricuspid valve structures [105].

Timing

Due to the high risk of early subaortic tunnel obstruction in newborns [106] and need for reintervention, anatomical correction of DORV «non-committed» «» type is recommended in patients at least 3 months old [107]. In symptomatic patients as a first stage a systemic-to-pulmonary shunt or pulmonary artery banding may be indicated, depending on the presence or absence of pulmonary artery stenosis, respectively.

Surgical Strategy

The main factors that influence choosing the type of surgical repair are the following:

- presence of pulmonary artery stenosis;
- arterial valves relationship;
- tricuspid-to-pulmonary valve distance.

Repair of DORV with non-committed VSD primarily depends on the proximity of VSD to any of the arterial trunks and the presence or absence of pulmonary artery stenosis. The several surgical options are available:

- aortic tunneling;
- aortic tunneling with RVOT reconstruction;
- pulmonary artery tunneling with ASO.

The tunnel is constructed with the arterial valve that is closer to VSD. Usually, if VSD is significantly remote from the aorta, it is likely to be closer to the pulmonary valve [105]. Tunneling of the pulmonary artery should always be supplemented with ASO to restore ventricular-arterial concordance, which does not require construction of a long tunnel (as it does when tunneling aortic valve), may be performed regardless of tricuspid-to-pulmonary valve distance and anomalous attachment of the tricuspid valve chordae. If VSD is equally remote from both arterial valves, then an intraventricular tunnel is constructed with aorta if arterial trunks relationship is normal or L-malposed, and with pulmonary artery in case of D-malposition (Fig. 31).

In the presence of uncorrectable pulmonary artery stenosis, an intraventricular tunnel is constructed with the aorta, since ASO cannot be performed in such a situation. With a sufficient tricuspid-to-pulmonary valve distance, aortic tunneling is supplemented by RVOT reconstruction. If the latter is not possible due to abnormal coronary artery crossing RVOT, an extracardiac conduit implantation is required [103]. If tricuspid-to-pulmonary valve distance is less than the diameter of the aorta, then Rastelli/REV operation may be considered with aortic tunneling, switching off the pulmonary valve from circulation and an extracardiac conduit implantation [104]. Factors complicating aortic tunneling include the significant remoteness of VSD, the tricuspid valve anomalous chordae interfering tunnel projection, the presence of subaortic obstruction etc. [104].

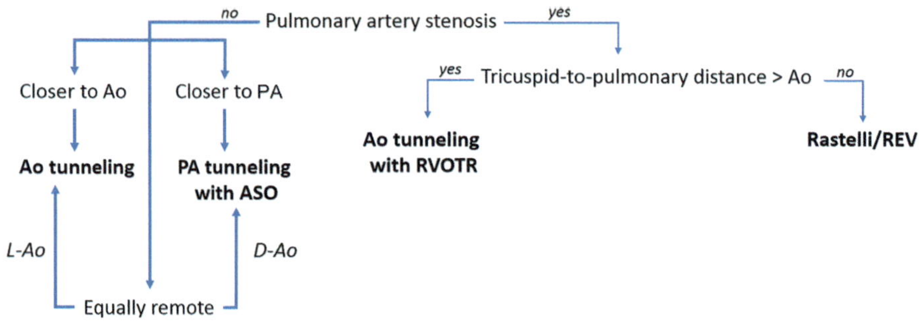

Fig. 31 Surgical strategy for DORV with non-committed VSD. See text. *Ao—aorta; PA—pulmonary artery; ASO—arterial switch operation; RVOTR—right ventricular outflow tract reconstruction*

Approach

Regardless of type of surgical option, a combined atrial and ventricular approaches is necessary for adequate exposure of all right ventricular structures [105].

Revision

Structures to be assessed:

- morphological type, size and proximity of VSD to the arterial valves;
- pulmonary artery stenosis;
- anomalous attachment of tricuspid valve chordae;
- subaortic obstruction;
- tricuspid-to-pulmonary valve distance;
- OS.

Determination the morphological type of non-committed VSD is important both in terms of surgical aspects and understanding of conduction system anatomy. With perimembranous inlet VSD His bundle follows its postero-inferior rim, while in muscular inlet VSD—along superior rim. Accordingly, in the presence of restrictive inlet perimembranous VSD, it can be safely enlarged in anterior–superior fashion.

Anomalous attachment of the tricuspid valve chordae to the OS complicates aortic tunneling, since the chordae cross the tunnel projection. In this case, anomalous insertion can be detached from the OS and subsequently reimplanted onto an intraventricular patch [12, 14]. When tunneling the pulmonary artery, the presence of anomalous chordae, as a rule, does not affect the tunnel construction.

Subaortic obstruction is represented by hypertrophied VIF and the OS [108], as well as the presence of abnormal muscle bands in subaortic infundibulum [105]. For nonobstructive blood flow all muscular elements contributing to subaortic obstruction should be excised.

Very often, during anatomical repair it is necessary to enlarge VSD, even if it is nonrestrictive in order to reduce the length of intraventricular tunnel [52].

4.1 Standard Surgical Techniques

Barbero-Marcial et al. developed an original technique of anatomical repair of DORV with inlet perimembranous and muscular VSDs using multiple patches for tunneling the aorta [104] (Fig. 32). In all cases the procedure is supplemented by VSD enlargement in antero-superior direction even if it is initially nonrestrictive. At the first stage of the operation, a semilunar-shaped patch is sewn to the inlet part of IVS through the right atrium. If necessary, the papillary muscles can be detached and subsequently reimplanted onto a patch (Fig. 32B). Next, an oval-shaped patch is sewn to the subaortic infundibulum (Fig. 32C). As a result, the longitudinal axes of both patches should be oriented at an angle of approximately 45°. The tunnel is completed by the third trapezoidal patch connecting the previous two ones (Fig. 32D). The main disadvantage of the operation is formation of a long and curved tunnel, which is associated with the high risk of subaortic obstruction.

Tchervenkov et al. proposed another technique of inlet VSD "translocation" to the subaortic area [109] (Fig. 33). The essence of translocation consists in tunnel construction with the only difference that during VSD patching its anterior rim (approximately 4 mm) is left open. Then through the right ventriculotomy, VSD is enlarged (translocated) toward the subaortic area through the open anterior rim, and the aorta is tunneled to the left ventricle.

To construct as straight exit from the left ventricle as possible, VSD should be enlarged in the direction of one of the arterial valves (taking care not to injure elements of conduction system) with resection of the subaortic/subpulmonary infundibulum and/or the OS and IVS. In some cases, the papillary muscle of the tricuspid valve is attached to the OS crossing the tunneling projection. In such cases the papillary muscle can be cut off and subsequently reimplanted onto an intraventricular patch [10, 12, 23, 103, 104, 107].

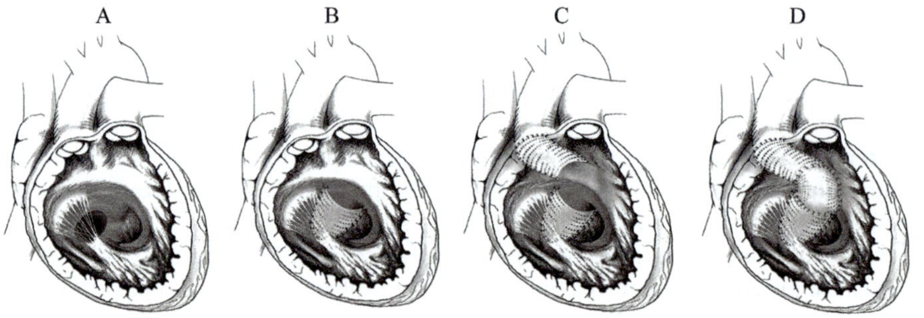

Fig. 32 Repair of DORV «non-committed» type by aortic tunneling with a multiple-patch technique. See text

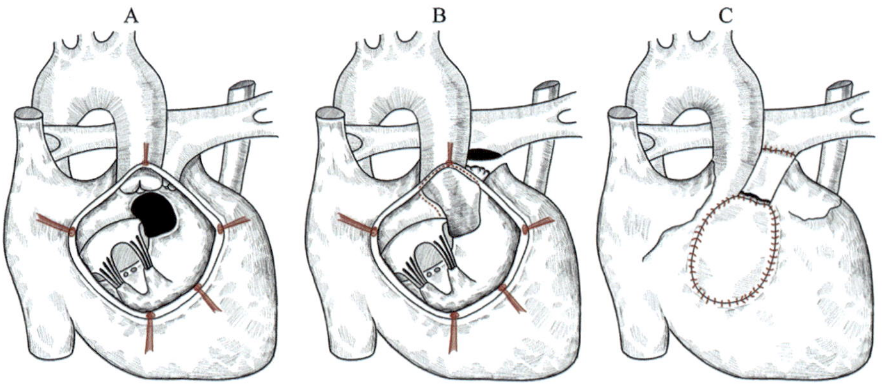

Fig. 33 Inlet VSD translocation to the subaortic area

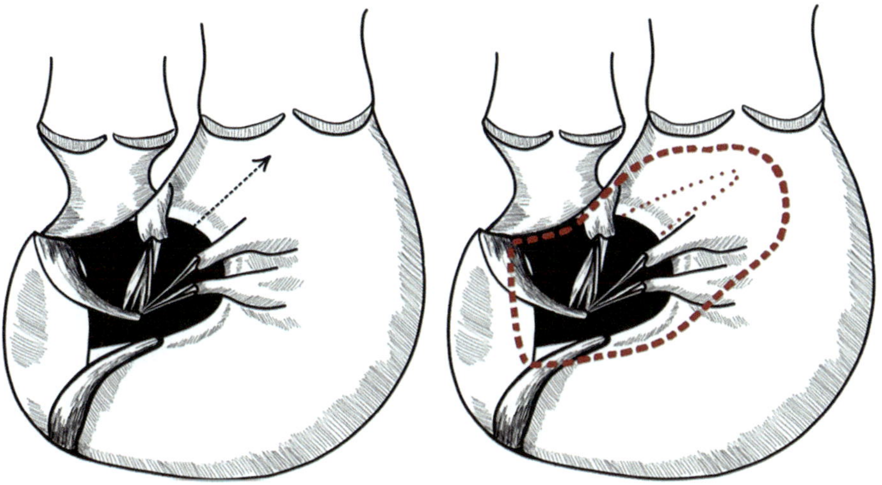

Fig. 34 Inlet VSD enlargement to the subpulmonary area

If VSD is closer to the pulmonary valve, then it can be enlarged antero-superiorly through the posterior limb of TS and TS itself. The incision line is carried out between the attachments of the papillary muscles of the tricuspid valve (Fig. 34). Tunneling of the pulmonary artery to the left ventricle is followed by ASO to restore ventriculo-arterial concordance [105, 110].

4.2 Alternative Surgical Techniques

Double Root Translocation

The main stages of the operation are similar to those described for DORV «TGA» type. Taking into account the presence of bilateral conus in DORV «non-committed» type the harvesting of the pulmonary root may be done more safely without the risk of damage to the anterior leaflet of the mitral valve.

Intraventricular Conduit Implantation

Intraventricular conduit implantation is tunneling of D- or L-aorta to the left ventricle using an intraventricular conduit [111] (Fig. 35).

Indications: DORV «non-committed» type.

Timing. Because itraventricular conduit occupies large space of the right ventricle, the operation in indicated in patients older than 2 years or weighing more than 10 kg.

Approach. Atriotomy combined with ventriculotomy below the aortic valve.

Technique. After intracardiac revision all the muscle elements that cause subaortic or subpulmonary obstruction should be excised. If VSD is restrictive, it should be

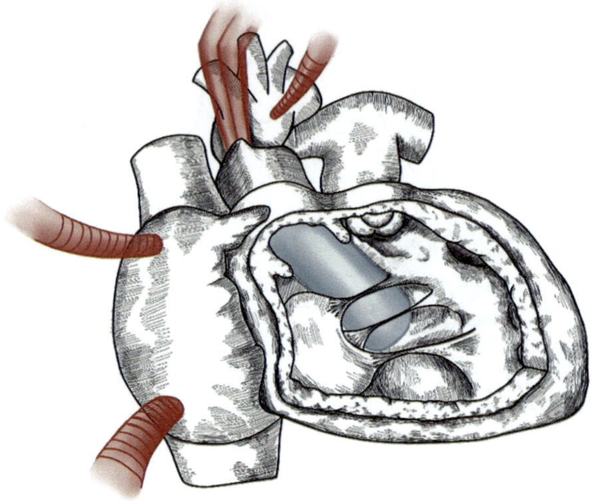

Fig. 35 Technique of intraventricular conduit implantation for aortic tunneling to the left ventricle in DORV «non-committed» type

enlarged through the TS. One of the most important parts of the operation is determination of optimal length of the conduit. Its lesser curvature corresponds to the distance between the superior rim of VSD and medial aspect of the subaortic conus, while the greater curvature corresponds to the distance between the inferior rim of VSD and lateral aspect of the subaortic conus. The authors of the method suggest using a conduit $\geq$ 16 mm in patients younger than 5 and $\geq$ 19 mm in patients older than 5 years. The proximal anastomosis is performed by interrupted sutures, and the distal one by continuous suture. In case of D-aorta the intraventricular conduit is placed under the infundibular papillary muscle, while in L-aorta above it.

Advantages: no influence of the infundibular papillary muscle and subvalvular structures of the tricuspid valve on conduit placement; no need for coronary arteries reimplantation; the operation is feasible in the presence of pulmonary artery stenosis as an alternative to ASO; relatively simple surgical technique.

Disadvantages: cannot be done in patients younger than 2 years and less than 10 kg.

5 DORV and «Straddling» Atrioventricular Valves

Straddling of atrioventricular valves represent a great challenge for the surgeon during the anatomical correction of all types of DORV [112]. First of all, during the intraoperative revision it is necessary to determine the type of abnormal attachment of an atrioventricular valve according to the Tabry classification (see Chap. 2). Anatomical correction can be performed in any type of anomaly, but in the presence of straddling of both atrioventricular valves it is recommended to proceed with univentricular palliation due to high surgical risk [14].

Tecnhiques of correction of straddling atrioventricular valves can be divided into translocation, penetration and reimplantation methods [113].

5.1 Translocation Method

Tricuspid Valve. In straddling type «A» the chordae and papillary muscle of the tricuspid valve are maximally stretched towards the right ventricle that allows to fix a patch to the crest of IVS without any difficulties. In straddling type «B» IVS should be partially dissected between the rim of VSD and the level of anomalous insertion of the papillary muscle, converting the straddling into type «A» with subsequent use of translocation technique. Also, anomalous chordae may be stretched towards the right ventricle like in «A» type as well as a patch may be sewn to IVS below the level of anomalous attachment of the papillary muscle on the side of the contralateral ventricle [52] (Fig. 36). In type «C» the papillary muscle is detached from the wall of the contralateral left ventricle and reimplanted onto a patch for intraventricular tunneling.

Mitral Valve. Abnormal attachment of the mitral valve chordae to the crest of VSD does not interfere with the tunnel construction and therefore such chordae are left intact, though it can cause LVOT obstruction after repair. In type «B» a patch for aortic tunneling is placed below the level of abnormal chordal attachment.

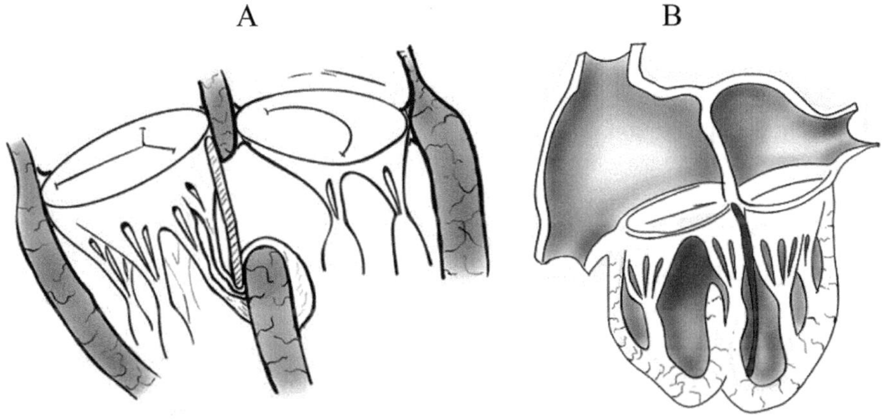

Fig. 36 Translocation methods of straddling tricuspid valve. The techniques of stretching the chordae towards the right ventricle (A) and placement a patch below the level of anomalous attachment of the papillary muscle (B) in straddling type «B»

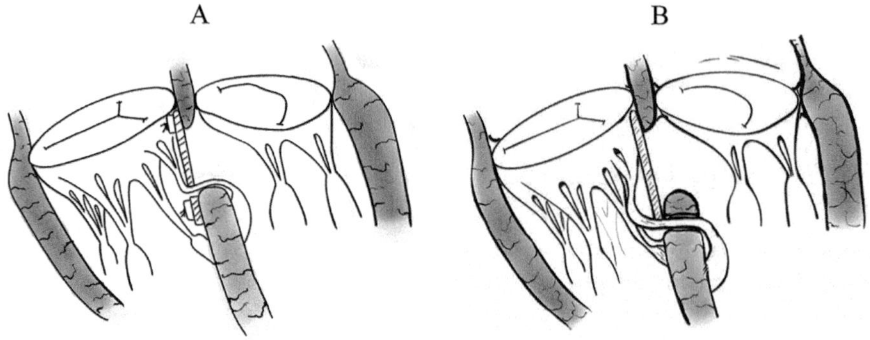

Fig. 37 Methods of patch (**A**) and IVS (**B**) penetration for straddling tricuspid valve

5.2 *Penetration Method*

With this method abnormally attached chordae are passed through the incision on a patch or IVS (Fig. 37).

5.3 *Reimplantation Method*

Reimplantation method is used in «C» type of straddling atrioventricular valves. Sometimes resection of the abnormal chordae without disruption of the valve function. If abnormal chordae are fixed to only one papillary muscle and significantly remote from the VSD crest, it is possible to cut off the papillary muscle with its subsequent reimplantation on IVS from the side of the corresponding ventricle or onto a patch for the intraventricular tunnel (in case of tricuspid valve).

6 DORV/AVSD

In the early stages of the development of congenital heart surgery, the treatment of patients with DORV/AVSD was accompanied by extremely high mortality due to the lack of effective surgical techniques [114, 115]. Only with the beginning of the anatomical correction the results significantly improved [116].

Danielson et al. in 1978 were the first to perform physiological correction of DORV/AVSD with situs inversus [117], while in 1980 anatomical correction was done by Pacifico et al. in situs solitus [115].

Because in the vast majority of cases DORV/AVSD is associated with heterotaxy syndrome, its surgical repair represents a big challenge due to high frequency of abnormal drainage of the systemic, hepatic and pulmonary veins. That is why in such cases univentricular palliation is done more frequently than biventricular repair.

Indications. Surgical correction of DORV/AVSD mainly depends on anatomical type of VSD.

Timing. Optimal time for surgery is similar to isolated AVSD.

Approach. Usually, combined atriotomy and ventriculotomy are used to expose all intracardiac structures. In some cases, for better exposure of VSD it is reasonable to temporarily detach the anterior bridging and anterolateral (right lateral) leaflets from the fibrous annulus [118].

Technique

Subaortic and Subatrerial VSD. In case of subaortic and subarterial VSD ventricular septation is performed using a comma-shaped patch which differs from a semicircular patch used for repair of isolated AVSD (Fig. 38A) [115]. In fact, such a patch divides the common atrioventricular valve into tricuspid and mitral components, eliminates interventricular communication and translocates the aorta to the left ventricle. In this regard, in an intraventricular patch can be distinguished the «septal» and «aortic» parts (Fig. 38B). When trimming a patch, it is necessary to take into consideration the degree of aortic dextraposition—the larger it is, the longer the «aortic» part of a patch needed [119].

Subpulmonary VSD. When aorta locates more anteriorly than the pulmonary artery, tricuspid-to-pulmonary valve distance is less than the diameter of the aorta as a rule, and therefore aortic tunneling is not feasible. In this case, the pulmonary valve is closer to VSD than the aortic valve. In such a situation biventricular repair may be performed by tunneling of pulmonary artery to the left ventricle (converting anatomy to hemodynamic TGA) after which ventricular-arterial concordance is restored by ASO [120, 121] (Fig. 39).

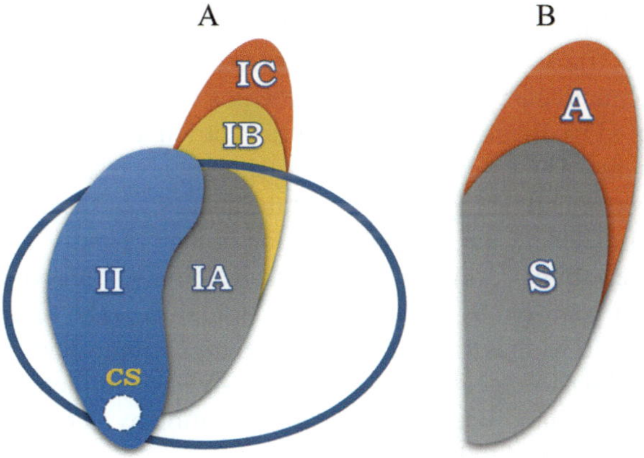

Fig. 38 The shape of an intraventricular patch depending on malformation: **A**—for repair of isolated AVSD (IA) and its association with Tetralogy of Fallot (IB) and DORV (IC); **B**—«septal» («S») and «aortic» («A») parts of a patch used for DORV/AVSD repair. *I—patch for ventricular septation; II—patch for atrial septation; CS—coronary sinus*

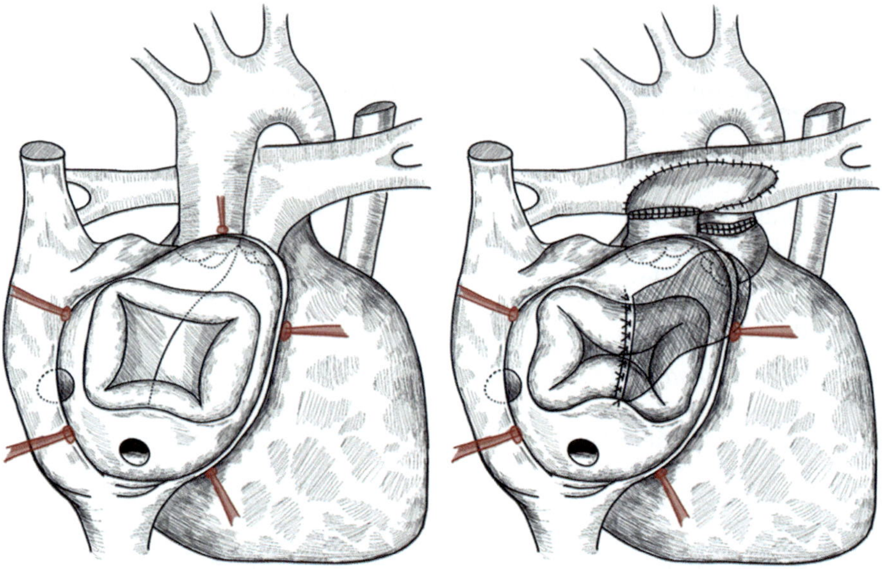

Fig. 39 Surgical technique for DORV/AVSD with pulmonary artery tunneling followed by arterial switch procedure

Non-committed VSD. Repair of this type of DORV is extremely complex own to difficulties in tunnel construction along with necessity to separate common atrioventricular valve. There are anatomical [109, 122] and physiological [123] methods of repair for this malformation.

The VSD «translocation» technique allows performing an anatomical repair by dissecting IVS towards the subaortic infundibulum followed by aortic tunneling to the left ventricle [109].

The two-patch technique allows to perform correction with any types of the arterial trunks relationship [124]. At the first stage of the operation through atriotomy a semicircular patch is sewn to the posterior rim of VSD. The upper part of a patch is used to divide the common atrioventricular valve into tricuspid and mitral components. The anterior part of a patch remains free (Fig. 40A). Next, atrial septation is performed taking into account the anatomy of the drained veins. At the second stage of the operation optimal resection of the OS and VSD translocation to the subaortic area are performed through ventriculotomy, after which the aorta is tunneled to the left ventricle by a second patch (Fig. 40B). The reduction of right ventricle cavity due to wide intraventricular tunnel necessitates RVOT reconstruction.

Physiological repair of DORV/AVSD with heterotaxy syndrome and DA-aorta implies modified double-switch operation by a combination of Musturd and Rastelli procedures [123].

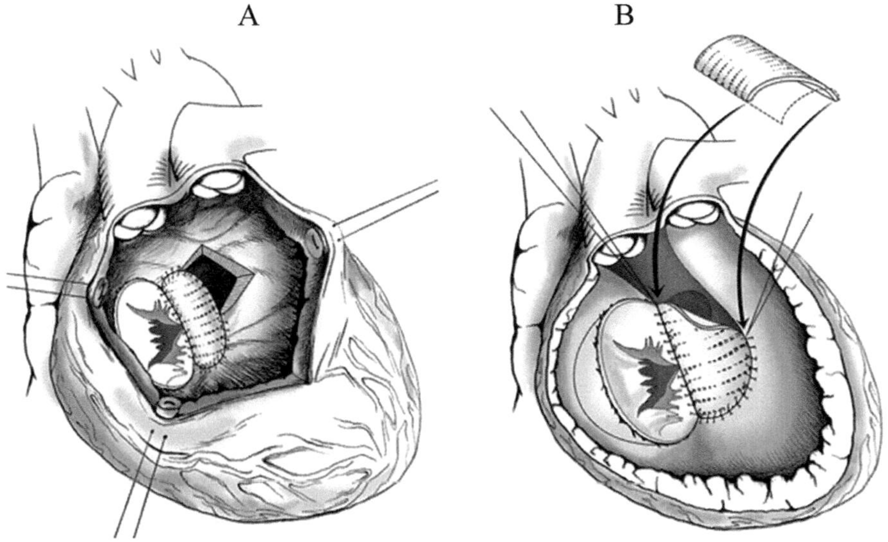

Fig. 40 Two-patch technique for repair of DORV/AVSD with non-committed VSD. See text

7 Subaortic Obstruction After Biventricular Repair

Subaortic obstruction is a serious and one of the most frequent complications after aortic tunneling. The incidence of tunnel obstruction is up to 5% [106, 125], and more often reveals in patients with DORV «non-committed» type.

The criterion of significant subaortic obstruction requiring surgical intervention is a pressure gradient between the left ventricle and the aorta $\geq$ 50 mmHg [125, 126]. Despite this, it is also necessary to take into account clinical symptoms, such as dyspnea, syncope, arterial hypoxemia etc. [106].

Subaortic obstruction develops after average 45 $\pm$ 66 months (from 1 to 213 months) after anatomical repair [106] and according to Kim et al. after 9.5 $\pm$ 6.3 years [125].

Belli et al. distinguished three different anatomical levels at which subaortic stenosis may develop [106] (Fig. 41):

- VSD level;
- tunnel level;
- aortic annulus level.

Depending on the morphological substrate subaortic obstruction can be divided into local or diffuse forms.

Local Obstruction. Local obstruction is usually observed under the aortic valve and may be represented by fibrous and/or muscular membrane. When local obstruction the pressure gradient between the left ventricle and the aorta usually does not exceed 30 mmHg, and reintervention is performed due to other intracardiac issues

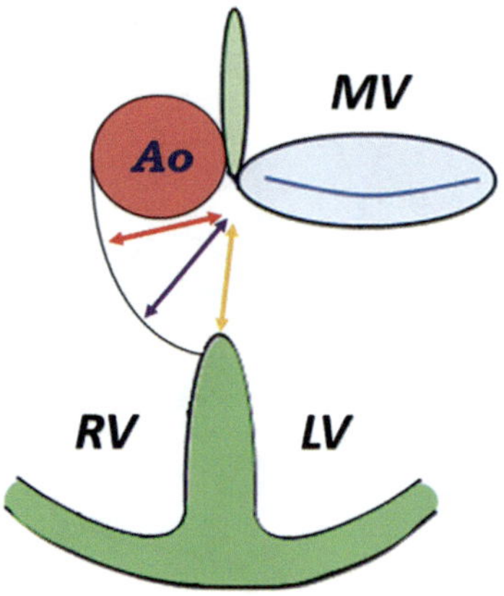

Fig. 41 Levels of subaortic (tunnel) obstruction after anatomical repair of DORV with aortic tunneling: VSD level (orange arrow), tunnel level (violet arrow), aortic annulus level (red arrow)

[125]. The stenotic area is approached through the ascending aorta and membrane resection technically does not differ from the isolated lesion.

Diffuse Obstruction. To understand the essence of diffuse subaortic muscular obstruction it is necessary to consider the following technical features of tunnel construction during anatomical repair of DORV. In order to avoid damage to the conduction tissue sutures are placed on IVS from right ventricular side, which involuntarily involves the remaining left ventricular part of IVS into the lumen of the tunnel. In addition, in the area of posterior-inferior rim of VSD closer to the septal leaflet of the tricuspid valve, the suture line goes some millimeters apart from the edge of VSD thereby contributing to inclusion of IVS muscular tissue in the tunnel. Similarly, the muscular elements of the OS and subaortic conus can be involved in the tunnel, which are potential substrates for subaortic obstruction in the future.

Superiorly the real exit from the left ventricle in DORV is limited by VIF, which is completely muscular structure, while in tetralogy of Fallot this area is fibrous (mitral-aortic fibrous continuity). This feature serves as a certain restriction of the exit from the left ventricle and contributes to the development of subaortic obstruction after repair.

According to Li et al. in patients with DORV and subarterial VSD (without OS) freedom from any reinterventions including for subaortic obstruction made up 100% [2]. Taking into account that in this type of DORV the OS as a muscular structure is completely absent, such results support the role of the OS in the development of subaortic obstruction after repair. In addition, in the study conducted by Uemura et al. none of the patients with subarterial VSD and absence of the OS developed subaortic obstruction after surgery [127].

Summarizing the above-mentioned, as muscle substrates of diffuse subaortic stenosis can be hypertrophied IVS (in other words, the rims of VSD involved in the tunnel lumen), the OS and muscular elements of subaortic conus. Also, tunnel obstruction may be caused by patient-patch mismatch.

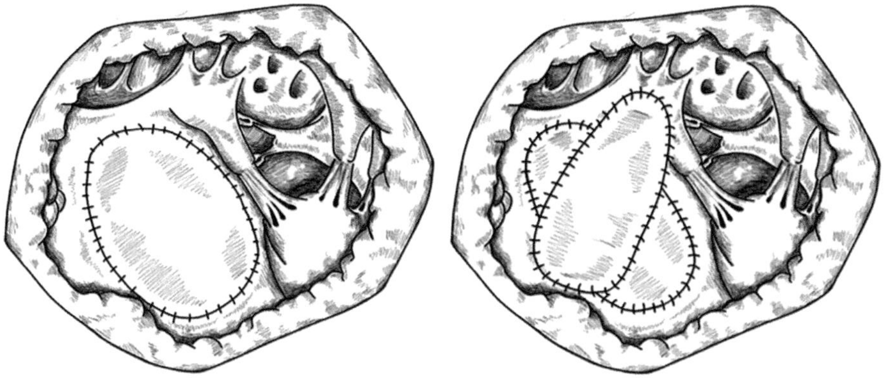

Fig. 42 Extended septoplasty for elimination of tunnel obstruction after previous anatomical correction of DORV

When determining the optimal time for surgical correction of tunnel obstruction, the most important indicators are the degree of systolic pressure gradient, performance of the left ventricle, as well as the presence and severity of clinical symptoms. It is advisable to perform operation in the presence of a hemodynamically significant gradient before decompensation of the left ventricle occurs (decrease in ejection fraction, increase in left ventricle end-diastolic diameter, mitral valve regurgitation, pulmonary hypertension, increased right ventricle pressure, heart failure).

Elimination of diffuse subaortic obstruction is performed by extended septoplasty technique (Fig. 42). For optimal exposure of all necessary structures, approach through the aortic valve should be combined with ventriculotomy. A short incision is made in the center of the previous patch, which then is extended toward both aortic fibrous annulus and the TS. Therefore, the incision extends beyond the patch and involves the subaortic infundibulum and IVS. After this, a new patch is used to reconstruct a tunnel. When extending an incision, it is necessary to avoid damage to the aortic valve, papillary muscles of the mitral valve, as well as large septal arteries near the anterior limb of TS [106].

An alternative technique in patients with severe subaortic obstruction is Konno-Rastan procedure with anterior enlargement of the aortic root [126].

8 Univentricular Repair

Preservation of biventricular anatomy in some cases may be impossible or is accompanied by unreasonably high surgical risk. The decision in favor of univentricular palliation is very likely with severe hypoplasia of one of the ventricles, the presence of non-committed VSD, especially in association with «straddling» atrioventricular valves type «C». Biventricular repair is also not recommended when straddling both atrioventricular valves take place, especially in association with abnormal attachment of additional chordae [14].

A special group are patients with heterotaxy syndrome, who are also considered mainly as candidates for univentricular palliation due to complex intracardiac anatomy and frequent associated anomalies, including anomalies of systemic, pulmonary and hepatic venous returns. Presence of abnormal attachment of the tricuspid valve chordae to the OS, infundibular stenosis or subaortic obstruction, a small tricuspid-to-pulmonary vale distance and restrictive VSD are not absolute contraindications for biventricular repair.

Absolute contraindications for biventricular repair are cases with unbalanced ventricles, heterotaxy syndrome and complex abnormal attachments of atrioventricular valves. Serraf et al. consider that the limitation to biventricular repair is only cases with unbalanced ventricles, as well as complex abnormal attachment of atrioventricular valve chordae to the rim of VSD [14]. In turn, non-committed nature of VSD is not a contraindication, but a limitation to biventricular repair, depending on the surgeon's experience, since such operations can be performed with acceptable results [104]. Moreover, if in DORV/AVSD subvulvular structures of the tricuspid component do not cross VSD projection, then biventricular repair is also possible [120].

According to other authors, absolute indications for univentricular palliation are severe hypoplasia of the left ventricle and «straddling» of the mitral valve type «C» [105, 128]. In addition, biventricular repair in patients with inlet VSD, heterotaxy syndrome and atrioventricular discordance is associated with a high surgical risk, so univentricular palliation is more preferable [129].

In the study of Ruzmetov et al. univentricular palliation was indicated in the following cases: unbalanced ventricles, atrial isomerism, «straddling» atrioventricular valve, total anomalous drainage of the pulmonary veins, "swiss cheese" non-committed VSD and «criss-cross» of the heart [130].

In some cases, if an intraventricular tunnel significantly occupies the cavity of the right ventricle, then one and a half ventricle repair may be effective.

References

1. Wu Q, Li D, Zhang M, Xu Z, Zue H. Surgical treatment of double-outlet right ventricle complicated by pulmonary hypertension. Chin Med J. 2017;4:409–13.
2. Li S, Ma K, Hu S, Hua Z, Yang K, Yan J, Chen Q. Surgical outcomes of 380 patients with double outlet right ventricle who underwent biventricular repair. J Thorac Cardiovasc Surg. 2014;147:817–24.
3. Tchervenkov CI, Marelli D, Beland MJ, Gibbons JE, Paquet M, Dobell ARC. Institutional experience with a protocol of early repair of double-outlet right ventricle. Ann Thorac Surg. 1995;60:S610-613.
4. Lecompte Y, Batisse A, DiCarlo D. Double-outlet right ventricle: a surgical synthesis. Adv Card Surg. 1993;4:109–36.
5. Walters HL III, Mavroudis C, Tchervenkov CI, Jacobs JP, Lacour-Gayet F, Jacobs ML. Congenital heart surgery nomenclature and database project: double outlet right ventricle. Ann Thorac Surg. 2000;69:S249-263.
6. Capuani A, Uemura H, Ho SY, Anderson RH. Anatomic spectrum of abnormal ventriculoarterial connections: surgical implications. Ann Thorac Surg. 1995;59:352–60.
7. *Рагимов Ф.Р.* Анатомия, диагностика, радикальное хирургическое лечение отхождение аорты и легочной артерии от правого желудочка. *Дисс. докт. мед. наук. АМН СССР ИССХ им. А.Н. Бакулева.* 1990.337 с.
8. Sakamoto K, Charpentier A, Popescu S, Geeter BD, Eisenmann B. Transaortic approach in double-outlet right ventricle with subaortic ventricular septal defect. Ann Thorac Surg. 1997;64:856–88.
9. Goor DA, Massini C, Shen-Tov A, Neufeld HN. Transatrial repair of double-outlet right ventricle in infants. Thorax. 1982;37:371–5.
10. Takeushi K, del Nido JP. Surgical management of double-outlet right ventricle with subaortic ventricular septal defect. Pediatric Cardiac Surgery Annual of the Seminar in Thoracic and Cardiovascular Surgery. 2000;3:34–42.
11. Goldberg SP, McCanta AC, Campbell DN, Carpenter EV, Clarke DV, da Cruz E, Ivy DD, Lacour-Gayet FG. Implications of incising ventricular septum in double-outlet right ventricle and in the Ross-Konno operation. Europ J Cardiothoracic Surgery. 2009;35:589–93.
12. Sakata R, Lecompte Y, Batisse A, Borromee L, Durandy Y. Anatomic repair of anomalies of ventriculoarterial connection associated with ventricular septal defect. I. Criteria of surgical decision. J Thoracic and Cardiovascular Surgery. 1988;95:90–95.
13. Aoki M, Forbess JM, Jonas RA, Mayer JE, Castaneda AR. Results of biventricular repair for double-outlet right ventricle. J Thorac Cardiovasc Surg. 1994;2:338–50.
14. Serraf A, Nakamura T, Lacour-Gayet F, Piot D, Bruniaux J, Touchot A, Sousa-Uva M, Houyel L, Planche C. Surgical approach for double-outlet right ventricle or transposition of the great arteries associated with straddling atrioventricular valves. J Thorac Cardiovasc Surg. 1996;111:527–35.
15. Burakovsky VI, Podzolkov VP, Ivanitsky AV, Ragimov FR. Surgical treatment of double outlet right ventricle. Cardiol Young. 1997;7:22–30.
16. Mason DT, Morrow AG, Elkins RC, Friedman WF. Origin of both great vessels from the right ventricle associated with severe obstruction to left ventricular outflow. Am J Cardiol. 1967;24:118–24.
17. Sridaromont S, Feldt RH, Ritter DG, Davis GD, Edwards JE. Double-outlet right ventricle: hemodynamic and anatomic correlations. Am J Cardiol. 1976;38:85–94.
18. Thanopoulos BD, Dubrow IW, Fisher EA, Hastreiter AR. Double outlet right ventricle with subvalvular aortic stenosis. Br Heart J. 1979;41:241–4.
19. Freed M, Rosenthal A, Plauth WH, Nadas AS. Development of subaortic stenosis after pulmonary artery banding. Circulation. 1973;48:S7-10.
20. Kirklin JW, Barratt-Boyes BG. Cardiac surgery, 4 edn. New York:Churchill Livingstone; 2013.

21. *Джонас Р.А.* Хирургическое лечение врожденных пороков сердца. *Пер. с англ. Под ред. М.В. Борискова. – М.: ГЭОТАР-Медиа.* 2017.736 с.
22. *Бокерия Л.А., Беришвили И.И.* Хирургическая анатомия сердца. Т.3. Врожденные пороки сердца – пороки конотрункуса и патофизиология кровообращения. *М.: НЦССХ им. А.Н. Бакулева РАМН.* 2006;312 с.
23. Serraf A, Belli E, Lacour-Gayet F, Zoghbi J, Planche C. Biventricular repair for double-outlet right ventricle. Pediatric Cardiac Surgery Annual of the Seminar in Thoracic and Cardiovascular Surgery. 2000;3:43–56.
24. Preminger TJ, Sanders SP, Van der Velde ME, Castaneda AR, Lock JE. "Intramural" residual interventricular defects after repair of conotruncal malformations. Circulation. 1994;89:236–42.
25. Patel JK, Glatz AC, Chosh RM, Jones SM, Natarajan S, Ravishankar C, Mascio CE, Spray TL, Cohen MS. Intramural ventricular septal defect is a distinct clinical entity associated with postoperative morbidity and mortality in children after repair of conotruncal anomalies. Circulation. 2015;132:1387–94.
26. Patel JK, Glatz AC, Chosh RM, Jones SM, Ravishankar C, Mascio CE, Cohen MS. Accuracy of transesophageal echocardiography in the identification of postoperative intramural ventricular septal defects. J Thorac Cardiovasc Surg. 2016;152:688–95.
27. Fujiia Y, Kotania Y, Takagakia M, Araia S, Kasaharaa S, Otsukib S, Sanoa S. The impact of the length between the top of the interventricular septum and the aortic valve on the indications for a biventricular repair in patients with a transposition of the great arteries or a double outlet right ventricle. Interact Cardiovasc Thorac Surg. 2010;10:900–5.
28. Awori MN, Mehta NP, Mitema FO, Kebba N. Optimal use of z-scores to preserve the pulmonary valve annulus during repair of tetralogy of Fallot. World J Pediatric and Congenital Heart Surgery. 2018;9:285–8.
29. Petterson MD, Skeens ME, Humes RA. Regression equations for calculation of Z score of cardiac structures in a large cohort of healthy infants, children, and adolescents: an echocardiographic study. J Am Soc Echocardiogr. 2008;21:922–34.
30. Lacour-Gayet F, Bove EL, Hraska V, Morell VO, Spray TL. Surgery of conotruncal anomalies. Springer;2016. p. 627.
31. Zhao J, Cai X, Teng Y, Nie Z, Ou Y, Zhuang J, Wen S, Cen J, Xu G, Cui H, Chen J. Value of pulmonary annulus area index in predicting transannular patch placement in tetralogy of Fallot repair. J Card Surg. 2020;35:48–53.
32. Tchervenkov CI, Pelletier MP, Shum-Tim D, Beland MJ, Rohlicek C. Primary repair minimizing use of conduits in neonates and infants with tetralogy of Fallot or double-outlet right ventricle and anomalous coronary arteries. J Thorac Cardiovasc Surg. 2000;119:314–23.
33. Turrentine M, McCarthy RP, Vijay P, McConell K, Brown J. PTFE monocusp valve reconstruction of the right ventricular outflow tract. Ann Thorac Surg. 2002;73:871–80.
34. Fermandes FP, Manlhiot C, Roche SL, Wortmann LG, Slorach C, McCrindle BW, Mertens L, Kantor PF, Friedberg MK. Impaired left ventricular myocardial mechanics and their relation to pulmonary regurgitation, right ventricular enlargement and exercise capacity in asymptomatic children after repair of tetralogy of Fallot. J Am Soc Echocardiogr. 2012;25:494–503.
35. Egbe AC, Pellikka PA, Miranda WR, Bonnichsen C, Reddy YNV, Borlaug BA, Connolly HM. Echocardiographic predictors of severe right ventricular diastolic dysfunction in tetralogy of Fallot: relations to patient outcomes. Int J Cardiol. https://doi.org/10.1016/j.ijcard.2020.02.067
36. Olive MK, Fraser CD, Kutty S, McKenzie ED, Hammel JM, Krishnamurthy R, Dobb NA, Maskatia SA. Infundibular sparing versus transinfundibular approach to the repair of tetralogy of Fallot. Congenit Heart Dis. 2019;14:1149–56.
37. Arafat AA, Elatafy EE, Elshedoudy S, Zalat M, Abdallah N, Elmahrouk A. Surgical strategies protecting against right ventricular dilatation following tetralogy of Fallot. J Cardiothorac Surg. 2018;13:14. https://doi.org/10.1186/s13019-018-0702-0.
38. Bautista-Hernandez V, Martinez-Bendayan I, Rueda F. Valve-sparing tetralogy of Fallot repair with intraoperative dilation of the pulmonary valve. Pediatr Cardiol. 2013;34:918–23.

39. Vida VL, Guariento A, Zucchetta F, Padalino M, Castaldi B, Milanesi O, Stellin G. Preservation of the pulmonary valve during early repair of tetralogy of Fallot: surgical technique. Seminars in Thoracic Cardiovascular Surgery. 2016;19:75–81.
40. Kwak JG, Kim W, Kim ER, Lim JH, Min J. One-year follow-up after tetralogy of Fallot total repair preserving pulmonary valve and avoiding right venticulotomy. Circ J. 2018;12:3064–8.
41. Bockeria LA, Makhachev OM, Gordeeva MV, Panova MS, Philippkina TY, Khiriev TK, Zaets SB. Quantitative anatomy of Taussig-Bing anomaly. Anatomy and Physiol: Currents Res. 2014;4:158–216. https://doi.org/10.4172/2161-0940.1000158.
42. Howell CE, Ho SY, Anderson RH, Elliot MJ. Fibrous skeleton and ventricular outflow tracts in double-outlet right ventricle. Ann Thorac Surg. 1991;51:394–400.
43. Williams WG, Freedom RM, Culham G, Duncan WJ, Olley PM, Rowe RD, Trusler GA. Early experience with arterial repair of transposition. Ann Thorac Surg. 1981;32:8–15.
44. Yacoub MH, Radley-Smith R. Anatomic correction of the Taussig-Bing anomaly. J Thorac Cardiovasc Surg. 1984;88:380–8.
45. Kanter K, Anderson R, Lincoln C, Firmin R, Rigby M. Anatomic correction of double-outlet right ventricle with subpulmonary ventricular septal defect (the "Taussig-Bing" anomaly). Ann Thorac Surg. 1986;41:287–92.
46. Wetter J, Sinzobahamvya N, Blaschzok HC, Cho M, Brecher AM, Granvinghoff LM, Urban AE. Results of arterial switch operation for primary total correction of the Taussig-Bing anomaly. Ann Thorac Surg. 2004;77:41–7.
47. Feng B, Liu Y, Hu S, Shen X, Wang X, Wang H, Ming B. Arterial switch for transposition of the great vessels and Taussig-Bing anomaly after six month of age. Ann Thorac Surg. 2009;88:1948–51.
48. Fricke TA, Donaldson S, Schneider JR, Menahem S, d'Udekem Y, Brizard CP, Konstantinov IE. Outcomes of the arterial switch operation in patients with aortic arch obstruction. The J Thoracic and Cardiovascular Surgery. 2020;159:592–599.
49. Alsoufi B, Cai S, Williams WJ, Coles JG, Caldarone CA, Redington AM, Van Arsdell GS. Improved results with single-stage total correction of Taussig-Bing anomaly. Europ J Cardiothoracic Surgery. 2008;33:244–50.
50. Comas JV, Mignosa C, Cochrane AD, Wilkinson JL, Karl TR. Taussig-Bing anomaly and arterial switch operation: aortic arch obstruction does not influence outcome. Europ J Cardiothoracic Surgery. 1996;10:1114–9.
51. Luo K, Zheng J, Wang S, Zhu Z, Gao B, Xu Z, Liu J. Single-stage correction for Taussig-Bing anomaly associates with aortic arch obstruction. Pediatric Cariology. 2017;38:1548–55.
52. Mavroudis C, Backer CL, Muster AJ, Rocchini AP, Rees AH, Gevitz M. Taussig-Bing anomaly: arterial switch versus Kawashima intraventricular repair. Ann Thorac Surg. 1996;61:1330–8.
53. Hayes DA, Jones S, Quaegebeur JM, Richmond ME, Andrews HF, Glickstein JS, Chen JM, Bacha E, Liberman L. Primary repair switch operation as a strategy for total correction of Taussig-Bing anomaly. A 21-year experience. Circulation. 2013;128:S194–198.
54. Griselli M, McGuirk SP, Ko C, Clarke AJB, Barron DJ, Brawn WJ. Arterial switch operation in patients with Taussig-Bing anomaly—influence of staged repair and coronary anatomy on outcome. European J Cardiothoracic Surgery. 2007;31:229–35.
55. Soszyn N, Fricke TA, Wheaton GR, Ramsay JM, d'Udekem Y, Brizard CP, Konstantinov IE. Outcomes of the arterial switch operation in patients with Taussig-Bing anomaly. Ann Thorac Surg. 2011;92:673–9.
56. Masuda M, Kado H, Shiokawa Y, Fukae K, Kaneqae Y, Kawachi Y, Morita S, Yasui H. Clinical results of arterial switch operation for double-outlet right ventricle with subpulmonary VSD. European J Cardiothoracic Surgery. 1999;15:283–8.
57. Wauthy P, Demanet H, Sanoussi A, Deuvaert F. Ventricular septal defect closure in Taussig-Bing heart: the «Pulmonic rule». Ann Thorac Surg. 2009;88:313–4.
58. Al-Muhaya MA, Ismail SR, Abu-Sulaiman RM, Kabbani MS, Najm HK. Short- and mid-term outcomes of total correction of Taussig-Bing anomaly. Pediatr Cardiol. 2012;33:258–63.

59. Sinzobahamvya N, Blaschzok HC, Asfour B, Arenz C, Jussli MJ, Schnidler E, Photiadis J, Yrban AE. Right ventricular outflow tract obstruction after arterial switch operation for Taussig-Bing anomaly. Eur J Cardiothorac Surg. 2007;31:873–8.
60. Brawn WJ, Mee RB. Early results for anatomic correction of transposition of the great arteries and for double-outlet right ventricle with subpulmonary ventricular septal defect. J Thorac Cardiovasc Surg. 1988;95:230–8.
61. Kawashima Y, Fujita T, Miyamoto T, Manabe H. Intraventricular rerouting of blood for the correction of Taussig-Bing malformation. J Thorac Cardiovasc Surg. 1971;62:825–9.
62. Kawahira Y, Yagihara T, Uemura H, Ishizaka T, Yoshikawa Y, Yoshizumi K, Kitamura S. Ventricular outflow tracts after Kawashima intraventricular rerouting for double outlet right ventricle with subpulmonary ventricular septal defect. Eur J Cardiothorac Surg. 1999;16:26–31.
63. Urban AE, Brecher AM. The arterial switch repair and the obstructive right ventricular outflow tract: does it matter? Thoracic and Cardiovascular Surgery. 1991;39:S170-175.
64. Patrick DL, McGoon DC. An operation for double-outlet right ventricle with transposition of the great arteries. J Cardiovasc Surg. 1968;9:537–42.
65. Rastelli GC. A new approach to “anatomic” repair of transposition of the great arteries. Mayo Clin Proc. 1969;44:1–12.
66. Snoody JW, Parr EL, Robertson LW, Mauck HP, McCue CM, Lower RR. Successful intracardiac repair of the Taussig-Bing malformation in 2 children. Ann Thorac Surg. 1978;25:158–63.
67. Kalfa DM, Lambert V, Baruteau AE, Stos B, Houyel L, Garcia E, Ly M, Belli E. Arterial switch for transposition with left outflow tract obstruction: outcomes and risk analysis. Ann Thorac Surg. 2013;95:2097–103.
68. Brown JW, Ruzmetov M, Huynh D, Rodefeld MD, Turrentine MW, Fiore AC. Rastelli operation for transposition of the great arteries with ventricular septal defect and pulmonary stenosis. Ann Thorac Surg. 2011;91:188–94.
69. Lecompte Y, Neveux JY, Leca F, Zannini L, Tu TV, Duboys Y, Jarreau MM. Reconstruction of the pulmonary outflow tract without prosthetic conduit. J Thorac Cardiovasc Surg. 1982;84:727–33.
70. Borromee L, Lecompte Y, Batisse A, Lemoine G, Vouhe P, Sakata R, Leca F, Zannini L, Neveux J. Anatomic repair of anomalies of ventriculoarterial connection associated with ventricular septal defect. II. Clinical results in 50 patients with ventricular septal defect. J Thoracic and Cardiovascular Surgery. 1988;95:96–102.
71. Lim H, Kim W, Lee JR, Kim YJ. Twenty-five years’ experience of modified Lecompte procedure for the anomalies of ventriculoarterial connection with ventricular septal defect and pulmonary stenosis. J Thorac Cardiovasc Surg. 2014;3:825–31.
72. Hightower BM, Barcia A, Bargeron LM, Kirklin JW. Double-outlet right ventricle with transposed great arteries and subpulmonary ventricular septal defect The Taussig-Bing malformation. Circulation. 1969;39:S207-213.
73. Piccoli G, Pacifico AD, Kirklin JW, Blackstone EH, Kirklin JK, Bargeron LM. Changing results and concepts in the surgical treatment of double-outlet right ventricle: analysis of 137 operations in 126 patients. Am J Cardiol. 1983;52:549–54.
74. Kirklin JW, Pacifico AD, Blackstone EH, Bargeron LM. Current risks and protocols for operations for double-outlet right ventricle. Derivation from an 18 year experience. J Thoracic and Cardiovascul Surgery. 198;92:913–930.
75. Luber JM, Castaneda AR, Lang P, Norwood WI. Repair of double-outlet right ventricle: early and late results. Circulation. 1983;62:144–7.
76. Musumeci F, Shumway S, Lincoln C, Anderson RH. Surgical treatment for double-outlet right ventricle at the Brompton Hospital, 1973 to 1986. J Thorac Cardiovasc Surg. 1988;96:278–87.
77. Stewart RW, Kirklin JW, Pacifico AD, Blackstone EH, Bargeron LM. Repair of double-outlet right ventricle. An analysis of 62 cases. J Thoracic and Cardiovascul Surgery. 1979;78:502–514.

78. Smith EEJ, Pucci JJ, Walesby RK, Oakley CM, Sapsford RN. A new technique for correction of the Taussig-Bing anomaly. J Thorac Cardiovasc Surg. 1982;83:901–4.
79. Binet JP, Lacour-Gayet F, Conso JF, Dupuis C, Bruniaux J. Complete repair of the Taussig-Bing type of double-outlet right ventricle using the arterial switch operation without coronary translocation. Report of one successful case. J Thoracic and Cardiovascular Surgery. 1983;85:272–275.
80. Ceithaml EL, Puga FJ, Danielson GK, McGoon DC, Ritter DG. Results of the Damus-Stansel-Kaye procedure for transposition of the great arteries and for double –outlet right ventricle with subpulmonary ventricular septal defect. Ann Thorac Surg. 1984;38:433–7.
81. Brown JW, Ruzmetov M, Okada Y, Vijay P, Turrentine MW. Surgical results in patients with double outlet right ventricle: a 20-year experience. Ann Thorac Surg. 2001;72:1630–5.
82. Abe T, Sugiki K, Izumiyama O, Komatsu S. A successful procedure for correction of the Taussig-Bing malformation. J Thorac Cardiovasc Surg. 1984;87:403–9.
83. Doty DB. Correction of Taussig-Bing malformation by intraventricular conduit. J Thorac Cardiovasc Surg. 1986;91:133–8.
84. Nikaidoh H. Aortic translocation and biventricular outflow tract reconstruction. A new surgical repair for transposition of the great arteries associated with ventricular septal defect and pulmonary stenosis. J Thoracic and Cardiovascular Surgery. 1984;88:365–372.
85. Yeh T, Ramaciotti C, Leonardo SR. The aortic root translocation (Nikaidoh) procedure: midterm results superior to the Rastelli procedure. J Thorac Cardiovasc Surg. 2007;133:461–9.
86. Yacoub MH, Radley-Smith R. Anatomy of the coronary arteries in transposition of the great arteries and methods for their transfer in anatomical correction. Thorax. 1978;33:418–24.
87. Morell VO, Jacobs JP, Quintessenza JA. Surgical management of transposition with ventricular septal defect and obstruction to the left ventricular outflow tract. Cardiol Young. 2005;15:S102-105.
88. Morell VO. Nikaidoh Procedure—how I teach It. Ann Thorac Surg. 2017;104:1446–9.
89. Raju V, Myers PO, Quinonez LG, Emani SM, Mayer JE, Pigula FA, del Nido P, Baird CW. Aortic root translocation (Nikaidoh procedure): intermediate follow-up and impact of conduit type. J Thorac Cardiovasc Surg. 2015;149:1349–55.
90. Ventosa-Fernandez G, Perez-Negueruela C, Mayol J, Paradela M. The Nikaidoh procedure for complex transposition of the great arteries: short-term follow-up. Cardiol Young. 2017;7:945–50.
91. Honjo O, Kotani Y, Bhatucha T, Mertens L, Caldarone CA, Redington AN, Arsdell GV. Anatomical factors determining surgical decision-making in patients with transposition of the great arteries with left ventricular outflow tract obstruction. Eur J Cardiothorac Surg. 2013;44:1085–94.
92. Hazekamp M, Portela F, Bartelings M. The optimal procedure for the great arteries and left ventricular outflow tract obstruction. An anatomic study. Europ J Cardio-Thoracic Surgery. 2007;31:879–887.
93. Hongu H, Yamagishi M, Miyazaki T, Maeda Y, Taniguchi S, Asada S, Fujita S, Yaku H. Late results of half-turned truncal switch operation for transposition of the great arteries. Ann Thorac Surg. 2018;106:1421–8.
94. Yamagishi M, Shuntoh K, Matsushita T, Fujiwara K, Shinkawa T, Miyazaki T, Kitamura N. Half-turned truncal switch operation for complete transposition of the great arteries with ventricular septal defect and pulmonary stenosis. J Thorac Cardiovasc Surg. 2003;125:966–8.
95. Sologashvili T, Myers PO, Deghetti M, Pretre R. Rotation of the outflow tracts. Interact Cardiovasc Thorac Surg. 2018;27:463–4.
96. Mair R, Sames-Dolzer E, Innerhuber M, Tulzer A, Grohman E, Nulzer G. Anatomic repair of complex transposition with en bloc rotation of the truncus arteriosus: 10-year experience. Eur J Cardiothorac Surg. 2016;49:176–82.
97. Prandstetter C, Tuzler A, Mair R, Sames-Dolzer E, Tulzer G. Effect of surgical en block rotation of the arterial trunk on the conduction system in children with transposition of the great arteries, ventricular septal defect and pulmonary stenosis. Cardiol Young. 2016;26:516–20.

98. Mair R, Sames-Dolzer E, Vondrys D, Lechner E. En block rotation of the truncus arteriosus—an option for anatomic repair of transposition of the great arteries, ventricular septal defect, and left ventricular outflow tract obstruction. J Thorac Cardiovasc Surg. 2006;131:740–1.
99. Hu S, Li S, Wang X, Wang L, Xiong H, Li l, Yan F, Wang X. Pulmonary and aortic root translocation in the management of transposition of the great arteries with ventricular septal defect and left ventricular outflow tract obstruction. The J Thoracic and Cardiovascular Surgery. 2007;133:1090–1092.
100. Hu S, Xie Y, Li S, Wang X, Yan F, Li Y, Hua Z, Li Y. Double-root translocation for double-outlet right ventricle with noncommited ventricular septal defect of double-outlet right ventricle with subpulmonary ventricular septal defect associated with pulmonary stenosis: an optimized solution. Ann Thorac Surg. 2010;89:1360–5.
101. Hu S, Li S, Li Y, Wang L. The double-root translocation technique. Operative Techniques in Thoracic and Cardiovascular Surgery. 2009;14:35–44.
102. Villemain O, Damien BD, Houyel L, Vergnat M, Ladouceur M, Lambert V, Jalal Z, Vouhé P, Belli E. Double-outlet right ventricle with noncommitted ventricular septal defect and 2 adequate ventricles: is anatomical repair advantageous? Semin Thorac Cardiovasc Surg. 2016;28:69–77.
103. Belli E, Serraf A, Lacour-Gayet F, Hubler M, Zoghby J, Houyel L, et al. Double-outlet right ventricle with non-committed ventricular septal defect. European Journal of Cardiothoracic Surgery. 1999;15:747–52.
104. Barbero-Marcial M, Tanamati C, Atik E, Ebaid M. Intraventricular repair of double-outlet right ventricle with non-committed ventricular septal defect: advantages of multiple patches. J Thorac Cardiovasc Surg. 1999;118:1056–67.
105. Lacour-Gayet F. Biventricular repair of double outlet right ventricle with noncommitted ventricular septal defect. Pediatric Cardiac Surgery Annual of the Seminars in Thoracic and Cardiovascular Surgery. 2002;5:163–72.
106. Belli E, Serraf A, Lacour-Gayet F, Inamo J, Houyel L, Bruniaux J, Planché C. Surgical treatment of subaortic stenosis after biventricular repair of double-outlet right ventricle. J Thorac Cardiovasc Surg. 1996;6:1570–8.
107. Li S, Ma K, Hu S, Hua Z, Yan J, Pang K, Wang X, Yan F, Liu J, Zhang S, Chen Q. Biventricular repair for double outlet right ventricle with non-committed ventricular septal defect. Eur J Cardiothorac Surg. 2015;48:580–7.
108. Stellin G, Ho SY, Anderson RH, Zuberbuhler JR, Siewers RD. The surgical anatomy of double-outlet right ventricle with concordant atrioventricular connection and noncommitted ventricular septal defect. J Thorac Cardiovasc Surg. 1991;102:849–55.
109. Tchervenkov CI, Korkola SJ, Be´land MJ. Single-stage anatomical repair of complete atrioventricular canal, double-outlet right ventricle and cor-triatriatum using ventricular septal defect translocation. Annals of Thoracic Surgery. 2002;73:1317–1320.
110. Ishibashi N, Aoki M, Fujiwara T. Successful extensive enlargement of a non-committed ventricular septal defect in double outlet right ventricle. Cardiol Young. 2005;15:431–3.
111. Lu T, Li J, Hu J, Huang C, Tan L, Wu Q, Wu Z. Biventricular repair of double-outlet right ventricle with noncommitted ventricular septal defect using intraventricular conduit. J Thorac Cardiovasc Surg. 2020;159:2397–403.
112. Geva T, Van Praagh S, Sanders SP, Mayer JJ, Van Praagh R. Straddling mitral valve with hypoplastic right ventricle, crisscross atrioventricular relations, double-outlet right ventricle and dextrocardia: morphologic, diagnostic and surgical considerations. J Am Coll Cardiol. 1991;17:1603–12.
113. Kupryashov AA. Straddling and overriding atrioventricular valves. Bockeria LA, Shatalov KV, editors. A chapter in the book pediatric cardiac surgery. Moscow:Bakulev Scientific Center of Cardiovascular Surgery; 2016. p. 864.
114. Sridaromont S, Feldt RH, Ritter DG, Davis GD, McGoon DC, Edwards JE. Double-outlet right ventricle associated with persistent common atrioventricular canal. Circulation. 1975;52:933–42.

115. Pacifico AD, Kirklin JW, Bargeron LM. Repair of complete atrioventricular canal associated with tetralogy of Fallot or double-outlet right ventricle: report of 10 cases. Ann Thorac Surg. 1980;4:351–6.
116. He G, Mee RBB. Complete atrioventricular canal associated with tetralogy of Fallot or double-outlet right ventricle and right ventricular outflow tract obstruction: a report of successful surgical treatment. Ann Thorac Surg. 1986;41:612–5.
117. Danielson GK, Tabry IF, Ritter DG, Maloney JD. Successful repair of double-outlet right ventricle, complete atrioventricular canal, and atrioventricular discordance associated with dextrocardia and pulmonary stenosis. J Thorac Cardiovasc Surg. 1978;76:710–7.
118. Ong J, Brizard CP, d'Udekem Y, Weintraub R, Robertson T, Cheung M, Konstantinov IE. Repair of atrioventricular septal defect associated with tetralogy of Fallot of double-outlet right ventricle: 30 years of experience. Ann Thorac Surg. 2012;94:172–8.
119. Karl T. Atrioventricular septal defect with tetralogy of Fallot or double-outlet right ventricle: surgical considerations. Semin Thorac Cardiovasc Surg. 1997;9:26–34.
120. Imamura M, Drummond-Webb JJ, Sarris GE, Murphy DJ, Mee RBB. Double-outlet right ventricle with complete atrioventricular canal. Ann Thorac Surg. 1998;66:942–4.
121. Takeuchi K, McGowan FX, Moran AM, Zurakowski D, Mayer JE, Jonas RA, del Nido PJ. Surgical outcome of double-outlet right ventricle with subpulmonary VSD. Ann Thorac Surg. 2001;71:49–53.
122. Tchervenkov CI, Hill S, Del Duca D, Korkola S. Surgical repair of atrioventricular defect with common atrioventricular junction when associated with tetralogy of Fallot or double-outlet right ventricle. Cardiol Young. 2006;16:S59-64.
123. Caffarena JM, Gomez-Ullate JM. Biventricular repair of complete atrioventricular canal, double-outlet right ventricle and common atrium using a modified double switch technique. A valid alternative to univentricular procedure. Interactive Cardiovascular and Thoracic Surgery. 2005;4:200–202.
124. Devaney EJ, Lee T, Gelehrter S, Hirsch JC, Ohye RG, Anderson RH, Bove EL. Biventricular repair of atrioventricular septal defect with common atrioventricular valve and double-outlet right ventricle. Ann Thorac Surg. 2010;89:537–43.
125. Kim CY, Kim W, Kwak JG, Jang W, Lee C, Kim DJ, Lim C, Chang WI. Surgical management of left ventricular outflow tract obstruction after biventricular repair of double outlet right ventricle. J Korean Med Sci. 2010;3:374–9.
126. Meng H, Pang K, Li S, His D, Yan J, Hu S, Hua Z, Wang H. Biventricular repair of double-outlet right ventricle: preoperative echocardiography and surgical outcomes. World J Pediatric and Congenital Heart Surgery. 2017;3:354–60.
127. Uemura H, Yagihara T, Kadohama T, Kawahira Y, Yoshikawa Y. Repair of double-outlet right ventricle with doubly-committed ventricular septal defect. Cardiol Young. 2001;11:415–9.
128. Artrip JH, Sauer H, Campbell DN, Mitchell MB, Haun C, Almodovar MC, Hraska V, Lacour-Gayet F. Biventricular repair in double outlet right ventricle: surgical results based on the STS-EACTS international nomenclature classification. European J Cardio-Thoracic Surgery. 2006;29:545–50.
129. Freedom RM, Van Arsdell GS. Biventricular hearts not amenable to biventricular repair. Ann Thorac Surg. 1988;66:641–3.
130. Ruzmetov M, Rodefeld MD, Turrentine MW, Brown J. Rational approach to surgical management of complex forms of double outlet right ventricle with modified Fontan operation. Congenital Heart Diseases. 2008;3:397–403.

Results

K. V. Shatalov and K. M. Dzhidzhikhiya

Abstract Surgical treatment of all types of DORV primarily depends on VSD location, presence of pulmonary artery stenosis and associated cardiac lesions. Surgical results of DORV with subaortic VSD are comparable to tetralogy of Fallot with 95% survival and almost 100% freedom from redo intervention. Contrary, DORV with non-committed VSD represents the most extreme and complex type of the malformation and is characterized by the highest risk of subaortic obstruction and redo intervention. ASO is nowadays considered to be the gold standard for patients with Taussig–Bing anomaly and shows good short-term and long-term results. Overall, nowadays all types of DORV are reparable, and their surgical treatment may be performed relatively safely with acceptable clinical results, but non-committed type remains a big challenge for the congenital cardiac surgeons. Surgical results of DORV are described in this chapter in accordance with arbitrary division into simple forms, complex forms (associated with AVSD and other complex atrioventricular valve abnormalities, and heterotaxy syndrome), DORV with non-committed VSD and results of ASO for Taussig–Bing anomaly.

Keywords Double-outlet right ventricle · Results

Results of surgical treatment of patients with DORV depend on many factors, among which the most important ones are VSD location and age at the time of operation. In addition, unbalanced ventricles, AVSD, heterotaxy syndrome, aortic arch obstruction, straddling atrioventricular valves, etc., significantly affect surgical results.

In the recent decades, the surgical approaches to DORV have changed markedly. These changes become obvious when comparing the results in the early (1980s) and the late (2000s) periods. Thus, in the early period biventricular repair was performed only in 53% of patients and univentricular repair in 13%, while in the late period these

K. V. Shatalov · K. M. Dzhidzhikhiya (✉)
Departement of Emergency Surgery of Congenital Heart Diseases, A. N. Bakulev National Medical Investigation Center for Cardiovascular Surgery, Moscow, Russia
e-mail: d.m.konstantine@mail.ru

K. V. Shatalov and K. M. Dzhidzhikhiya (eds.), *Double-Outlet Right Ventricle*,
https://doi.org/10.1007/978-3-031-49707-0_11

Table 1 Mortality rate of patients with DORV operated on before and after 1980 according to the different authors

Period	Vogt [2] (%)	Piccoli* [3] (%)	Musumeci [4] (%)
Before 1980	41	35	42
After 1980	13	17	14

*before and after 1977

approaches were implemented in 97% and 1% of patients, respectively. In addition, there is a significant difference in the number non-operated patients (33% in the early period *vs* 2% in the late period) [1].

The improvement of surgical results is also noticeable when comparing patients operated on before and after 1980, which may be explained by the expansion of indications for biventricular repair, as well as improvement of surgical, anesthesiological and perfusion aspects (Table 1).

To date, the results of surgical treatment of all types of DORV are satisfactory with a five-year survival rate approaching 95%. Patients with non-committed VSD represent a separate group and are characterized by the highest mortality and reintervention rate. In non-committed VSD, it is impossible to construct a straight exit from the left ventricle to the aorta, and therefore, residual subaortic stenosis after repair (i.e., tunnel obstruction) is always expected especially in the young children. At the same time, there is a correlation between the age at the time of surgery and the risk of severe subaortic stenosis: the lesser the age the more the risk. Although in the study of Villemain et al. [5] reintervention rate after biventricular repair of DORV with non-committed VSD was significantly higher compared to univentricular palliation, the decision-making regarding whether to proceed with any of the surgical options remains up to the surgeon.

One of the most difficult categories of patients are those with DORV and AVSD and/or heterotaxy syndrome. When associated with AVSD, the choice between univentricular or biventricular repair depends on the surgeon's experience and can be performed with similar results [6]. In turn, in the presence of heterotaxy syndrome, frequent association with anomalies of the systemic, pulmonary and hepatic venous drainage severely complicate or even preclude biventricular repair.

The advent of ASO in clinical practice in 1976 [7] revolutionized not only surgical approaches to TGA, but later also to DORV with subpulmonary VSD. Mortality rate of DORV «TGA» type after ASO decreased to 14.3% compared to 60% for atrial switch (Musturd procedure) with pulmonary artery tunneling (a technique used earlier) [4]. According to Kawashima et al. [8], mortality rate of Taussig–Bing anomaly before and after 1985 was 32% and 18%, respectively, and today does not exceed 3.7–9% [9–12].

Of particular interest are patients with DORV and subarterial VSD without the OS, which according to some reports are characterized by 100% freedom from reinterventions [13, 14]. This fact may provide some clarity in understanding the cause of tunnel obstruction in patients with other types of DORV. It is known that in case of spiraling arterial trunks and subarterial VSD the OS is absent and is represented by a fibrous structure to which an intraventricular patch is sewn. This anatomical point takes part in formation of the exit from the tunnel into the aortic valve. Probably due to fibrous nature of the OS remnants such patients are unlikely to develop tunnel obstruction. In contrast, in DORV with the muscular OS (e.g., «tetralogy» type) a tunnel construction is accompanied by risk of its obstruction in the future. Taken together, these data may indicate a particular role of the OS in development of subaortic obstruction after repair.

Due to wide anatomical variability of DORV, patients with different types of the malformation may belong to completely different clinical categories. Accordingly, results of surgical treatment of the disease in this chapter will be described in accordance with the following division:

- results of simple DORV;
- results of complex DORV;
- results of DORV non-committed type;
- results of Taussig–Bing anomaly after ASO.

1 Results of Simple DORV

Simple forms of DORV are those anatomical variants of the malformation which are not associated with AVSD, heterotaxy syndrome and complex anomalies of the atrioventricular valves and as a rule which are treated with biventricular approach.

1.1 Survival

Early mortality after biventricular repair of simple forms of DORV is 3–7% [5, 13, 15–17]. Actuarial survival of the patients after 1, 5 and 10 years following biventricular repair is 87.7%, 87.2% and 86.2%, respectively, while the highest mortality rate is observed in patients with non-committed VSD [5]. Sudden cardiac death is the main reason of mortality after biventricular repair which occurs in the first year after surgery [18]. Actuarial survival of patients with DORV depending on the type of VSD is shown in Table 2.

Table 2 Actuarial survival rate of patients with DORV after biventricular repair depending on the type of VSD according to Li et al. [13]

VSD type	6 months (%)	1 year (%)	5 years (%)
Subarterial	100	100	100
Subaortic	96.3	95.3	95.3
Subpulmonary	94.8	94.8	94.8
Non-committed	89.5	86.2	86.2
Total survival rate	94.4	93.5	93.5

Table 3 Freedom from subaortic obstruction after biventricular repair of DORV depending on the type of VSD according to Li et al. [13]

VSD type	1 year (%)	3 years (%)	5 years (%)
Subarterial	–	–	100
Subaortic	99.1	98	98.0
Subpulmonary	–	–	95.8
Non-committed	94.0	84.4	72.3
Overall freedom	98.4	96.3	92.8

1.2 Reinterventions

The main reasons for reintervention after repair of simple forms of DORV are residual VSD, RVOT obstruction (including dysfunction of an extracardiac conduit) and subaortic stenosis.

Freedom from any reinterventions after 1, 5 and 10 years following biventricular repair is 86.5%, 74.1% and 61.4%, respectively. DORV «non-committed»type is associated with a significantly higher rate of reinterventions [5]. Subaortic stenosis (i.e., tunnel obstruction) develops in 3.8% of patients after 44–55 months after repair [16] and is more typical for «non-committed» type [13]. Overall freedom from subaortic obstruction after 1 and 3 years is 98.1% and 87.9%, respectively [15]. Freedom from subaortic obstruction depending on the type of VSD is shown in Table 3.

Tough patients with staged repair have more complex intracardiac anatomy (non-committed VSD, multiple VSDs, totally anomalous pulmonary venous drainage, left ventricle hypoplasia and anomalies of the atrioventricular valves), and there is no significant difference in survival, subaortic obstruction rate and reintervention rate compared to patients with one-stage approach [15].

1.3 Risk Factors

For early mortality: Restrictive VSD, cleft of the mitral valve, coronary artery anomalies [5], preoperative pulmonary hypertension [13], AVSD and aortic arch obstruction [17].

For late mortality [5]:

- *aortic tunneling*: AVSD, concomitant surgical procedures, cleft of the mitral valve, mitral valve abnormalities, non-committed VSD and coronary artery anomalies;
- *aortic tunneling with RVOT reconstruction*: subaortic obstruction, early reoperation, long ventilation and cardio-pulmonary bypass time;
- *pulmonary artery tunneling with ASO*: early reoperation, concomitant surgical procedures, non-committed VSD, cleft of the mitral valve, long ventilation and cardio-pulmonary bypass time;

- *overall*: early reoperation, cleft of the mitral valve, non-committed VSD, concomitant surgical procedures, restrictive VSD, coronary artery anomalies, pulmonary artery tunneling followed by ASO, long ventilation and cardio-pulmonary bypass time and low body weight.

For late reinterventions [5]:

- *aortic tunneling*: AVSD, subaortic obstruction and restrictive VSD;
- *aortic tunneling with RVOT reconstruction*: non-committed VSD and implantation of an extracardiac conduit [15];
- *pulmonary artery tunneling with ASO*: AVSD, subaortic obstruction, restrictive VSD, concomitant surgical procedures, long ventilation and cardio-pulmonary bypass time.

For subaortic obstruction [13]: age less than 1 year, non-committed VSD and presence of subaortic conus.

2 Results of Complex DORV

Complex forms of DORV are associated with AVSD and/or heterotaxy syndrome as well as complex anomalies of the atrioventricular valves. In the study conducted by Takeuchi et al. on 96 cases of DORV associated with AVSD and/or heterotaxy syndrome univentricular and biventricular repair were performed in 88 (91.6%) and 8 (8.4%) patients, respectively [19]. Neonatal age, common atrioventricular valve regurgitation greater than moderate and pulmonary veins obstruction were identified as independent risk factors for death.

According to the results of Brown et al., mortality rate in patients with complex DORV, most of which undergo univentricular palliation, is higher compared to patients with simple DORV [17]. Comparative actuarial survival after 15 years in patients with simple DORV, Taussig–Bing anomaly and complex DORV was 95.8%, 89.7% and 89.5%, respectively, while freedom from reinterventions was 87%, 72% and 100%, respectively.

Ong et al. showed that early and late mortality after biventricular repair in the general group of patients with DORV/AVSD and tetralogy of Fallot/AVSD was 13.6% and 8.3%, respectively [20]. Actuarial survival after 2, 5 and 20 years was 82%, 76% and 71%, respectively, and freedom from reinterventions was 65% after 2 years and 55% after 5 and 20 years.

In the comparative study conducted by Raju et al. [6] actuarial survival of patients with DORV/AVSD after 1, 5 and 15 years following biventricular repair was 92%, 77% and 77%, respectively, and following univentricular repair—83%, 79% and 70%, respectively. Freedom from reinterventions after 1, 5, 10 and 15 years was 95%, 85%, 74%, 67%, respectively, in the biventricular group and 96%, 91%, 82.4%, 82.4%, respectively, in the univentricular group. The authors revealed no statistically significant difference in survival rate ($p = 0.9$) and freedom from reinterventions ($p = 0.1$) between the groups.

The main reasons for reinterventions after biventricular repair of DORV/AVSD are: regurgitation of the mitral component of the common atrioventricular valve, residual VSD, residual RVOT obstruction, subaortic obstruction, and dysfunction of an extracardiac conduit.

3 Results of DORV «Non-committed» Type

Among all morphological types DORV with non-committed VSD is associated with the highest rate of mortality and reintervention, in particular due to development of subaortic obstruction [21–24].

According to Li et al. [24], overall actuarial survival rate of patients with DORV «non-committed» type (without heterotaxy or AVSD) after 6 months was 90.6% and after 1 and 5 years was 87.1%. Survival rate did not differ significantly between patients with aortic tunneling (87.5% after 6 months, 1 and 5 years) and pulmonary artery tunneling (94.2%, 86.6% and 86.6% after 6 months, 1 and 5 years, respectively).

Despite no difference in long-term mortality, tunnel construction with the aortic valve was accompanied by more frequent subaortic obstruction compared to tunneling of the pulmonary artery, which may be explained by a shorter tunnel in the latter [23]. With equally remote VSD, tunnel construction with any of the arterial trunks does not affect long-term mortality, reintervention rate and functional status of the heart [24].

Villemain et al. [21] compared results of biventricular (24/36) and univentricular (12/36) correction of DORV with non-committed VSD. Overall survival after 5 and 10 years was 81.2% and 73.1%, respectively, and freedom from reoperations was 95% and 63.9%, respectively. Survival rate between the groups did not differ—74.7 ± 5% in the biventricular group versus 71 ± 7% the univentricular group. However, freedom from reintervention differed significantly between the groups—58 ± 5% in the biventricular group *vs* and 70 ± 7% in the univentricular group. The presence of AVSD and cleft of the mitral valve were identified as independent risk factors for death and reinterventions.

4 Results of Taussig-Bing Anomaly After ASO

Although the Kawashima operation shows acceptable clinical results and does not increase the risk of reintervention [25], ASO remains the «gold standard» for surgical treatment of patients with Taussig–Bing anomaly.

Surgical results of ASO for TGA are much better compared to Taussig–Bing anomaly [26, 27]. This can be explained by more frequent association of Taussig–Bing anomaly with aortic arch and RVOT obstructive lesions as well as coronary artery anomalies.

4.1 Survival

Early mortality after Taussig–Bing repair by ASO is 3.7–9% [9–12]. Actuarial survival according to different authors is presented in Table 4.

Types «B», «C» and «E» of coronary arteries are the risk factors for early mortality [11, 12]. Mortality rate in patients with «C» and «E» types is 21%, while in «A» and «D» types only 3%. At the same time, the risk of death in «C» and «E» types is 12 times higher compared to «A» and «D» types [12].

Six-year survival of patients with and without concomitant aortic arch obstruction is 100% and 81%, respectively ($p > 0.05$) [28]. According to other data, survival rate of patients with aortic arch obstruction after 20 years is 94% [29].

One-stage repair of Taussig–Bing anomaly with aortic arch obstruction is more preferable and can be performed with good results with five-year survival of 89.7% [30].

In the presence of concomitant hypoplasia of one of the ventricles or in some complex cases of biventricular attachment of atrioventricular valves, univentricular palliation is indicated. In the study provided by Takeuchi et al. [35], mortality among such patients after univentricular and biventricular repair was 0% and 20%, respectively ($p = 0.11$).

Table 4 Actuarial survival of patients with Taussig–Bing anomaly after ASO according to different authors

Author	1 year (%)	3 years	5 years (%)	10 years (%)	15 years (%)	20 years (%)
Vergnat [12]	86	–	–	86	–	–
Soszyn [31]	–	–	–	–	94.6 ± 3.1	–
Griselli [11]	88	–	88	–	88	–
Fricke* [29]	–	–	–	–	–	94
Sinzobahamvya [32]	–	–	85.1	–	–	–
Patwary** [33]	83.3	–	83.3	–	–	–
Alsoufi [34]	100	–	–	–	–	–

*including patients with Taussig–Bing anomaly and aortic arch obstruction and patients with TGA
**including patients with TGA

4.2 Reinterventions

The most common complications after ASO requiring reinterventions are RVOT obstruction and pulmonary artery stenosis. In the long-term after correction, subaortic obstruction, recurrent aortic arch obstruction and aortic insufficiency may also develop.

Reinterventions after 10 years of biventricular repair are required in 42% of patients [12]. Freedom from all reinterventions according to different authors is presented in Table 5.

The presence of aortic arch obstruction is a risk factor for reintervention [12]. According to Fricke et al. [29], freedom from reintervention in the general group of patients with Taussig–Bing anomaly and TGA with aortic arch obstruction after 5, 10 and 20 years is 77%, 71% and 68%, respectively, while in patients without obstruction—89%, 89% and 81%, respectively ($p = 0.006$).

According to most studies, relationship of arterial trunks does not affect early and late results [11, 12, 36]. However, in the study conducted by Takeuchi et al., it has been shown that side-by-side relation is a risk factor for death after ASO, which is associated with more frequent coronary artery anomalies and concomitant aortic arch obstruction [35]. Another group of authors observed a positive correlation between side-by-side position and reintervention rate [11].

Small age at the time of surgery, aortic arch obstruction, body weight <3 kg, prolonged circulatory arrest, as well as aortic Z-score <−2.5 are risk factors for reinterventions [10].

Table 5 Actuarial freedom from reinterventions after ASO in patients with Taussig–Bing anomaly according to different authors

Author	1 year (%)	3 years (%)	5 years (%)	10 years (%)	15 years (%)	20 years (%)
Soszyn [31]	95 ± 3.5	–	75.3 ± 7.2	75.3 ± 7.2	75.3 ± 7.2	–
Hayes [10]	73	–	64	60	–	–
Luo [30]	94.3	85.7	77.1		–	
Fricke* [29]	–	–	89	89	–	81
Fricke** [29]	–	–	77	71	–	68
Rodefeld [36]	93	–	80	–	75	–
Schwarz [37]	–	–	–	–	67.3	–
Alsoufi [34]	88 ± 11	–	–	–	–	–

*without aortic arch obstruction
**with aortic arch obstruction

Table 6 Actuarial freedom from reinterventions on RVOT after ASO for Taussig-Bing anomaly according to different authors

Author	5 years (%)	10 years (%)	15 years (%)	20 years (%)
Fricke* [29]	98	97	–	95
Fricke** [29]	88	86	–	83
Griselli [11]	88 ± 7	81 ± 9	–	–
Schwarz [37]	–	–	80.3	–

*without interrupted aortic arch
**with interrupted aortic arch

4.2.1 Reinterventions on the Right Heart

The main reason for reinterventions on the right heart after ASO is mainly development of subvalvular and/or supravalvular pulmonary artery stenosis, the mechanism of which is different. Subvalvular stenosis may develop as a consequence of initial subaortic obstruction before ASO. The elements of obstruction are represented by the same anatomical structures, i.e., the OS and the right half of the VIF. In turn, the mechanism responsible for supravalvular stenosis is mainly the tension of the pulmonary arteries after the Lecompte maneuver.

According to Sinzobahamvya et al. [32], RVOT obstruction >30 mmHg was observed in 39% of patients (11/28) in the long term after ASO, while 80% of them had no gradient at the time of discharge. In 82% of cases, there was a combined stenosis at the valvular and subvalvular levels.

Reinterventions on the right heart are required in 25% of patients with Taussig–Bing anomaly and 8% with TGA after ASO. The presence of aortic arch obstruction before the surgery significantly affects the rate of complications. Thus, freedom from reinterventions on the right heart after 5, 10 and 20 years is 98%, 97% and 95%, respectively, and with concomitant arch obstruction is 88%, 86 and 83%, respectively ($p < 0.001$) [29].

Actuarial freedom from reinterventions on the right heart after ASO according to different authors is presented in Table 6.

4.2.2 Reinterventions on the Left Heart

Reinterventions on the left heart after ASO are required in 13.6% of patients [37] due to subvalvular neoaortic stenosis, neoaortic valve regurgitation (6.8%) and recurrent aortic arch obstruction (5.4%) [29].

According to Griselli et al. [11], freedom from subaortic stenosis and recurrent arch obstruction at 1, 5 and 10 years after ASO is 97 ± 3%, 90 ± 7% and 90 ± 7%, respectively.

According to Soszyn et al. [31], freedom from moderate and severe aortic regurgitation at 5 and 10 years after surgery is 97.8 ± 2.2% and 91.1 ± 4.9%, respectively.

References

1. Bradley TJ, Karamlou T, Kilik A, Mitrovic B, Vigneswaran T, Jaffer S, Glasgow PD, Williams WG, Van Arsdell GS, McCrindle BW. Determinants of repair type, reintervention, and mortality in 393 children with double-outlet right ventricle. J Thorac Cardiovasc Surg. 2007;134:967–73.
2. Vogt PR, Carrel T, Pasic M, Arbenz U, von Segesser LK, Turina MI. Early and late results after correction for double-outlet right ventricle: uni- and multivariate analysis of risk factors. Eur J Thoracic Cardiovasc Surg. 1994;8:301–7.
3. Piccoli G, Pacifico AD, Kirklin JW, Blackstone EH, Kirklin JK, Bargeron LM. Changing results and concepts in the surgical treatment of double-outlet right ventricle: analysis of 137 operations in 126 patients. Am J Cardiol. 1983;52:549–54.
4. Musumeci F, Shumway S, Lincoln C, Anderson RH. Surgical treatment for double-outlet right ventricle at the Brompton Hospital, 1973 to 1986. J Thorac Cardiovasc Surg. 1988;96:278–87.
5. Villemain O, Belli E, Ladouceur M, Houyel L, Jalal Z, Lambert V, Ly M, Vouhe P, Bonnet D. Impact of anatomic characteristics and initial biventricular surgical strategy on outcomes in various forms of double-outlet right ventricle. J Thorac Cardiovasc Surg. 2016;152:698–706.
6. Raju V, Burkhart HM, Hedberg NR, Eidem BW, Li Z, Connolly H, Schaff HV, Dearani JA. Surgical strategy for atrioventricular defect and tetralogy of Fallot or double-outlet right ventricle. Ann Thorac Surg. 2013;95:2079–85.
7. Jatene AD, Fontes VF, Paulista PP, Souza LCB, Heger F, Galantier M, Sousa JE. Anatomic correction of transposition of the great vessels. J Thorac Cardiovasc Surg. 1976;72:364–70.
8. Kawashima Y, Matsuda H, Yagihara T, Shimazaki Y, Yamamoto F, Miura T, Uemura H. Intraventricular repair for Taussig-Bing anomaly. J Thorac Cardiovasc Surg. 1993;105:591–7.
9. Masuda M, Kado H, Shiokawa Y, Fukae K, Kaneqae Y, Kawachi Y, Morita S, Yasui H. Clinical results of arterial switch operation for double-outlet right ventricle with subpulmonary VSD. Eur J Cardiothorac Surg. 1999;15:283–8.
10. Hayes DA, Jones S, Quaegebeur JM, Richmond ME, Andrews HF, Glickstein JS, Chen JM, Bacha E, Liberman L. Primary repair switch operation as a strategy for total correction of Taussig-Bing anomaly. A 21-year experience. Circulation. 2013;128:S194–S198.
11. Griselli M, McGuirk SP, Ko C, Clarke AJB, Barron DJ, Brawn WJ. Arterial switch operation in patients with Taussig-Bing anomaly - influence of staged repair and coronary anatomy on outcome. Eur J Cardiothorac Surg. 2007;31:229–35.
12. Vergnat M, Baruteau A, Houyel L, Ly M, Roussin R, Capderou A, Lambert V, Belli E. Late outcomes after arterial switch operation for Taussig-Bing anomaly. J Thorac Cardiovasc Surg. 2015;149:1124–32.
13. Li S, Ma K, Hu S, Hua Z, Yang K, Yan J, Chen Q. Surgical outcomes of 380 patients with double outlet right ventricle who underwent biventricular repair. J Thorac Cardiovasc Surg. 2014;147:817–24.
14. Uemura H, Yagihara T, Kadohama T, Kawahira Y, Yoshikawa Y. Repair of double-outlet right ventricle with doubly-committed ventricular septal defect. Cardiol Young. 2001;11:415–9.
15. Oladunjoye O, Piekarski B, Baird C, Banka P, Marx G, del Nido PJ, Emani SM. Repair of double outlet right ventricle: midterm outcomes. J Thorac Cardiovasc Surg. 2019. https://doi.org/10.1016/j.jtcvs.2019.06.120.
16. Meng H, Pang K, Li S, His D, Yan J, Hu S, Hua Z, Wang H. Biventricular repair of double-outlet right ventricle: preoperative echocardiography and surgical outcomes. World J Pediatr Congenital Heart Surg. 2017;3:354–60.

17. Brown JW, Ruzmetov M, Okada Y, Vijay P, Turrentine MW. Surgical results in patients with double outlet right ventricle: a 20-year experience. Ann Thorac Surg. 2001;72:1630–5.
18. Shen W, Holmes DR, Porter CJ, McGoon DC, Ilstrup DM. Sudden death after repair of double-outlet right ventricle. Circulation. 1990;81:128–36.
19. Takeuchi K, McGown FX, Bacha EA, Mayer JE, Zurakowski D, Otaki M, del Nido PJ. Analysis of surgical outcome in complex double-outlet right ventricle with heterotaxy syndrome or complete atrioventricular canal defect. Ann Thorac Surg. 2006;82:146–52.
20. Ong J, Brizard CP, d'Udekem Y, Weintraub R, Robertson T, Cheung M, Konstantinov IE. Repair of atrioventricular septal defect associated with tetralogy of Fallot of double-outlet right ventricle: 30 years of experience. Ann Thorac Surg. 2012;94:172–8.
21. Villemain O, Damien BD, Houyel L, Vergnat M, Ladouceur M, Lambert V, Jalal Z, Vouhé P, Belli E. Double-outlet right ventricle with noncommitted ventricular septal defect and 2 adequate ventricles: is anatomical repair advantageous? Semin Thorac Cardiovasc Surg. 2016;28:69–77.
22. Belli E, Serraf A, Lacour-Gayet F, Hubler M, Zoghby J, Houyel L, et al. Double-outlet right ventricle with non-committed ventricular septal defect. Eur J Cardiothorac Surg. 1999;15:747–52.
23. Lacour-Gayet F, Haun C, Ntalakoura K, Belli E, Houyel L, Marcsek P, et al. Biventricular repair of double outlet right ventricle with non-committed ventricular septal defect (VSD) by VSD rerouting to the pulmonary artery and arterial switch. Eur J Cardiothorac Surg. 2002;21:1042–8.
24. Li S, Ma K, Hu S, Hua Z, Yan J, Pang K, Wang X, Yan F, Liu J, Zhang S, Chen Q. Biventricular repair for double outlet right ventricle with non-committed ventricular septal defect. Eur J Cardiothorac Surg. 2015;48:580–7.
25. Mavroudis C, Backer CL, Muster AJ, Rocchini AP, Rees AH, Gevitz M. Taussig-Bing anomaly: arterial switch versus Kawashima intraventricular repair. Ann Thorac Surg. 1996;61:1330–8.
26. Losay J, Touchot A, Serraf A, Litvinova A, Lambert V, Piot JD, Lacour-Gayet F, Capderou A, Planche C. Late outcome after arterial switch operation for transposition of the great arteries. Circulation. 2001;104:121–126.
27. Pretre R, Tamisier D, Bonhoeffer P, Mauriat P, Pouard P, Sidi D, Vouhe P. Results of the arterial switch operation in neonates with transposed great arteries. Lancet. 2001;357:1826–30.
28. Comas JV, Mignosa C, Cochrane AD, Wilkinson JL, Karl TR. Taussig-Bing anomaly and arterial switch operation: aortic arch obstruction does not influence outcome. Eur J Cardiothorac Surg. 1996;10:1114–9.
29. Fricke TA, Donaldson S, Schneider JR, Menahem S, d'Udekem Y, Brizard CP, Konstantinov IE. Outcomes of the arterial switch operation in patients with aortic arch obstruction. J Thoracic Cardiovasc Surg. 2020;159:592–599.
30. Luo K, Zheng J, Wang S, Zhu Z, Gao B, Xu Z, Liu J. Single-stage correction for Taussig-Bing anomaly associates with aortic arch obstruction. Pediatric Cariology. 2017;38:1548–55.
31. Soszyn N, Fricke TA, Wheaton GR, Ramsay JM, d'Udekem Y, Brizard CP, Konstantinov IE. Outcomes of the arterial switch operation in patients with Taussig-Bing anomaly. Ann Thorac Surg. 2011;92:673–9.
32. Sinzobahamvya N, Blaschzok HC, Asfour B, Arenz C, Jussli MJ, Schnidler E, Photiadis J, Yrban AE. Right ventricular outflow tract obstruction after arterial switch operation for Taussig-Bing anomaly. Eur J Cardiothorac Surg. 2007;31:873–8.
33. Patwary ME, Khan MS, Marwah A, Singh V, Shekhawat S, Sharma R. Arterial switch for transposition of the great arteries with large ventricular septal defect and for Taussig-Bing anomaly: experience from a tertiary care center in the developing world. World J Pediatr Congenital Heart Surg. 2015;6:413–21.
34. Alsoufi B, Cai S, Williams WJ, Coles JG, Caldarone CA, Redington AM, Van Arsdell GS. Improved results with single-stage total correction of Taussig-Bing anomaly. Eur J Cardiothorac Surg. 2008;33:244–50.
35. Takeuchi K, McGowan FX, Moran AM, Zurakowski D, Mayer JE, Jonas RA, del Nido PJ. Surgical outcome of double-outlet right ventricle with subpulmonary VSD. Ann Thorac Surg. 2001;71:49–53.

36. Rodefeld MD, Ruzmetov M, Vijay P, Fiore AC, Turrentine MW, Brown JW. Surgical results of arterial switch operation for Taussig-Bing anomaly: is position of the great arteries a risk factor? Ann Thorac Surg. 2007;83:1451–7.
37. Schwarz F, Blaschzok H, Sinzobahamvya N, Sata S, Korn F, Weber A, Asfour B, Hraska V. The Taussig-Bing anomaly: long-term results. Eur J Cardiothorac Surg. 2013;44:821–7.

Index

K. V. Shatalov and K. M. Dzhidzhikhiya (eds.), *Double-Outlet Right Ventricle*, https://doi.org/10.1007/978-3-031-49707-0

GPSR Compliance

The European Union's (EU) General Product Safety Regulation (GPSR) is a set of rules that requires consumer products to be safe and our obligations to ensure this.

If you have any concerns about our products, you can contact us on ProductSafety@springernature.com

In case Publisher is established outside the EU, the EU authorized representative is:

Springer Nature Customer Service Center GmbH
Europaplatz 3
69115 Heidelberg, Germany

Batch number: 10726060

Printed by Printforce, the Netherlands